Justice in Oral Health Care

Justice in Oral Health Care
Ethical and Educational Perspectives

Jos V.M. Welie, Editor

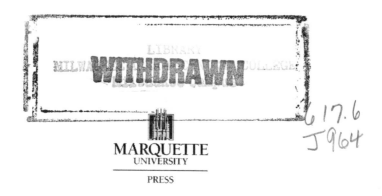
MARQUETTE
UNIVERSITY
PRESS

Library of Congress Cataloging-in-Publication Data

Justice in oral health care : ethical and educational perspectives /
Jos V.M. Welie, Editor.
  p. cm. — (Marquette studies in philosophy ; no. 47)
Includes bibliographical references and index.
ISBN-13: 978-0-87462-670-4 (pbk. : alk. paper)
ISBN-10: 0-87462-670-6 (pbk. : alk. paper)
  1. Dental ethics—United States. 2. Dental care—Social aspects
—United States. 3. Dental health education—United States.
  I. Welie, Jos V. M. II. Series: Marquette studies in philosophy ; # 47.
[DNLM: 1. Ethics, Dental—United States. 2. Dental Care—ethics
—United States. 3. Socioeconomic Factors—United States. 4. Insurance,
Dental—ethics—United States. 5. Health Services Accessibility—ethics
—United States. 6. Social Responsibility—United States. 7. Health
Policy—United States. WU 50 J96 2006]
RK52.7.J87 2006
617.6—dc22
                                                    2006008210

Photo front cover: John Windmueller
(fragment of geodesic dome of the Epcot Center, Orlando, USA).
Photo back cover: Urban Wiesing. Reprinted with permission.

♾ The paper used in this publication meets the minimum requirements of the
American National Standard for Information Sciences—
Permanence of Paper for Printed Library Materials, ANSI Z39.48-1992.

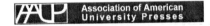

Association of American
University Presses

MARQUETTE UNIVERSITY PRESS
MILWAUKEE

The Association of Jesuit University Presses

Table of Contents

Part III: Educational and Policy Perspectives

Part IV: Appendices

Jos V.M. Welie

Are Oral Health Disparities Merely Unfortunate or Also Unfair? An Introduction to the Book

Oral Health Disparities

The United States spends a greater part of its national gross product on health care than any other nation. It can boost some of the finest hospitals and clinics worldwide and is generally acknowledged to be at the forefront of innovative biomedical research. Indeed, a 2000 World Health Organization (WHO) report on health care systems notes that Americans themselves believe the US system to best respond to the needs of the country when compared to systems elsewhere (WHO 2000). But the same WHO report also ranks the US health care system 37th in overall performance. This low ranking is due in large part to the unequal distribution of care. Approximately one in seven US citizens still has no health care insurance and approximately twice that many are inadequately insured. Consequently, millions of Americans, including many children, are underserved. The problem of unequal access and the resulting disparities is not limited to medical care. It also plagues many other domains of health care, in some cases even more painfully than in medicine. Most notably, 108 million people lack dental insurance, which is more than 2½ times the number who lack medical insurance. More than one third of the US population (or some 100 million people) have no access to community water fluoridation, one of the most important components of preventive oral care.

As is often the case, some sections of the population are much harder hit than others. Institutionalized elderly are a notable example. At any given time 5 percent of Americans aged 65 and older (some 1.7 million people) are living in long-term care facilities where dental care is problematic (US Dept. of Health and Human Services 2000, p. 3). People living in rural areas are likewise affected. Only 6 percent of the dental needs in the designated Health Professional Shortage Areas are presently met by the 306 dental care providers working in these areas. It is estimated that an additional 4,873 dental care providers are needed to meet the current demand (see US Dept. of Health and Human Services 2000, p. 237). Yet another group suffering severely are children. Over 14 percent of children under 18 years of age have no form of private or public medical insurance, but more than twice that many, some 23 million children, have no dental insurance (US Dept. of Health and Human Services 2000, p. 231). Insurance is a strong predictor of access to dental care. Uninsured children are 2½ times less likely than insured children to receive dental care (US Dept. of Health and Human Services 2000, p. 2). Whereas some 70 percent of individuals with private dental insurance reported seeing a dentist, only half of those without dental insurance did (US Dept. of Health and Human Services 2000, p. 229).

The failure of the uninsured to access dental care is probably caused at least in part by the relative lack of public funding for dental care. Only 4 percent of dental services is financed publicly versus 32.2 percent of medical care, and state Medicaid frequently provides lower reimbursement for dental than for medical services (see US Dept. of Health and Human Services 2000, p. 229). In turn, these lower reimbursement rates render dentists hesitant to accept Medicaid patients into their practices. Fewer than one in five Medicaid-covered children received a single dental visit in a recent year-long study period (US Dept. of Health and Human Services 2000, p. 2). And the end is not in sight yet. For the prices for dental services have increased at a rate faster than those for physicians and all medical services combined. Average dental graduate student debt now is $84,000, which is 14 percent more than medical school debt. (See US Dept. of Health and Human Services 2000, p. 237)

It should be emphasized that these problems are not new, nor is it clear that the situation is becoming worse. McCluggage reported that in the mid-1920, "dentists served only about twenty percent of the population during the course of a year" (1959, p. 407). Statistics from the early 1930s already "linked economic status with dental need – the lower the income the greater the need for dental care" (p. 419).

Moreover, health economists, administrators and policy makers are acutely aware of the startling oral health disparities and many reports have been written of late that address this problem, identifying a variety of activities that will have to be undertaken. An example in point is the 2002 report from the National Institute of Dental and Craniofacial Research entitled *A Plan to Eliminate Health Disparities* (NIDCR 2002). It advocates scientific research about physiological, genetic and pathological factors that may contribute to the disparities in certain populations, as well as preventive and therapeutic modalities. Psychosocial, legal, administrative and other systemic conditions that cause members of certain populations to become patients in disproportionate numbers must be identified. And financial barriers to the provision of equitable care must be examined and where possible relieved.

In short, there appears to be widespread agreement that the startling oral health disparities are truly unfortunate. But are they also unfair? There is a crucial ethical difference between, on the one hand, a situation which is merely unfortunate and, on the other hand, a situation which is also unfair. In the former case, it would certainly be good and laudable to do something about the situation, to try to make things better. And many dentists do. More than half of private dentists provide some charitable care (US Dept. of Health and Human Services 2000, p. 239). But nobody is morally obligated to do something. After all, the situation is merely unfortunate, not unfair. If, on the other hand, the situation is both unfortunate and unfair, a moral obligation arises to do something about it. Something ought to be done about the situation. Non-engagement would be morally wrong. If oral health disparities are unfair, the profession of dentistry as a whole as well as its individual members are called to take action, to strive for better access to oral health care services for all in need of such dental care.

Unfortunate and unfair

A strong argumentative case can be made *against* such an alleged professional duty to increase access. History and sociology proves that professions were established foremost to serve the interests of the service providers themselves. The widespread adoption of the "professional" label by just about every occupation today underscores this point. Kultgen (1988) has argued that professional altruism is simply a myth. More recently, Bertolami (2004) has seconded this view, arguing that dentists (like their patients) will always give priority to their *own* interests. Altruism not only is a myth; according to Bertolami this ethical principle is actually untrue. Indeed, the very fact that more than half of private dentists provide some form of charitable care also means that nearly half of all dentists do *not* provide any form of charitable care. More than likely, these dentists do not consider such charitable care an essential professional duty. This also explains why most (inter)national codes of dental ethics do not specify a professional duty to increase access (see the Digest of Codes appended to this volume).

But I venture to guess that few dentists consider the multimillion dollar practice, notwithstanding its appealing lure, their ultimate goal and the defining hallmark of their professional career as an oral health care provider. Granted, there is an ever present tension between being a caring oral health care provider and being a successful entrepreneur. But the very fact that there is a tension also underscores that dentistry is not merely a business but always also a professional health care practice. Indeed, most dentists consider dentistry first and foremost to be a professional health care practice, even if they also have to be entrepreneurs and, in many cases like it that way.

Professionalism implies the moral duty to be altruistic. For the very root of the word "profession" is the joint public promise not to capitalize on the need-induced vulnerability of those served but to give priority to the relief of their needs. This "profession" is the basis of the public's unconditional trust in every member of the profession (Welie 2004a, 2004b, 2004c).

At the risk of being an overly hasty historian, one could argue that in the early days of the profession of dentistry, that is, the late 18th and 19th century, the primary risk to the "profession" was the existence of many quacks who did not hesitate to engage in fraudulent practices. The monopolization of all dental services into a single dental profession effectively protected the public from such quacks. In the early 20th century, the remaining variance in competence even among licenced dentists became a primary source of concern for the profession. But the rapidly advancing science of dentistry and the accreditation of dental schools effectively addressed this threat to public trust. At the dawn of the 21st century, now that each dentist is licensed and qualified to provide effective care, the main threat is disparities in access. The "social contract" between the profession and the public is endangered when the needs of a large segment of the public are not met.

If many people have no access to legal counsel when tried in court, the legal profession *qua* profession is at risk. If children, even a few, are sexually abused by ministers, the integrity of the whole profession of ministry is at risk. If many patients suffering from genuine oral health care needs do not receive even basic dental care, the integrity of the whole profession of dentistry is at risk. This endangerment occurs even if many individual members of the profession strive to serve without discriminating. For the "social contract" is not between the public and individual dentists but between the public and the dental profession as a whole.

Justice in Oral Health Care

If we acknowledge as both unfortunate and unfair the inability of many people in dire need of dental care to access such services, a new series of questions immediately arises. What exactly is the duty of the profession of dentistry to address this problem? How much are individual dentists obligated to do? What is the theoretical basis for distributing scarce oral health care services? And what practical relief strategies are feasible?

These are all complex questions. The contributions to this book do not provide final answers. However, they hopefully will inform and enrich the discussion. In the first section, a variety of theoretical perspectives are presented. Given the magnitude of the problem, as aptly described by Garcia in the first chapter, the only realistic solution is one that focuses on basic oral health care for all in need. But what exactly is basic oral health care? The definition of oral health care is the topic of the subsequent chapter by McNally. Dharamsi follows with a constructivist analysis of the various ways in which dentists and their allies in education, business and government address disparities in dental care systems, and what shapes their practices. The next four chapters each address the issue from a different ethical perspective. Winslow makes a plea for a system in which all citizens at least have access to basic oral health care. Referencing the social historian Bellah, he argues that the religious and political traditions of the United States, notwithstanding the country's apparent embrace of the free market, actually contains the moral roots for a consistent concern about people on the margin of society. Winslow underscores the importance of sharing with students stories about the lives of virtuous members of the profession, about the colleagues we most admire. Such stories can help new members envision the embodiment of what moral excellence means. Welie and Rule follow Winslow in his defense of virtue ethics. Unlike many rival ethical concepts, virtues are by definition practical. They are, in modern educational jargon, moral competencies. Welie and Rule argue that strengthening the moral competencies of future dentists will foster connectedness and communal engagement. In the subsequent chapter, Welie presents an ethical theory – or rather, a theological perspective – that most radically focuses on the plight of the poor and marginalized. The so-called "preferential option for the poor" stems from the moral conviction that the poor have a fundamental claim on our resources not because we could have been the unlucky ones (as game theories essentially would have it), but because the inhumane conditions of their lives are a violation of their essential humanity. Finally, Chambers argues that classical theories based on universal principles and on rights are of limited application and uncertain usefulness. Instead, he examines game theory solutions because they offer the most promise and have been most widely developed.

In Part II, four authors from four different countries broaden our perspective. McFarland focuses on oral health care of Native-American patients. Referencing her own experiences as a care giver for these peoples, she emphasizes the importance of cultural competence lest well-intended care of patients turns into unjust care. Görkey provides a sweeping overview of the oral health care system in Turkey. He shows how in a country with an extraordinarily long history of excellence in dental science and discovery, questions about justice are nevertheless relatively new and equally challenging. Salo and Pöyry describe the Finish oral health care system, which has undergone a series of structural changes in the recent past in order to keep oral health care available to all Finish citizens. Finally, Nordenram from neighboring Sweden focuses on the unintended and potentially harmful consequences of a national oral health care system, specifically overtreatment and undertreatment. She concludes that dentists must be willing to share in the burden of allocating scarce resources justly, which is a new challenge for Swedish dentists who traditionally have left such decisions to governmental agencies.

In Part III, the contributing authors attempt to propose various remedies, or at least partial remedies, to the problem of oral health disparities. Niessen makes a plea for innovative leadership, both in the area of policy development and in education. Dental education is also the principal theme of the subsequent chapters. Rule and Welie focus on the internal culture of the dental school and propose a stepwise strategy for achieving a culture of connectedness. Henshaw discusses a particular pedagogical approach, that is, service-learning. Service-learning differs both from community-based education (which focuses on the educational needs of the students only), and voluntary service activities (which focus on the health care needs of the patients only) by ensuring that service activities are integrated into the academic curriculum. Because service-learning requires that community representatives are involved in the educational planning process and, conversely, that students gain insight in the relevant cultural and policy aspects of those communities, service-learning programs increase not only students' clinical competencies but also their sense of civic responsibility and socio-cultural skills, in short, their moral competencies. Finally, Zarkowski, former President of the American Dental Education Association, broadens the perspective yet again by looking at the education not only of future dentists, but also of other oral health care providers, as well as continuing education programs. She concludes that nobody on the dental team can afford to remain morally indifferent in the face of the many injustices that have yet to be overcome.

The book concludes with two appendices. First, the excellent 2003 report on *Improving the Oral Health Status of All Americans: Roles and Responsibilities of Academic Dental Institutions. The Report of the ADEA President's Commission* is reprinted with permission of the American Dental Education Association (ADEA). This report, though well-known among American dental educators, and rightly so, is perhaps less familiar to dental educators elsewhere in the world. I therefore wish to thank the ADEA for generously allowing the reprint. Finally, a digest of fragments of justice related sections from various codes of dental ethics is presented. It should be emphasized that the purpose of this digest is not to provide a comprehensive overview of codes of ethics from around the world, but rather to provide the reader with yet more food for thought. For in final resort, increasing justice in oral health care is a challenge that will require the creative insights of many more thinkers than the contributors to this volume.

Indeed, this volume is merely the result of two related events. The 5th International Congress on Dental Ethics and Law, co-sponsored by the International Dental Ethics and Law Society and Creighton University

Medical Center, took place in 2003 in Omaha, USA, and was devoted to the topics of Justice, Rights and Access to Oral Health Care. A number of the chapters included here were first presented there. At about the same time, a three-year Planning Grant (2002-2005) on the "Impact of Education on Oral Health Disparities" (1 R21 DE014969-01) was awarded by the National Institute of Dental and Craniofacial Research (NIDCR) to Creighton University Medical Center. The remaining chapters in this book have been written in conjunction with this project and I therefore wish to thank the NIDCR for its generous support.

Bibliography

Bertolami CN. Why our ethics curricula don't work. *Journal of Dental Education* 2004; 68(4): 414–25

Kultgen J. *Ethics and Professionalism*. Philadelphia: University of Pennsylvania Press, 1988

McCluggage RW. *A History of the American Dental Association*. Chicago: ADA, 1959

National Institute of Dental and Craniofacial Research. *A Plan to Eliminate Health Disparities*. Washington DC: NIDCR, February 2002. Available on-line at: http://www.nidcr.nih.gov/NR/rdonlyres/54B65018-D3FE-4459-86DD-AAA0AD51C82B/0/hdplan.pdf (access verified on 11/3/05)

U.S. Dept. of Health and Human Services. Oral Health in America: A Report of the Surgeon General. Rockville, MD: USDHHS, NIDCR, NIH, 2000 Available on-line at: http://www.surgeongeneral.gov/library/oralhealth/ (access verified on 11/3/05)

Welie JVM. Is Dentistry a Profession? Part I: Professionalism Defined. *Journal of the Canadian Dental Association* 2004a, 70(8): 529–32. Also on-line at http://www.cda-adc.ca/jcda/vol-70/issue-8/529.html (access verified on 31/10/05)

Welie JVM. Is Dentistry a Profession? Part II: Hallmarks of Professionalism. *Journal of the Canadian Dental Association* 2004b, 70(9): 599-602. Also on-line at http://www.cda-adc.ca/jcda/vol-70/issue-9/599.html (access verified on 31/10/05)

Welie JVM. Is Dentistry a Profession? Part III: Future Challenges. *Journal of the Canadian Dental Association* 2004c, 70(10): 675-678. Also on-line at http://www.cda-adc.ca/jcda/vol-70/issue-10/675.html (access verified on 31/10/05)

World Health Organization. *The World Health Report 2000. Health Systems: Improving Performance*. WHO: 2000. Available on-line at http://www.who.int/whr/en/ (access verified on 11/3/05)

Part I

Theoretical Perspectives

Raul I. Garcia

Oral Health Disparities:
Health Care and Resource Allocation in the U.S.

Introduction

A society that does not view health as a basic human right is likely to experience disparities in health status that parallel other societal disparities in access to economic resources, goods and services. In the developed world, the United States is a prime example of the health consequences to a society where access to health care is not readily available to all without regard to their ability to pay. In 2003, the first U.S. National Healthcare Disparities Report was issued by the Federal Agency for Healthcare Research and Quality (AHRQ 2003). It presented a comprehensive national overview of disparities, including oral health disparities, in access to health care services and insurance, in health outcomes, and in the quality of care among U.S. racial, ethnic, and socioeconomic groups. It is now well documented in the U.S. that African Americans, Hispanics, American Indians/Alaska Natives, and various Asian subpopulation groups, bear a disproportionate burden of disease and disability, and that these health disparities result in "lower life expectancy, decreased quality of life, loss of economic opportunities, and perceptions of injustice" (Centers for Disease Control and Prevention 2004). Importantly, disparities in health care and health outcomes also significantly affect the developmentally disabled and other special needs populations.

These problems have been recognized by policymakers and the reduction of health disparities has been set as a national goal for the United States. In "Healthy People 2010," the detailed enumeration of health goals for the U.S., "all differences among populations in measures of health and health care are considered evidence of disparities" (US Dept. of Health and Human Services 2000a). In 2002, the Institute of Medicine, in its report "Unequal Treatment," refined the definition of health disparities as those differences among population groups that

Table 1a. Health insurance (dental and/or medical) of U.S. adults, by education and family income

Characteristics	With Dental Insurance		With Any Health Insurance*	
	BRFSS 1997	BRFSS 2001	BRFSS 1997	BRFSS 2001
	N=28,504 Percent (95% CI)	N=30,549 Percent (95% CI)	N=118,650 Percent (95% CI)	N=185,895 Percent (95% CI)
Total	55.70 (55.06, 56.35)	61.02 (60.38, 61.66)	85.88 (85.56, 86.20)	86.19 (85.91, 86.47)
Education				
< 12th grade	32.85 (31.11, 34.58)	40.00 (37.91, 42.09)	73.60 (72.39, 74.80)	70.46 (69.26, 71.65)
12th grade	53.51 (52.38, 54.64)	56.84 (55.69, 57.99)	83.90 (83.32, 84.47)	84.14 (83.64, 84.64)
> 12th grade	63.15 (62.32, 63.98)	67.65 (66.85, 68.44)	90.22 (89.86, 90.58)	91.00 (90.71, 91.29)
Family annual income				
< $15,000	31.52 (29.66, 33.38)	38.94 (36.41, 41.48)	69.57 (68.23, 70.91)	71.69 (70.47, 72.91)
$15,000-$24,999	40.60 (39.09, 42.12)	40.61 (38.96, 42.27)	76.47 (75.58, 77.36)	74.23 (73.33, 75.14)
$25,000-$34,999	54.07 (52.40, 55.75)	56.70 (54.97, 58.42)	85.62 (84.80, 86.44)	84.15 (83.37, 84.93)
$35,000-$49,999	67.78 (66.35, 69.22)	68.91 (67.52, 70.30)	92.30 (91.71, 92.88)	90.39 (89.82, 90.97)
> $50,000	74.90 (73.81, 76.00)	78.62 (77.66, 79.58)	96.10 (95.74, 96.46)	95.72 (95.43, 96.02)

* Any health insurance includes medical or dental insurance.

Data source: 1997 and 2001 Behavioral Risk Factor Surveillance System, Centers for Disease Control and Prevention.

remain after taking into consideration patients' individual needs and preferences and the availability of health care (Smedley et al. 2002). However, Moy and colleagues (2005) have recently noted that data limitations at the national level are insufficient to permit a rigorous assessment of such preferences and that analyses of differences in health

Table 1b. Health insurance (dental and/or medical) of U.S. adults, by race/ethnicity

Characteristics	With Dental Insurance		With Any Health Insurance*	
	BRFSS 1997	BRFSS 2001	BRFSS 1997	BRFSS 2001
	N=28,504 Percent (95% CI)	N=30,549 Percent (95% CI)	N=118,650 Percent (95% CI)	N=185,895 Percent (95% CI)
Total	55.70 (55.06, 56.35)	61.02 (60.38, 61.66)	85.88 (85.56, 86.20)	86.19 (85.91, 86.47)
Race/ethnicity				
Non-Hispanic white	56.39 (55.69, 57.09)	60.70 (60.01, 61.39)	89.07 (88.77, 89.37)	90.00 (89.76, 90.25)
Non-Hispanic black	60.83 (58.86, 62.81)	66.34 (63.97, 68.72)	81.77 (80.70, 82.83)	81.59 (80.63, 82.55)
Hispanic	46.20 (44.10, 48.30)	54.10 (50.45, 57.76)	69.25 (67.66, 70.84)	69.76 (68.41, 71.10)

* Any health insurance includes medical or dental insurance.

Data source: 1997 and 2001 Behavioral Risk Factor Surveillance System, Centers for Disease Control and Prevention.

Note: The health insurance data shown in Tables 1a and 1b were obtained from the U.S. Behavioral Risk Factor Surveillance System (BRFSS) core survey and thus comes from all states. However, the dental insurance data for 1997 come from only the following 20 self-selected states and is thus not nationally representative: Alabama, California, Colorado, Florida, Idaho, Indiana, Maryland, Mississippi, Missouri, Montana, Nevada, New Jersey, New Mexico, New York, Ohio, Tennessee, Texas, Utah, Virginia, and West Virginia. The 2001 dental insurance data come from only the following 14 self-selected states: Arizona, Idaho, Iowa, Missouri, Nebraska, New Hampshire, North Carolina, North Dakota, Pennsylvania, Rhode Island, South Carolina, Virginia, Washington, and Wisconsin

status, outcomes, and quality of and access to care, remain the focus of current disparities research and policy.

The study of oral health disparities similarly suffers from a paucity of national sample data that comprehensively capture health status, access, quality and patient preference variables. In addition, a full understanding of oral health disparities among various racial/ethnic subgroups is also constrained by the lack of national data on Asian and Hispanic

Table 2. Use of preventive dental services during 2000 by U.S. children
aged 18 years and younger living above the federal poverty level

Characteristics	% with No preventive dental services	% with Basic preventive dental services[a]	% with Any preventive dental services[b]
Total percent	49.9 (47.5, 52.4)	47.1 (44.7, 49.6)	50.1 (47.6, 52.5)
Race/ethnicity			
Hispanic	65.3 (60.7, 69.8)	31.6 (27.2, 36.0)	34.7 (30.2, 39.3)
Black	68.4 (63.4, 73.5)	30.5 (25.4, 35.5)	31.6 (26.5, 36.6)
White and other	43.8 (40.8, 46.7)	53.0 (50.0, 56.1)	56.3 (53.3, 59.2)
Insurance status			
Any private[c]	45.6 (42.9, 48.2)	51.3 (48.6, 54.0)	54.4 (51.8, 57.1)
Any public	64.6 (59.1, 70.2)	34.0 (28.4, 39.5)	35.4 (29.8, 40.9)
Uninsured	72.4 (67.2, 77.6)	24.4 (19.4, 29.4)	27.6 (22.4, 32.8)

* All variables are age-adjusted to the year 2000 U.S. standard population, except
those for age subgroups.

a. Includes general exam or consultation; cleaning, prophylaxis, or polishing;
   x-rays, radiographs, or bitewings; or fluoride treatment.
b. Includes general exam or consultation; cleaning, prophylaxis, or polishing;
   x-rays, radiographs, or bitewings; fluoride treatment; fillings; or orthodontia.
c. Includes military-related coverage through CHAMPUS and CHAMPVA.

Data source: Agency for Healthcare Research and Quality, Rockville, MD:
Public Health Service. 2000 Medical Expenditure Panel Survey Household
Component (MEPS HC).

subgroups. Nevertheless, what data are available clearly show that, as
compared to non-Hispanic Whites, racial/ethnic minorities in the U.S.
have poorer access to oral health care services and have poorer oral
health status.

Insurance and Access to Care

The U.S. Census Bureau reported that in 2003, of 290 million Americans, there were over 45 million without health insurance, an increase
of 1.4 million from 2002, and of 5.2 million from 2000. Remarkably,

Table 3a. Visits to a dentist during a prior 12-monts among all Americans, aged 2 years and older, by selected demographic characteristics

Characteristics	NHANES III (1988-1994)	MEPS 2000	NHIS 2001
	Visits to a dentist during the past year *	At least one dental visit during the year 2000	Last saw or talked to a dentist or other dental professional in past year
Total	67.2 (65.7, 68.8)	43.1 (41.7, 44.5)	65.7 (65.1, 66.4)
Race/ethnicity[a]			
Non-Hispanic white	70.3 (68.4, 72.2)	N/A	69.2 (68.4, 70.0)
Non-Hispanic black	58.2 (55.9, 60.5)	N/A	58.6 (57.0, 60.2)
Mexican American	51.9 (49.6, 54.2)	N/A	N/A
Hispanic	N/A	26.9 (24.6, 29.2)	52.5 (51.0, 54.0)
Black	N/A	27.8 (25.2, 30.4)	N/A
White and other	N/A	48.2 (46.6, 49.8)	N/A
Federal poverty level (FPL)			
Below FPL	50.7 (47.8, 53.3)	27.6 (25.2, 30.1)	49.2 (47.1, 51.2)
At or above FPL	71.0 (69.4, 72.6)	45.0 (43.6, 46.5)	67.8 (67.1, 68.5)
Education[b]			
< 12th grade	49.8 (47.5, 52.1)	25.5 (23.5, 27.5)	43.3 (41.8, 44.8)
12th	65.8 (63.8, 67.8)	38.1 (36.5, 39.7)	60.6 (59.5, 61.6)
> 12th grade	79.2 (77.6, 80.9)	54.0 (52.4, 55.7)	75.1 (74.3, 75.9)

*   All variables are age-adjusted to the year 2000 U.S. standard population, except those for age subgroups

a   MEPS reports race/ethnicity as Hispanic, black-not Hispanic, and other (including whites)

b   Education in NHANES III represents the education of the head of the household for persons under 18; otherwise, it represents the education of the individual person. In MEPS, if the age is less than 18 years, then the education is referred to the highest education of either parent. In NHIS, the education categories are less than high school, high school graduate, and more than high school.

the number of Americans without dental insurance is three-fold higher; and, more than half of the children in America lack dental insurance.

It is well recognized that the lack of insurance has serious health consequences for Americans. The National Academy of Sciences (Smedley et al. 2002) has estimated that over 18,000 adults die each

Table 3b. Visits to a dentist during a prior 12-month period among all Americans, aged 2 years and older, by race/ethnicity and Federal poverty level

Characteristics	NHANES III (1988-1994) Visits to a dentist during the past year*	MEPS 2000 At least one dental visit during the year 2000	NHIS 2001 Last saw or talked to a dentist or other dental professional within past year
Total	67.2 (65.7, 68.8)	43.1 (41.7, 44.5)	65.7 (65.1, 66.4)
Below FPL			
Non-Hispanic white	52.2 (47.1, 57.2)	N/A	52.4 (49.3, 55.4)
Non-Hispanic black	50.7 (48.1, 53.3)	N/A	48.1 (44.2, 52.0)
Mexican American	40.9 (38.7, 43.1)	N/A	N/A
Hispanic	N/A	17.9 (14.6, 21.2)	42.5 (39.5, 45.4)
Black	N/A	24.2 (18.7, 29.7)	N/A
White and other	N/A	33.2 (29.6, 36.8)	N/A
Federal poverty level (FPL)			
Non-Hispanic white	72.6 (70.8, 74.4)	N/A	70.3 (69.5, 71.1)
Non-Hispanic black	62.7 (60.0, 65.4)	N/A	60.7 (58.7, 62.7)
Mexican American	61.0 (57.95, 64.1)	N/A	N/A
Hispanic	N/A	29.2 (26.8, 31.6)	57.2 (55.3, 59.0)
Black	N/A	28.8 (25.9, 31.6)	N/A
White and other	N/A	49.5 (47.9, 51.1)	N/A

* All variables are age-adjusted to the year 2000 U.S. standard population, except those for age subgroups.

Data sources for Tables 3a and 3b: The Third National Health and Nutrition Examination Survey (NHANES III: 1988-1994), 2001 National Health Interview Survey, National Center for Health Statistics, Centers for Disease Control and Prevention, and 2000 Medical Expenditure Panel Survey Household Component (MEPS HC), Agency for Healthcare Research and Quality

year specifically because they are uninsured and cannot get proper care. While providing access to health insurance is recognized as a necessary prerequisite to effectively reducing disparities, insurance status does not fully explain the mortality gap between White and Black Americans. For example, Satcher et al (2005) have estimated that there are over 83,000 excess deaths each year in African Americans.

Table 4. US Children and adolescents with dental sealants by age group
and selected demographic characteristics

Characteristics	Percentage of Children with Dental Sealants on 1st or 2nd Molars (95% C I)	
	Aged 8 - 10 (N=1,611)	Aged 14 - 16 (N=1,194)
Total	26.09 (20.02, 32.15)	22.18 (17.18, 27.18)
Race/ethnicity		
Non-Hispanic white	30.58 (22.87, 38.30)	29.06 (22.50, 35.62)
Non-Hispanic black	12.59 (9.84, 15.33)	8.13 (4.46, 11.80)
Mexican American	16.67 (11.48, 21.86)	9.35 (5.41, 13.30)
Federal poverty level (FPL)		
Below FPL	14.62 (6.05, 23.20)	14.89 (5.63, 24.15)
At or Above FPL	30.11 (23.79, 36.44)	24.96 (19.03, 30.89)
Below FPL		
Non-Hispanic white	16.48 (4.44, 28.53)	28.63 (9.33, 47.93)
Non-Hispanic black	12.38 (6.70, 18.07)	7.11 (3.64, 10.58)
Mexican American	10.71 (3.41, 18.01)	3.37 (0.81, 5.94)
At or Above FPL		
Non-Hispanic white	33.15 (25.46, 40.83)	29.56 (22.32, 36.80)
Non-Hispanic black	14.02 (10.39, 17.66)	9.45 (4.28, 14.62)
Mexican American	22.56 (12.94, 32.17)	13.82 (6.80, 20.85)

Data source: The Third National Health and Nutrition Examination Survey
(NHANES III) 1988-1994, National Center for Health Statistics, Centers for
Disease Control and Prevention.

In addition to racial disparities in Americans' health insurance coverage,
significant differences in coverage also exist related to socioeconomic
status, as measured by family income and the educational attainment
of the head of household (Table 1a). Interestingly, while many fewer
American have dental insurance than have medical
insurance, the racial disparities in dental insurance do not appear to be
as great (Table 1b). However, the key issue regarding dental insurance
and access to care is in whether persons have private dental insurance
as opposed to public (i.e., Medicaid) dental insurance coverage (Table
2).

Table 5. Increased disparities in U.S., 1971-1975 to 1988-1994, in untreated dental caries among children (aged 6-8 years) and adolescents (aged 12-15 years) by selected demographic characteristics

	Prevalence (& 95% Confidence Interval)			
	6-8 Year Old-Primary (ds)		12-15 Year Old-Permanent (DS)	
	NHANES I (1971-1975)	NHANES III (1988-1994)	NHANES I (1971-1975)	NHANES III (1988-1994)
Total	48.65 (44.36, 52.93)	26.52 (23.29, 29.76)	53.19 (48.95, 57.44)	16.91 (13.86, 19.96)
Race/ethnicity				
Non-Hispanic white	44.87 (40.09, 49.64)	20.69 (16.65, 24.72)	48.70 (43.81, 53.59)	13.64 (9.78, 17.49)
Non-Hispanic black	50.87 (43.72, 58.02)	33.48 (30.26, 36.67)	65.15 (58.91, 71.39)	27.35 (22.59, 32.12)
Mexican American	78.61 (64.48, 92.74)	44.75 (38.27, 51.24)	51.06 (40.80, 61.32)	28.34 (24.42, 32.25)
Federal poverty level (FPL)				
Below FPL	65.79 (58.42, 73.16)	45.24 (39.13, 51.35)	69.26 (64.17, 74.36)	29.42 (21.26, 37.59)
At or Above FPL	43.99 (39.39, 48.59)	19.74 (16.16, 23.33)	50.17 (45.59, 54.75)	13.54 (10.23, 16.84)
Education (head of household)				
<12th grade	63.31 (56.64, 69.97)	41.56 (35.00, 48.13)	67.15 (62.29, 72.00)	28.71 (23.73, 33.68)
12th grade	46.77 (40.37, 53.17)	28.12 (22.63, 33.61)	49.23 (43.21, 55.26)	20.09 (14.79, 25.39)
> 12th grade	31.28 (22.93, 39.62)	16.27 (11.39, 21.16)	35.68 (29.14, 42.21)	7.29 (4.22, 10.37)

Data source: The First National Health and Nutrition Examination Survey (NHANES I) 1971-1975, and the Third National Health and Nutrition Examination Survey (NHANES III) 1988-1994, National Center for Health Statistics, Centers for Disease Control and Prevention.

Dental insurance, in particular private insurance, and access to oral health care services are intimately linked. For example, in the year 2000 (Table 2), the differences in children's use of preventive dental services were greater between those with private vs. public insurance, than between those with public insurance vs. the uninsured. Furthermore, these differences by insurance status are similar in magnitude to the racial/ethnic

Table 6. Percent U.S. 3rd graders with untreated caries, by state

State	School Year	Percent with Untreated Tooth Decay[1]		Response Rate[2] (%)	Percent eligible for free and reduced-cost lunch program[3]		
					Sample		State
					Schools[4]	Students[5]	
Arkansas	2001-2002	%	42.1	86	55	NR	45
		CI	(38.4-45.8)				
		N	815				
Oklahoma	2002-2003	%	40.2	74	NR	NR	41
		CI	(35.8-44.7)				
		N	495				
Nevada	2002-2003	%	38.9	46	39	45	39
		CI	(37.0-40.9)				
		N	2470				
New Mexico	1999-2000	%	37.0	47	NR	NR	NR
		CI	(32.3-41.6)				
		N	2136				
Delaware	2001-2002	%	30.9	43	37	41	40
		CI	(26.0-35.7)				
		N	1032				
Wisconsin	2001-2002	%	30.8	67	39	NR	34
		CI	(29.3-32.5)				
		N	3307				
South Dakota	2002-2003	%	30.6	71	38	NR	41
		CI	(27.2-34.1)				
		N	710				
Kansas	2003-2004	%	27.6	32	NR	NR	NR
		CI	(24.9-30.4)				
		N	3375				
Massachusetts	2002-2003	%	26.6	53	NR	NR	29
		CI	(25.1-28.1)				
		N	3439				
Idaho	2000-2001	%	25.8	71	50	NR	39
		CI	(23.6-28.1)				
		N	3126				

disparities (Table 2). Comparable differences exist in adults' access to prevention and other treatments (Agency for Healthcare Research and Quality 2000). Manski et al (2002) conducted a detailed analysis of the role of private insurance on access to care, using national data from the 1996 Medical Expenditure Panel Survey. They found that non-Whites were less likely to have private dental coverage, and that poor and low-income persons were less likely to have private dental coverage than were

State	School Year	Percent with Untreated Tooth Decay[1]		Response Rate[2] (%)	Percent eligible for free and reduced-cost lunch program[3]		
					Sample		State
					Schools[4]	Students[5]	
Colorado	2003-2004	%	25.4	68	34	NR	33
		CI	(23.6-27.4)				
		N	2031				
Missouri	1999-2000	%	23.0	80	NR	NR	NR
		CI	(22.0-24.0)				
		N	3031				
Utah	2000-2001	%	23.0	51	NR	NR	NR
		CI	(21.0-25.0)				
		N	800				
New Hampshire	2000-2001	%	21.7	78	NR	NR	NR
		CI	(14.3-29.1)				
		N	410				
Washington	1999-2000	%	20.5	40	37	37	31
		CI	(18.3-22.8)				
		N	1217				
Maine	1998-1999	%	20.4	51	NR	31	32
		CI	(18.3-22.6)				
		N	1297				
Vermont	2002-2003	%	16.1	68	31	NR	31
		CI	(12.8-20.1)				
		N	409				

%   Percentage   N   Number of students in sample
CI 95% Confidence Interval   NR   Not Reported

1   The percent with untreated tooth decay shown here is not adjusted for nonresponse.
2   Survey response rates differ among states. Differential nonresponse can bias the
    estimates. Response rates, the percent of selected children who actually participated,
    are presented to help the reader judge the potential for bias.
3   Untreated tooth decay may be associated with income. Eligibility for the free and
    reduced-cost lunch program is presented to help the reader assess whether the survey
    sample is representative of all 3rd graders in the state.
4   The percent eligible for the free and reduced-cost lunch program among students
    attending schools that participated in the survey.
5   The percent eligible for the free and reduced-cost lunch program among students
    who participated in the survey.
Data source: National Oral Health Surveillance System, Centers for Disease Control and
Prevention

those with higher incomes. Interestingly, persons without private dental coverage, irrespective of their income levels, were less likely to report a dental visit than those with coverage. During 1996, over 40 percent of all dental expenditures were paid by private dental insurance, over half of expenditures were paid out of pocket by patients, while less than 4 percent was paid for by government programs.

Table 7a. US adults, aged 18 and older, with a self-assessed oral health status of good or better, by selected demographic characteristics

Characteristic	Percent (95% C I)*
Total	65.06 (63.15, 66.97)
Age	
18-24	70.99 (67.85, 74.13)
25-34	68.46 (65.58, 17.35)
35-44	66.74 (63.40, 70.07)
45-54	66.61 (62.57, 70.66)
55-64	58.65 (55.15, 62.15)
65-74	56.68 (53.85, 59.52)
75 and older	53.32 (48.71, 57.92)
Federal poverty level (FPL)	
Below FPL	44.25 (40.68, 47.82)
At or above FPL	68.01 (66.20, 69.83)
Education	
< 12th grade	45.80 (43.66, 47.94)
12th grade	62.84 (59.97, 65.71)
> 12th grade	76.28 (74.52, 78.03)

* Age standardized to the year 2000 U.S. population.

Data source: The Third National Health and Nutrition Examination Survey (NHANES III) 1988-1994, National Center for Health Statistics, Centers for Disease Control and Prevention

Disparities in Care and Oral Health Outcomes

Over the past decade, U.S. national survey data have consistently shown that large disparities exist in access to oral health care services by race/ethnicity, education and income (Table 3a). Interestingly, the racial/ethnic disparities persist irrespective of whether persons are poor or non-poor (Table 3b and Table 4). In regards to reported annual dental visits (Table 3a), multiple surveys show that Hispanics/Mexican

Table 7b. US adults, aged 18 and older, with a self-assessed
oral health status of good or better, by race/ethnicity and
Federal poverty level

Characteristic	Percent (95% C I)*
Total	65.06 (63.15, 66.97)
Race/ethnicity	
Non-Hispanic white	69.22 (66.97, 71.48)
Non-Hispanic black	50.99 (49.22, 52.76)
Mexican American	43.37 (41.30, 45.43)
Below FPL	
Non-Hispanic white	50.42 (43.67, 57.16)
Non-Hispanic black	41.30 (38.01, 44.59)
Mexican American	34.28 (31.85, 36.72)
At or above FPL	
Non-Hispanic white	70.76 (68.60, 72.92)
Non-Hispanic black	54.30 (51.77, 56.83)
Mexican American	49.93 (47.20, 52.65)

* Age standardized to the year 2000 U.S. population.

Data source: The Third National Health and Nutrition Examination
Survey (NHANES III) 1988-1994, National Center for Health
Statistics, Centers for Disease Control and Prevention

Americans and African Americans fare much worse than non-Hispanic
Whites. Similar differences are found in regards to access to children's
preventive services, such as dental sealants (Table 4).

Disparities in Children

Such disparities in access to preventive services are also reflected by
disparities in clinical measures of oral health status, such as presence of
untreated caries (Table 5). While much has been made of the extraordi-
nary improvements in children's oral health in the U.S. over the past four
decades, it is also now well recognized that the benefits in oral health
have not been equitably distributed among all population groups (US

Table 8. Untreated dental caries prevalence, 1988-1994, in US adults
(aged 35-44 years) by selected demographic characteristics

Characteristic	Percentage of Untreated Decay (dt/DT) (95% C I)
Total	26.12 (23.60, 28.65)
Race/ethnicity	
Non-Hispanic white	21.90 (18.87, 24.93)
Non-Hispanic black	45.92 (41.60, 50.25)
Mexican American	33.49 (29.91, 37.08)
American Indian / Alaska Native*	68 (NA)
Federal poverty level (FPL)	
Below FPL	50.74 (45.71, 55.76)
At or above FPL	23.07 (20.36, 25.78)
Education	
< 12th grade	47.57 (41.12, 54.01)
12th grade	33.14 (28.81, 37.48)
> 12th grade	15.50 (13.00, 18.00)
Below FPL	
Non-Hispanic white	48.60 (38.10, 59.10)
Non-Hispanic black	57.36 (49.55, 65.18)
Mexican American	54.02 (45.27, 62.77)
At or above FPL	
Non-Hispanic white	20.31 (17.14, 23.47)
Non-Hispanic black	42.39 (36.87, 47.91)
Mexican American	22.16 (18.27, 26.05)

* Data are for the Indian Health Service areas for 1999.
NA: Not available
Data source: The Third National Health and Nutrition Examination Survey
(NHANES III) 1988-1994, National Center for Health Statistics, Centers for
Disease Control and Prevention

Dept. of Health and Human Services 2000b). For example, from the
1970's to the 1990's the percentage of children with untreated caries has
declined dramatically, from 49 to 27 percent in the primary dentition,
and from 53 to 17 percent in the permanent dentition. However, the
disparities among racial/ethnic groups have actually increased over the

Table 9. Prevalence of gingivitis and periodontitis in U.S. adults aged 20 and older by selected demographic characteristics

Characteristic	Gingivitis (Total N=13,003)	Destructive periodontal disease (Total N=12,976)
	Percent (95% C I)	Percent (95% C I)
Total	52.90 (48.70, 57.10)	26.14 (24.41, 27.88)
Race/ethnicity		
Non-Hispanic white	50.14 (45.39, 54.89)	7.04 (25.18, 28.91)
Non-Hispanic black	58.19 (54.08, 62.30)	38.63 (36.48, 40.78)
Mexican American	66.47 (62.30, 70.65)	33.52 (31.89, 35.15)
Federal poverty level (FPL)		
Below FPL	64.63 (60.07, 69.20)	42.22 (39.20, 45.24)
At or above FPL	23.07 (20.36, 25.78)	27.39 (25.68, 29.10)
Education		
< 12th grade	60.93 (56.96, 64.89)	38.96 (36.72, 41.21)
12th grade	53.82 (48.66, 58.98)	30.80 (28.22, 33.37)
> 12th grade	48.30 (43.51, 53.10)	23.03 (20.70, 25.36)

Data source: The Third National Health and Nutrition Examination Survey (NHANES III) 1988-1994, National Center for Health Statistics, Centers for Disease Control and Prevention

same period of time (Table 5). While all groups experienced significant reductions in untreated caries over 20 years, the improvements in non-Hispanic Whites were much greater than for the minority groups, resulting in an exacerbation of the disparities. In the most recent U.S. national survey (NHANES III 1988-1994), African American and Mexican American adolescents were more than twice as likely to have untreated caries as non-Hispanic Whites. Similarly, the racial/ethnic disparities in untreated caries among 6 to 8 year olds also worsened over time (Table 5). In addition, within the U.S., there exist wide disparities among states in prevalence of untreated caries in children (Table 6). The best available state-level data from the CDC National Oral Health Surveillance System shows a wide range, from a low of 16 percent in Vermont to a high of 42 percent in Arkansas.

Table 10. Racial disparity in U.S. oral and pharyngeal cancer incidence and stage of diagnosis

SEER Historic Stage	Race/ethnicity		
	White	Black	All Races/ethnicities
	Rate per 100,000* (95%CI)		
In Situ	0.4 (0.3, 0.4) *	0.3 (0.3, 0.4)	0.3 (0.3, 0.4)
Localized	4.2 (4.2, 4.3)	3.0 (2.9, 3.2)	4.0 (4.0, 4.1)
Regional	4.4 (4.4, 4.5)	7.0 (6.8, 7.2)	4.7 (4.6, 4.7)
Distant	1.0 (1.0, 1.0)	2.1 (2.0, 2.2)	1.1 (1.1, 1.1)
Unstaged	1.1 (1.0, 1.1)	1.2 (1.1, 1.3)	1.1 (1.0, 1.1)
All Stages	**11.1 (11.0, 11.2)**	**13.6 (13.3, 13.9)**	**11.2 (11.1, 11.3)**

* The rates are per 100,000 and are age-adjusted to the 1970 U.S. standard population
Data source: Surveillance, Epidemiology, and End Results (SEER) 9 Registries Public-Use, November 2002 Submission (1973-2000), National Cancer Institute

Disparities in Adults

The extent of oral health disparities described in U.S. children is paralleled in adult Americans. Reports of poorer self-rated oral health status increase with increasing age, and are related to lower level of education attainment and to poverty status (Table 7a), and also to being non-White (Table 7b). While 69 percent of White adults rate their oral health status as good or better, significantly fewer Blacks (51%) and Hispanics (43%) rate their oral health status as good or better. This lower self-rating of oral health by racial/ethnic minority adults is also reflected in worse clinical measures of oral health status. When compared to minority adults, significantly fewer White American adults have untreated caries (Table 8), gingivitis and periodontitis (Table 9). As was noted earlier, private insurance status is a significant predictor of dental care utilization in adults, including elders, with fewer dentate older adults from minority groups having dental visits (Macek et al. 2004).

Table 11. Racial disparity in U.S. adults in rate of oral and pharyngeal cancer examinations

Characteristics	US Adults aged 40 years and older reporting having had Oral/Pharyngeal Cancer Examination in Past 12 months	
	Percent (95% C I)	
	1992	1998
Total	7.6 (6.8, 8.5)	14.7 (14.0, 15.4)
Race/ethnicity		
Non-Hispanic white	8.4 (7.5, 9.3)	16.6 (15.8, 17.4)
Non-Hispanic black	3.3 (1.7, 4.9)	7.2 (5.8, 8.6)
Mexican American	3.9 (2.1, 5.8)	6.6 (5.2, 7.9)
Federal poverty level (FPL)		
Below FPL	3.3 (1.6, 4.9)	5.7 (4.4, 7.0)
At or above FPL	8.5 (7.6, 9.4)	16.9 (16.0, 17.8)
Education		
< 12th grade	3.6 (2.5, 4.7)	5.7 (4.8, 6.6)
12th grade	6.2 (5.0, 7.3)	7.5 (3.9, 11.1)
> 12th grade	11.9 (10.2, 13.5)	17.1 (16.3, 17.9)

Data source: 1992 and 1998 National Health Interview Surveys, National Center for Health Statistics, Centers for Disease Control and Prevention.

Perhaps the most serious oral health disparity in the U.S. is that regarding oral cancer. Not only is the incidence of oral and pharyngeal cancer in Blacks significantly higher than in Whites, but the stage at which cancer diagnosis occurs in Blacks is less favorable (Table 10). Over 40 percent of the oral cancers in Whites are diagnosed when they are either in situ or localized lesions, as compared to 24 percent in Blacks; over two-thirds of oral cancers in Blacks have already metastasized at the time of diagnosis, while less than half of oral cancers in Whites have metastasized at the time of diagnosis. As may be expected, this delay in diagnosis is related to disparities in access to oral cancer examinations (Table 11). While the overall rates of oral cancer examinations in U.S. adults have increased for all racial/ethnic groups in the past decade, the rates remain disturbingly low. And, as was earlier noted regarding overall improvements over time in caries prevalence, the overall improvements

Table 12. Racial disparity in U.S. Oral and pharyngeal cancer deaths
(per 100,000)

Characteristics	Age-adjusted death rate* (95% CI)	
	Year 1998	Year 2001
Total	3.0 (2.9, 3.0)	2.7 (2.7, 2.8)
Race/ethnicity		
Non-Hispanic Whites	2.8 (2.8, 2.9)	2.6 (2.6, 2.7)
Non-Whites	4.0 (3.7, 4.2)	3.5 (3.3, 3.7)

* The rates are displayed as cases per 100,000 and are age-adjusted to the 2000
U.S. standard population.

Data source: Surveillance, Epidemiology, and End Results (SEER) Mortality -
All COD, Public-Use with State, National Cancer Institute.

in oral cancer examination rates have not lessened the racial/ethnic
disparities. Whites remain over twice as likely as Blacks to have oral
cancer examinations (Table 11). Given such data, it is thus not surprising that Blacks continue to have a significantly higher mortality rate for
oral and pharyngeal cancer than Whites (Table 12).

Discussion

The data clearly show that the burden of oral disease is unequally
distributed in American society. In large part, these disparities in oral
health status among population groups are related to financial barriers,
primarily lack of private dental insurance, that limit access to preventive
and therapeutic services. People with private dental insurance coverage
are more likely to visit a dentist, have a greater number of visits and
have higher expenditures than persons without coverage (Manski et al.
2002). While private dental insurance coverage is clearly not the only
determinant of dental care use, addressing the lack of such coverage
would seem to be a necessary step (though insufficient by itself) in
efforts to reduce disparities in oral health status.

The racial/ethnic groups disproportionately affected by oral diseases
are also those groups in America that are disproportionately poorer,

less well-educated, and lack private dental insurance. Social disparities in health that are independent of race have been recognized in the
U.S., where low-income Whites have worse health than more affluent
Americans, and similar situations exist in other developed nations
(Marmot 2004). Social class and race/ethnicity are intimately related
in the U.S. and the particular role of each in understanding the nature
of health disparities remains a matter of current controversy (Isaacs &
Schroeder 2004; Navarro 1990). These issues are directly relevant to
work on oral health disparities. Work to date would indicate that both
class and race matter. Where multivariate analyses are carried out to
control for various socioeconomic factors, there remain significant disparities in oral health status related to race and ethnicity. For example,
in a study comparing endodontic treatment versus extractions in VA
patients, where costs of care are not a barrier, it was found that Blacks
had significantly more extractions (Kressin et al. 2003).

Similar racial/ethnic disparities have been noted in analyses of systemic health outcomes and medical care utilization, in children and in
adults (Flores et al. 2005; Kressin et al. 2004). For example, a recent
U.S national study showed that there exist significant differences by
race and gender in the management of acute myocardial infarction,
leading to increased mortality (Vaccarino et al. 2005). Importantly,
an analysis of racial trends in the use of major medical procedures
among the elderly found no evidence that efforts over the prior decade
to eliminate racial disparities in procedure use were successful (Jha et
al. 2005). Such findings have led to calls for needed systems changes
in the structure and processes of health care in the U.S. (Lurie 2005).
In addition, there is growing recognition of the need to explore both
patient-based factors, such as patients' beliefs and preferences for care,
as well as provider-based factors, such as providers' expectations of
patient compliance and acceptance of care recommendations (Flores et
al. 2005; Kressin & Petersen 2001).

In the search for solutions to the health disparities problem, increasing
attention is being given to creating a provider workforce that is better
educated to be competent in providing care to a culturally diverse
patient population. Part of this effort has entailed cultural competence
education for both majority and minority health care providers, as
well as specific enhancements in the numbers of minority health care
providers (Smedley et al. 2004). An important impetus for the latter
efforts is the clear evidence showing that minority dentists are more
likely than white dentists to see minority patients (Brown et al. 2000).

While less than 25 percent of the average White dentist's patients are minorities, 73 percent of Black dentist's patients are minorities, 70 percent of Hispanic dentist's patients are minorities, and 52 percent of Asian dentist's patients are minorities (Brown et al 2000). It has also become recognized that changes in the dentist workforce alone may be insufficient to eliminate oral health disparities (Nash & Nagel 2005) and that other health care providers need to become engaged in oral health promotion (Mouradian et al. 2005).

Policy Implications

Various policy solutions have been proposed to address access to health insurance and care. These efforts have included programs targeted at the recruitment and retention of minority oral health care providers, to health care financing reforms that would extend dental insurance coverage more broadly. While the current political climate in the U.S. against "big government" and higher taxes has limited progress, the financial constraints posed by economic trends have also been a major obstacle to progress. Universal, government-financed health insurance is unlikely to occur in the foreseeable future in the U.S., in part given the country's foundational cultural norms of reliance on private enterprise and individual responsibility to address social needs.

As importantly, there is a growing realization that no single or simple solution may work for all (Garcia 2005). In the case of expansions of health insurance coverage, it is now understood that people are uninsured for a variety of reasons and thus different solutions may be required for different population groups. Lastly, the monumental failure in 1994 of the comprehensive national health care reform plan proposed by President Clinton has led many policy experts to conclude that it will not be politically or economically feasible to radically restructure the U.S. healthcare system nor provide health insurance to all through a single national program. Rather, reforms seem more likely to succeed when they are incremental, rely on the private sector, and build on existing Federal-state programs. For example, in 2005 U.S. health leaders made recommendations such as:

• Federal tax credits for low-income families to directly purchase insurance, and for small businesses to provide insurance to their employees;

• Expansion of Medicaid to all adults with annual income below the Federal poverty level ($9,000 in 2005), with Federal incentives for individual states to adopt such expansions of eligibility;
• Federal tax-favored individual health savings accounts, funded by individual contributions, for purchase of insurance or for direct health services.

It remains to be seen the extent to which oral health care would become an insured component of health care services in this mix of private insurers and pubic programs.

The "silent epidemic" of oral disease that the U.S. Surgeon General systematically described in his 2000 Report to the nation (US Dept. of Health and Human Services 2000b) was due to many causes and is not amenable to easy solutions. An important outcome of the Surgeon General's Report, however, was a "Call to Action" (US Dept. of Health and Human Services 2003) that specified a number of key policy initiatives whose overall aim was the elimination of oral health disparities in the U.S. An essential feature of such efforts, still being led by the Surgeon General of the United States, is the importance of public-private partnerships. Another important feature is the continuing need to educate the public and policymakers about the interactions between each person's general health and well being and their oral health, that people cannot be truly healthy unless they have good oral health. The important message is that "oral health matters." Oral problems may be related in important ways to a person's medical health status, and equally importantly is that oral health is an essential determinant of a person's quality of life, their functional abilities, their sense of well-being. Raising the "oral health literacy" of all Americans will be an essential component of any successful efforts to eliminate disparities (Horowitz et al. 2005).

While this message is being taken to the public and policymakers by our national health leaders, dental practitioners and dental educators have related roles to play within the profession in the overall efforts to eliminate oral health disparities. For example, as educators we need to instill in students that dental practice entails more than simply caring for the patients one sees in the private office setting. We need to instill in students that it is our professional obligation to promote the oral health of the entire community, not just taking responsibility for the oral health of the patients we see in our dental chair. We readily acknowledge the responsibility to provide the best quality care to "our own patients" but we do not seem to extend this sphere of responsibility to the level of the community. We need dentists to accept the responsibility of ensuring that all persons in a community have access to the best quality care.

A related factor is the need to inculcate in students a deeper understanding of the very important obligations that come together with the rights and privileges of being a Professional, in particular, the social responsibilities that being a professional entail. While some may question whether social responsibility, even social advocacy, fits within a concept of being a "dental professional" it is clearly accepted by the medical profession that social responsibility is an integral component of being a physician. For example, the American Board of Internal Medicine has identified the elements of professionalism to include: excellence, accountability, duty, honor and integrity, respect for others, and altruism. It is perhaps self-evident that a healing profession such as medicine or dentistry, that serves others, must value that service above personal reward. Although it has become fashionable to apply business models to health care and to consider patients as "customers" (and although there is clear value to such an approach), we must exercise great caution to not teach our students to apply such business models indiscriminately to all aspects of patient care. Unlike most business transactions involving customers, professionals have a fiduciary relationship with our patients. Dentists have the ethical responsibility to act in the best interests of our patients, not in our own best interests. Similarly, we also have a duty as professionals to act in the best interests of our community. The oral health care needs of the under-served are not "someone else's problems" but rather they are our collective problem. Dental professionals clearly have a responsibility to contribute to the elimination of oral health disparities.

Acknowledgments

Preparation of this review was supported in part by the Northeast Center for Research to Evaluate and Eliminate Dental Disparities, and by grants (U54 DE14264 and K24 DE00419) from the National Institute of Dental and Craniofacial Research and the National Center on Minority Health and Health Disparities, National Institutes of Health. The assistance of Dr. Martha Nunn, Janis Johnson and Brenda Heaton is gratefully acknowledged. An abridged version of the introduction

Bibliography

Agency for Healthcare Research and Quality. *National Healthcare Disparities Report – 2003*. Rockville, MD: US DHHS Pub. No. 04-0035, AHRQ, 2003

Agency for Healthcare Research and Quality. *2000 Medical Expenditure Panel Survey, Household Component*. Rockville, MD: AHRQ, Public Health Service, 2000

Brown LJ, Wagner KS, Johns B. Racial/Ethnic Variations of Practicing Dentists. *Journal of the American Dental Association* 2000, 131: 1750-1754

Centers for Disease Control and Prevention. Health Disparities Experienced by Racial/Ethnic Minority Populations. *MMWR* 2004, 53: 755

Flores G, Olson L & Tomany-Korman SC. Racial and Ethnic Disparities in Early Childhood Health and Health Care. *Pediatrics* 2005, 115: 183-193

Garcia RI. Addressing Oral Health Disparities in Diverse Populations. *Journal of the American Dental Association* 2005, 136: 1210-1212

Horowitz AM, Rudd RE, Kirsch IS, White KW, Comings J, Garcia RI, Strucker J, Taylor GW, Evans C, Ismail AI, Kenyon DM & Kleinman DV. The Invisible Barrier: Literacy and its Relationship with Oral Health. *Journal of Public Health Dentistry* 2005, 65: 174-182

Isaacs SL & Schroeder SA. Class – The Ignored Determinant of the Nation's Health. *New England Journal of Medicine* 2004, 351: 1137-1142

Jha AK, Fisher ES, Li Z, Orav EJ & Epstein AM. Racial Trends in the Use of Major Procedures among the Elderly. *New England Journal of Medicine* 2005, 353: 683-691

Kressin NR & Petersen LA. Racial Differences in the Use of Invasive Cardio-vascular Procedures: Review of the Literature and Prescription for Future Research. *Annals of Internal Medicine* 2001, 135: 352-366

Kressin NR, Boehmer U, Berlowitz D, Christiansen CL, Pitman A & Jones JA. Racial Variations in Dental Procedures: The Case of Root Canal Therapy Versus Tooth Extraction. *Med Care* 2003, 41: 1256-1261

Kressin NR, Chang BH, Whittle J, Peterson ED, Clark JA, Rosen AK, Orner M, Collins TC, Alley LG & Petersen LA. Racial Differences in Cardiac Catheterization as a Function of Patients' Beliefs. *American Journal of Public Health* 2004, 94: 2091-2097

Lurie N. Health Disparities – Less Talk, More Action. *New England Journal of Medicine* 2005, 353: 727-729

Macek MD, Cohen LA, Reid BC & Manski RJ. Dental Visits Among Older U.S. Adults, 1999: The Roles of Dentition Status and Cost. *Journal of the American Dental Association* 2004, 135: 1154-1162

Manski RJ, Macek MD n& Moeller JF. Private Dental Coverage: Who Has it and How Does it Influence Dental Visits and Expenditures? *Journal of the American Dental Association* 2002, 133: 1551-1559

Marmot M. *The Status Syndrome: How Social Standing Affects our Health and Longevity.* New York: Henry Holt, 2004; p. 319

Mouradian WE, Reeves A, Kim S, Evans R, Schaad D, Marshall SG & Slayton R. An Oral Health Curriculum for Medical Students at the University of Washington. *Academic Medicine* 2005, 80: 434–442

Moy E, Dayton E & Clancy CM. Compiling the Evidence: The National Healthcare Disparities Reports. *Health Affairs* 2005, 24: 376-387

Nash DA & Nagel RJ. Confronting Oral Health Disparities among American Indian/Alaska Native Children: the Pediatric Oral Health Therapist. *American Journal of Public Health* 2005, 95: 1325-1329

Navarro V. Race or Class Versus Race and Class: Mortality Differential in the U.S. *Lancet* 1990, 336: 1238-1240

Satcher D, Fryer GE Jr, McCann J, Troutman A, Woolf SH & Rust G. What If We Were Equal? A Comparison of the Black-white Mortality Gap in 1960 and 2000. *Health Affairs* 2005, 24: 459-464

Smedley BD, Butler AS & Bristow LR (Eds.). *In the Nation's Compelling Interest: Ensuring Diversity in the Health Care Workforce.* Washington: National Academies Press, 2004; p. 432

Smedley BD, Stith AY & Nelson AR (Eds.) *Unequal Treatment: Confronting Racial and Ethnic Disparities in Health Care.* Washington, DC: Institute of Medicine, National Academies Press, 2002

U.S Census Bureau, 2003. http://www.census.gov. Accessed April 19, 2005

U.S. Dept. of Health and Human Services. *Healthy People 2010: Understanding and Improving Health,* 2nd ed. Washington, DC: US DHHS, 2000a

U.S. Dept. of Health and Human Services. *Oral Health in America: A Report of the Surgeon General.* Rockville, MD: USDHHS, NIDCR, NIH, 2000b. Available on-line at: http://www.surgeongeneral.gov/library/oralhealth/ (access verified on 11/3/05)

U.S. Dept. of Health and Human Services. *A National Call to Action to Promote Oral Health.* Rockville, MD: USDHHS, NIH Publication No. 03-5303, 2003

Vaccarino V, Rathore SS, Wenger NK, Frederick PD, Abramson JL, Barron HV, Manhapra A, Mallik S & Krumholz HM. Sex and racial differences in the management of acute myocardial infarction, 1994 through 2002. *New England Journal of Medicine* 2005, 353: 671-682

Mary McNally

Defining Oral Health

Introduction

Examining social arrangements, evaluating the distribution of goods and services, and considering why some members of society are subjects of undue burdens of poor health are important starting points whenever questions about justice in healthcare are raised. Moreover, the pursuit of justice in healthcare also requires that the considered goals for health are, in some sense, defensible. Framing what we mean by "health" lays the groundwork for establishing its worth as a social good and as a resource allocation issue. Is there a correct measure of health and if so, what needs must be addressed in order to achieve health?

In examining worthy goals for the pursuit of justice in the realm of oral health care, we are faced with a number of significant conceptual challenges. Not only must we examine conceptions of health, but we must also explore the peculiarity of "oral health" itself. For various reasons, oral health is considered separately from general health – a reality most clearly emphasized by its absence from most publicly funded healthcare systems. This chapter arises from a Canadian perspective, but its relevance is not meant to be limited by geographical borders. While Canada is well known for its universal healthcare system, it is often surprising to international audiences that oral health services are virtually excluded from publicly funded healthcare.

In this chapter, the meaning of oral health and the consequences of its separation from general health are examined from a philosophical, clinical and political point of view. Of primary importance is a consideration of the contemporary usage and critiques of the meaning of health as defined by the World Health Organization (WHO). Its influence on how concepts of oral health are theoretically perceived within the overall context of health is also explored. This inquiry into the meaning and correct measure of oral health underlies the larger philosophical questions about justice.

Conceptions of Health

In 1948, the WHO expanded the definition of health from narrow conceptions such as "absence of disease" or "physical well being" to a more expansive notion describing health as "a state of complete, physical, mental, and social well-being and not merely the absence of disease or infirmity." According to the WHO, health is a right of every human being; is fundamental to peace and security; and is basic to the "happiness, harmonious relations and security of all people"[1]. In spite of much controversy and debate about this definition, it has not been officially revised in fifty-six years and it remains the dominant definition of health.

Much of the debate centers around the appropriateness of a definition of health that is evaluative in nature. If human judgments about what constitutes "complete social well-being" are part of a definition of health, how does this affect the scope of what we mean by "health" and ultimately, the provision of health care? Norman Daniels (1999), one of the most influential contemporary theorists of health care justice, suggests that the WHO definition treats "health as an idealized level of fully developed functioning …and seems to conflate notions of health with those of general well-being, satisfaction, or happiness, over-medicalizing the domain of social philosophy." In fact, Daniel Callahan reports that the WHO definition was motivated by the belief that the improvement of world health would make an important contribution to world peace since health was intimately related to economic and cultural welfare. And although Callahan himself denies that health problems have ever been a serious cause of war, in the vision of the WHO, "health and peace were seen as inseparable"(Callahan 1990). The over-ambitious and boundless scope of the WHO definition has motivated both Callahan and Christopher Boorse to argue for a more narrow definition of health that has, as its basis, the physical and objective measures of bodily integrity. We will next discuss these alternative accounts of health, followed by Tristram Engelhardt's who insists that definitions of health inevitably include social constructions and uses historical examples to illustrate how social values can determine what we mean by health.

Christopher Boorse's concept of health as a capacity "to function in species typical ways" is a theoretical conception that is meant to oppose the widely held view that health is an evaluative notion (1977). He maintains that analyses of health should occur within the rubric of physiological medicine, because "the functional normality that defines it is worth having" and ultimately, these functions contribute to a measurable goal (1999). Boorse argues that judgments about health need not – and should not – include value judgments as part of their meaning and to do so is to misrepresent what is meant by disease. By appealing to "species typical functions" as a baseline for what constitutes health, Boorse opposes the use of value laden normative ideals for formulating parameters of health (1999). On Boorse's account, it follows that the manifestation of disease is understood as a "type of internal state which impairs health" (i.e., reduces one or more functional abilities of a particular species below typical efficiency when compared to its particular age and gender cohort) (1977). For Boorse, confining a definition of health to statistically and biologically normal species functioning is value neutral and equally, judgments about disease (or disruptions to normal function) are value neutral. He argues that the WHO definition is too broad and disagrees with the caveat of the WHO that health is unconditionally worth promoting. "Health is functional normality, and as such is desirable exactly insofar as it promotes goals one can justify on independent grounds"(1999).

An important feature of Boorse's account of health is his recognition of the conflation of theoretical and practical concepts of health that muddy perceptions about value neutrality. Health care providers are caught up in both theory and practice, which leads to a conception of health that reflects what Boorse calls "weak normativism." He uses this term to refer to descriptive theoretical concepts that are under the influence of therapeutic values in the provision of health care. He believes that it is at this level that confusion arises about the evaluative nature of health. In other words, Boorse acknowledges that clinical practice involves practical judgments (that include value judgments) about how people ought to be treated in the face of illness. But for Boorse, it is the judgment about what counts as illness that carries with it evaluative baggage, not the theoretical concept of health itself. "There are, then, two senses of 'health'. In one sense it is a theoretical notion, the opposite of 'disease'. In another sense it is a practical or mixed ethical notion, the opposite of 'illness'" (1999).

This "mixed notion" captures more of what is meant by health in the day-to-day world of pragmatic health care professions than it does in the theoretical domain. Health care providers investigate signs and symptoms of physiological changes, discomfort and disturbances (as well as potential disturbances such as in the case of breast cancer screening) for comparison to statistical baselines and physical norms, and they make judgments and interpretations about how this information is used. The fact that clinicians must often move forward in the face of uncertainty about a particular diagnosis means that value judgments are inherently a part of the practical activities of health as it relates to treating illnesses, but not, says Boorse, as it relates to determining what does and does not count as disease. For Boorse, defining disease is a purely empirical enterprise about what counts as a legitimate disruption to species typical function. As mentioned, illness is a special category of the objective measure of disease. "An illness must be, first, a reasonably *serious* disease with incapacitating effects that make it undesirable... and ...secondly, to call a disease an illness is to view its owner as deserving special treatment and diminished moral accountability" (Boorse 1999).

Interestingly, Boorse uses dental caries in two different contexts to support his arguments about what is meant by a value neutral concept of disease. Since this chapter ultimately seeks to examine conceptions of oral health, it is important to point out that his notions about dental decay are rather misguided. He seriously considers dismissing dental caries from conceptions of both disease and of illness but ultimately situates caries under the rubric of disease.

First, Boorse argues that one of the limitations of his own concept of disease relates to the issue of "universal diseases." For instance, by his definition, conditions that affect all of a certain cohort at the same time should actually be considered "species typical" and therefore would not constitute disease. Nevertheless, he holds the view that certain conditions are universal (such as dental caries or environmentally induced lung irritation) and are conventionally accepted as diseases in spite of the fact that they are so widespread that they might be considered normal within a species. To account for environmentally induced universal conditions, Boorse expands his definition of disease to include "limitations on functional ability caused by environmental agents" and argues that the expanded account "covers conditions like lung irritation and provides an alternate explanation of tooth decay" (1977). In other words, tooth decay is a disease, in spite of its being species typical, because it is not in the nature of the species and is due to environmental causes.

Although it seems correct that dental caries must ultimately be considered in the realm of disease, his argument involves a misconception about the universality and environmental nature of dental caries. In fact, dental caries is not entirely environmental as Boorse has argued – nor is it universal. Although the prevalence of caries in North America was higher in the mid-1970s (when Boorse carried out this work) than it is now, this particular oral disease has been on a sharp decline for the general population of the western world over the past five decades. This decline has been a result of better management of the disease with greater availability of restorative therapy and disease management, the introduction of fluoride to water supplies as a public health measure in the middle of the last century and, even more profoundly, a consequence of the development and aggressive marketing of oral health care products such as fluoridated toothpastes in more recent decades. Although it could be argued that these interventions are largely a testimony to Boorse's position that dental caries is environmental and that these measures have essentially meant an improvement to the environment, I would argue that this is an incomplete account for the etiology of dental caries. It is known that the incidence of dental caries in young children can be correlated with the caries status of their mothers (environment factors such as diet, and fluoride being equal, genetic predisposition and physical contact with cariogenic bacteria are two possible explanations). It is also known that some individuals are simply resistant to caries in spite of environmental factors working against them (again, genetic predisposition and lack of exposure to infectious bacteria are two explanations). Elders provide a very interesting cohort to consider the environmental influences of dental caries. It is not unusual for an adult to reach their senior years having been caries free for decades. Yet, the onset of physical disabilities associated with aging (e.g., arthritis, deterioration of vision) can negatively impact oral health status because of a concomitant decline in oral hygiene practices. This could occur with little change (or even an improvement) in the environmental influences that have kept adults caries free. And, why do some members of this particular cohort remain disease resistant? It is therefore a mistake to label this etiological phenomenon as completely "environmental."

Boorse's definition of health has as its main elements, statistical normality of biological function within a species cohort and, essentially, a failure of normal function equals disease. Dental caries is not a statistically universal phenomenon of a species cohort. Quite simply, a lot of people don't have and never have had dental caries and of those who have a history of dental decay, it is inappropriate to assume that they will necessarily be affected by it in future. Like other infections, once treated and eradicated, it may recur but then again, it may not. Therefore, if it falls under any definition proposed by Boorse, it is an example of a failure of normal species function – which would be more in keeping with his functional definition of disease, not the universal species typical exception. It could be argued that this misconception about dental caries is simply an epidemiological error. For the purposes of this discussion, however, it is an oversight worth mentioning. It will become clear as this chapter unfolds that oral health is inappropriately dismissed rather frequently from the domain of health proper – even at a conceptual level. Boorse's perspectives contribute to misconceptions about the meaning of oral health.

Secondly, Boorse uses dental caries as an example of a condition that is pathologically inconsequential and does not count a "single dental cavity" as serious enough to count as illness (1999). Specifically, he refers to dental caries as the "vitiligo"[2] of the teeth, indicating that dental caries is a local pathology affecting teeth that is more or less inconsequential with no systemic affects (1977). Unlike vitiligo of the skin, caries even at a very early stage of a single lesion, can result in serious pain and discomfort affecting function. Furthermore and again unlike skin vitiligo, if allowed to progress on its natural course, infection originating as a carious lesion can propagate and develop into a condition that is systemic in nature and oral function can be permanently compromised. Dental caries is, in fact, a transmittable infectious disease that is influenced by many factors including diet, individual immunity, systemic diseases and oral hygiene practices in removing local bacteria.

Thus, Boorse is wrong both in discounting dental caries as "a reasonably serious disease" and in arguing that dental decay is a purely objective condition. Indeed, more sick-leave is attributed to dental problems than most other disorders and the Provincial Health Officer of British Columbia has recently disclosed that dental treatments are the most common hospital-based surgical procedures for children under 14 years of age (Dharamsi & MacEntee 2002). I would argue instead on the basis of dental caries being an undesirable condition and the fact that the condition requires the influence of therapeutic values in the provision of care to treat it, that it falls into the mixed ethical notion of health that Boorse has referred to as the opposite of "illness."

Why is this an important argument to make? First, the major disease seen and treated by dentists is dental caries, and it is important to the discussion to understand that dental caries can be both incapacitating and serious and that there is an evaluative and morally sensitive component to this disease in our overall conception of health. Second, the term "serious" that Boorse uses to distinguish between disease and illness is itself evaluative and a source of confusion about his meaning of health. A single dental cavity may cause people to take time off work if they interpret it as serious.

Finally, it should be pointed out that Boorse assumes that the attainment of empirical information is value free. But is it possible to measure "normal species function?" in an objective, value-free manner? Peer review journals in biological sciences are testimony to the fact that there is constant debate about what counts as valid in the determination of physiological function. Debates about validity are not purely empirical in nature. For example, influences of the free market (e.g., large drug manufacturers) are known to influence the path of scientific investigation. If Boorse is simply defending the possibility of determining universally agreed upon valid measures of normal species function, then his theory about the meaning of health has limited practical use. Besides the potential evaluative effects on the scientific method itself, there are influences of human values on the direction of investigations in medicine and biology. These issues will be raised later in the discussion with reference to the work of Tristram Engelhardt.

Like Boorse, Daniel Callahan favors a narrow definition of health, a physically adequate functional conception. Both authors are concerned with the appropriate ethical boundaries associated with the term "health." For Boorse, ethical questions arise not about the objective empirical parameters of health and disease but about what ought to be done in the face of the debilitating effects of illness. Callahan argues for a narrow conception of health based on his critical appraisal of the WHO definition and the substantive ethical, social and political implications arising from it. Callahan's central arguments against the broad WHO definition of health stem from his worry that accepting such a broad definition leads to grave misuses of the term health. For Callahan, it is important to distinguish between health as a norm and health as a moral, political and social ideal. To avoid misuses of the definition of health, Callahan narrows the definition to "a state of physical well-being." "That state need not be 'complete', but it must be at least adequate, i.e., without significant impairment of function" (2001).

Callahan develops his argument in favor of a narrow definition of health by analyzing common objections to the WHO definition that delineate its potential misuse. For Callahan, "the ethical problem in defining the concept of health is to determine what the implications are of the various uses to which a concept of health can be put" and the "real or possible abuses to which the WHO definition leads" (2001). One of the objections is that "including the notion of 'social well-being' under its rubric, it turns the enduring problem of human happiness into one more medical problem, to be dealt with by scientific means" (2001). "[B]y implication, it makes the medical profession the gatekeeper for happiness and social well-being" (2001). He elaborates on this point by noting a number of unexamined implications. For example, are the pragmatic clinicians of medicine interested in and capable of discerning underlying values associated with subjective aspects of well-being such as human happiness? And what is the implication of the word "complete" in the WHO definition, as it refers to various aspects of human well-being and associated subjective and infinite human desires? Callahan argues that the only condition under which "complete well-being" is attainable, is for people to decrease their expectations about what life has to offer. This seems unlikely in the current climate where human desires are virtually insatiable. Attempts by medicine to respond to these expectations through technological and other therapeutic means would be an abuse of the proper goals of health. Besides, "complete social well being" connotes the potential for value judgments about health that could not possibly be accounted for in any practical way. Says Callahan, "there is no particular reason to believe that medicine can do anything more than make a modest, finite contribution" (to human happiness) (2001).

Another of Callahan's worries is that the responsibility for human miseries is misplaced when this is seen as a matter of health. By placing the responsibility there, it removes such problems from other, more appropriate, areas of responsibility that lie outside of the medical arena. Although there are sometimes psychological and psychiatric ills that contribute to social strife, other overwhelming influences such as "political injustice, economic scarcity, food shortages, unfavorable physical environments, have a far greater historical claim as sources of failure to achieve social well-being" (2001). Rather than resolving social problems by addressing the political, economic and environmental injustices influencing them, medical solutions will inappropriately be sought. "Such an ideology has the practical effect of blurring the lines of appropriate authority and responsibility" (2001). For example, medical solutions (he uses the example of incarcerating criminals within mental institutions rather than prison) will be sought for social issues that do not belong within the tradition of health and health care.

Callahan notes that "it seems simply impossible to devise a concept of health which is rich enough to be nutritious and yet not so rich as to be indigestible"(2001). By defending a narrow definition of health, Callahan supports an equally narrow scope of responsibility within the purview of traditional medicine. He wants to see issues of social responsibility placed within their proper arenas. He does not want medicine to be the gatekeeper of social and moral issues that exceed its proper domain. While this move may be defensible in allaying the potential abuses and misuses that he outlines, the question remains whether his definition is "rich enough to be nutritious?" By focusing only on functional physical adequacy, does he capture enough? Callahan's definition includes the subjective phrases "well-being" and "adequate." How well? And how adequate? And what if physical manifestations of function underlie mental health issues? What about the physical manifestations of malnutrition that are the result of unemployment and poverty? How will significant impairments of physical function associated with spousal abuse be addressed without attention to contributing social patterns? Callahan would not deny that contributing social patterns need attention. But such moral and political concerns are not health concerns and treating them as such is misguided. This barrier between health and moral and political influences on health is a theme that will reappear in this discussion.

To counter the positions outlined by Boorse and Callahan, I will argue that we cannot situate health outside of moral and political domains. Moreover, I will argue that social values influence and ultimately shape conceptions of health and disease. Qualifying what we mean by health must precede our deciding upon appropriate responses to health issues, and I do not believe that the accounts of Boorse and Callahan will allow for an adequate and just response.

Unlike Boorse and Callahan, Tristram Engelhardt recognizes that socially preferred functional norms encompass a great deal of what we mean by health. Engelhardt argues that humans set their own standards of health and disease which impact on the definition, evaluation and treatment of disease. Engelhardt acknowledges that "[a] 'disease entity' operates as a conceptual form organizing phenomena in a fashion deemed useful for certain goals. The goals, though, involve choice by man and are not objective facts, data 'given' by nature. They are ideals imputed to nature" (Engelhardt1999).[3] Callahan wants to avoid giving too much power to the "high priests of medicine" by limiting health to empirically justified physical measures. Engelhardt argues that this is misguided. Rather than narrow the scope of what we mean by health to physical parameters that can be managed by medicine, he favors expansion of the management domains concerned with health and disease. His suggestion that disease entities are not reducible to objective facts necessitates a multidisciplinary approach to issues of health. If health is indeed a social construct, it cannot remain the exclusive domain of medicine.

> Humans are animals which make their own nature, set their own standards of health and disease, and thus raise core issues concerning the directions and goods of life....Surely much awaits an interdisciplinary effort by philosophers, medical sociologists, and anthropologists (Engelhardt 1976).

In addition to Engelhardt's support of a conception of health that recognizes the influence of social values and the inclusion of disciplines other than medicine, he responds to the WHO definition by providing a scope of "well-being" for specific consideration by medicine. Engelhardt (1976) calls a state of affairs an illness if it is characterized as "being in some sense bad." He proposes that the types of evaluative judgments involved in such selections of clusters of phenomena as syndromes (illnesses) are diverse. They can, however, be arrayed into at least three groups: the teleological (i.e., preclude the goals chosen as integral to the general life of humans); the algesic (i.e., cause pain) and; the aesthetic (i.e., preclude a physical form that other humans would hold to be normal, not deformed) (1976). Accordingly, "the delineation of the scope of health depends on what one judges to be the elements of normal human life" (1976).

I believe Engelhardt's account provides a conception of disease and illness that should be of great interest to dentistry. His characterization of health and illness may be especially useful in establishing a meaningful scope of oral health needs that warrant some measure of social response.

Situating Oral Health

Diseases of the mouth, in spite of measurable morbidity and justifiability within even the narrowest conceptions of health, are curiously excluded from the scope of publicly funded health care in Canada as well as in many other countries with universal and public health care systems. Moreover, matters of oral health are not routinely included as a basic health consideration in private systems. Somewhere in the evolution of both public and private health care programs, deliberate decisions have been made about the meaning of oral health.

As mentioned, the consideration of a definition of health is important to understanding how theoretical concepts and practical activities can be understood relative to each other. Oral health is an interesting anomaly to our general conceptions of health (be they broad or narrow conceptions) for a number of reasons. In spite of the oral cavity being part of our overall physique, it is largely ignored by the medical profession that Callahan refers to as the gatekeeper of health. The duality of mouth and body is of practical importance in the provision of health care, but it is also an interesting conundrum that has received little if any attention in the philosophical literature. Beyond the philosophical interest, this separation of mouth from body has important ramifications within the arena of social justice where health issues concerning the mouth – because of its separation from the body (and hence from health care systems) – do not garner public interest or resources. The practical activities facing professionals responding to oral health care needs are profoundly influenced by this separation. David Locker suggests that

> ...[I]n dentistry, there has been a tendency for us to treat the oral cavity as if it were an autonomous anatomical structure that happens to be located within the body but is not connected to it (the body) or the person in any meaningful way. That is, the mouth as an object of enquiry has usually been isolated from both the body and the person (1997).

In this section, I will outline the peculiarities behind oral health's distinction from health and will present arguments to support my claim that it is an inappropriate distinction.

The most comprehensive scientific report in contemporary dentistry to take aim at the duality of mouth and body is the 2000 United States Public Health Service Surgeon General's first ever report on "Oral Health in America" (US Department of Health and Human Services, 2000). This report was meant to alert citizens to the "full meaning of oral health and its importance to general health and well-being" and is organized around a number of important themes. The first theme draws specific attention to expanding the meaning of oral health to be more in keeping with the broader definition of health defended by the World Health Organization (WHO) and furthermore, "oral health means much more than healthy teeth." This particular theme in the 2000 Surgeon General's Report is meant not only to expand the meaning of health to include a broader perception of well-being, but also to expand the physiological basis of oral health to include what is collectively known as the craniofacial complex. Well-being associated with oral health would be under the influence of conditions affecting all aspects of the craniofacial complex including the teeth, gingiva, their underlying supporting structures such as connective tissue and bone, the hard and soft palate, the tongue and floor of the mouth, the throat, the mucosa of the oral cavity and underlying salivary glands, the lips, muscles of mastication, and jaws (the mandible and maxilla). Conditions and dysfunction associated with this complex go far beyond the conventional perception that teeth and gums encompass all that is meant by "oral." Hence, the physiological scope of oral health is exemplified by tooth decay and periodontal disease as well as oral-facial pain conditions such as temporo-mandibular dysfunction (TMD); oral and pharyngeal cancers; oral soft tissue lesions; birth defects such as cleft lip and palate; to name a few of the conditions that are under the influence of the determinants of health.

The second theme, "oral health is integral to general health," is meant to express a reciprocal interconnectedness of these two. Simply put, general health affects oral health and oral health affects general health. The report has coined the phrase "the mouth is a mirror of health or disease" to describe the impact of assessing oral structures as a means to diagnosing underlying systemic problems (i.e., how general health affects oral health). Signs of nutritional deficiencies, immune dysfunction and even metastatic cancers often manifest in the oral cavity which can provide a means of early detection. For example, dysfunction and disease symptoms arising from the oral cavity (e.g., limited opening due to TMD, necrotizing ulcerative gingivitis) can affect the ability to eat and swallow thereby affecting overall nutrition status. Blood borne oral bacteria have long been implicated as a causative agent in life threatening bacterial endocarditis for people afflicted with heart valve defects.

That the health of the mouth and body are considered as separate concepts is perplexing but not inexplicable. There is a long history of professional separation between the realms of oral health care and general medicine (i.e., dentists and physicians). In addition to its absence from health service plans, education and clinical practice occur in entirely separate institutions and settings, and there is dearth of collaboration in academic research. David Locker (1997) therefore concludes that the idea of oral health is a "historical accident":

> We do not attach the concept of health to any body part other than the oral cavity and, indeed, it seems ludicrous to do so. According to the definitions (of health), oral cavities as anatomical structures cannot be healthy or unhealthy only people can. Consequently, the distinction that is often made or implied between general health and oral health is unwarranted; it has no underlying biological or theoretical logic. Rather, it should be seen as nothing more than an organizational distinction that arose through historical accident (1997).

Locker's suggestion that the question "what is oral health" should be reduced to "what is health?" (1997) seems right. Moreover, this point of view is also clearly emphasized in the Surgeon General's Report: "just as we now understand that nature and nurture are inextricably linked, and mind and body are both expressions of our human biology, so, too, we must recognize that oral health and general health are inseparable" (2000).

While these positions are convincing, the political and structural realities that separate the concepts of oral health from general health are very influential and cannot be ignored. Recognizing this, Locker asks, "what then should we do with the concept of oral health, given that it is somewhat anomalous and yet so central to our research and practical activities?" (1997). It seems that, for practical reasons, we must formulate a defensible concept of oral health.

There is no universally accepted definition of oral health. Prior to the recent adoption of a formal definition of oral health by the Canadian Dental Association, the closest expressed commitment appeared in the CDA Code of Ethics (CDA 1991) as a central value for Canadian dentists that patients should be entitled to "appropriate and pain free oral functioning." This expression is taken from the work of David Ozar (1988) and expresses a view of oral health akin to Callahan's narrow definition of health. In more recent work by Ozar and Sokol (2002), it is clearly recognized that oral health defined as "appropriate and pain free oral functioning" is an oversimplification. Specifically, Ozar and Sokol argue that we must be mindful that health is an evaluative concept and not merely factual. For them, the evaluative concept of health is necessary "to identify certain characteristics and conditions of humans as the ones that humans are better off having" (2002). They challenge members of the dental profession to think carefully about the meaning of oral health and its implications to professional practice.

Like Ozar and Sokol, I argue that a narrow physiological definition of oral health that excludes values is inconsistent with common perceptions about oral health and what it means to have a healthy dentition. For instance, losing one tooth may not have serious physiological consequences. But the social consequences of losing a central incisor are considerable. Indeed, social service agencies sometimes pay more for the restoration of a front teeth than the retention of posterior teeth, even though the posterior teeth are crucial to the proper function of mastication. I once asked a social worker why their policy allowed significantly more resources to be directed toward anterior teeth. The answer was quite simply: "Our clients will have better opportunities when seeking employment if they aren't missing front teeth." This social priority has little to do with oral functioning and more with moving people off welfare. The example underscores the need of a conception of oral health that goes beyond physical parameters.

The British National Health Services (NHS) for dentistry, which allots more resources to oral health are than its North American counterparts, defines oral health as "such a standard of health of the teeth, their supporting structures and any other tissues of the mouth, and of dental efficiency, as in the case of any patient is reasonable, having regard to the need to safeguard his general health" (Burke & Wilson, 1995). Clearly this definition makes the connection between oral health and general health. However, Yewe-Dyer (1993) argues that the NHS definition, by referring to general health as the primary goal, still excludes services related to esthetics and is therefore too narrow. To cover these perceived inadequacies, he proposes a broader definition: "oral health is the state of the mouth and associated structures where disease is contained, future disease is inhibited, the occlusion is sufficient to masticate food, and the teeth are of a socially acceptable appearance"(1993). Yewe-Dyer's criticism of the definition is grounded in observations of the practical limitations of treatment that the NHS definition affords. But Locker notes that while Yewe-Dyer's definition "makes reference to functional and social concerns, and in so doing attempts to cross the divide between medical and socioenvironmental paradigms of health, ultimately it remains largely within the former. That is, health is equated with the absence of disease and the focus remains predominantly on the mouth rather than the person" (Locker 1997).

Much like the WHO definition of health in general, so Yewe-Dyer's work reveals the impact of justice concerns on attempts to define oral health. Yewe-Dyer proposed a broader definition out of concern that the scope of treatment provided by the British NHS did not provide for enough publicly funded oral health service. Conversely, as Norman Daniels has pointed out, in order to "specify a notion of health care needs, we need clear notions of health and disease" (1999). Daniels examines conceptions of health in order to frame a theory of health needs. This theory then provides the basis for what he perceives as the most appropriate range of needs that will guarantee an individual a reasonable share of certain basic social goods. Thus, in the interest of distributive justice and in response to the scarcity of public resources, Daniels wants to identify which health care needs can be justifiably characterized as social goods. In March of 2001, the Canadian Dental Association formally developed and approved the following definition: "Oral health is a state of the oral and related tissues and structures that contribute positively to physical, mental and social well-being and the enjoyment of life's possibilities, by allowing the individual to speak, eat and socialize unhindered by pain, discomfort or embarrassment"(CDA 2001). This definition is modeled in part by the work of David Locker, the WHO definition of health, and the British Health Department's definition of oral health. The Canadian Dental Association (CDA) sought to reinforce to Canadians the importance of oral health to general health and to incorporate the subjective perception of the importance of oral health to function, socialization and well being. The CDA serves as a central voice for the dental profession and speaks to issues of policy, professional and public responsibility, responsible marketing of oral health products, dental education, and priorities for research.

This new definition of oral health provides a useful and defensible point from which to speak to this broad range of issues. Indeed, a broad definition of health is attractive to the extent that it captures aspects of health and health care that are not only characterized by "typical species functioning" or "appropriate and pain free oral function." However, unless the Canadian public is willing to provide limitless resources for the provision of oral health care, the CDA definition may not provide useful parameters for elucidating a range of needs that justify a reasonable share of public resources toward oral health care.

Concluding Observations

In keeping with Locker's concerns and the findings of the US Surgeon General, the CDA – even in its definition of oral health – ultimately gives priority to the health of the person, not just the mouth. Like the WHO, the CDA definition is committed to "physical, mental and social well-being" as the proper domain of oral health by referring to a status of oral health that "contributes positively" to these ideals. Note, however, that the definition does not stipulate the attainment of "complete" well-being but only that oral health "contributes positively" to that end. The second part of the definition refers to functions dependent upon the craniofacial complex (i.e., speaking, eating and socializing) without which "life's possibilities" might not be enjoyed. In tracking the evolution of the CDA definition of oral health, it is difficult to determine the exact rationale for the specific inclusion of the "enjoyment of life's possibilities" within the meaning of oral health although it is likely that the notion stems from perceptions about how quality of life impacts on personal well-being. Clearly, what constitutes "life's possibilities" is subjective and evaluative. However, the CDA definition circumvents the potential interpretation of "life's possibilities" as being infinite human desires by clarifying that the definition is related to the functional activities associated with speech, eating, and socializing. More problematic is the reference to "embarrassment." How does one assess "embarrassment" and how can we reasonably assess what will contribute positively to "mental well-being" and "enjoyment of life's possibilities"?

The Surgeon General's Report would seem to support a broad definition such as the CDA's by recognizing multiple "oral health quality of life" issues that include an individual's ability to function normally in the routines of daily living (e.g., speech, eating, swallowing), experience symptom relief from disease and disability, and fulfill usual roles in personal relationships and social interactions as important and measurable parameters of quality of life and well-being (US Department of Health and Human Services 2000). Research must be undertaken to focus priorities and identify oral health needs that are worthy of public support. Sensitivity to human values and the impact of quality of life determinants are as important to research and education in health care as understanding pathological and physiological manifestations of illness. In keeping with Engelhardt's view, there is no reason to exclude these subjective aspects of health from the purview of health care providers nor does this require that the health care profession becomes the sole proprietor of all aspects of health. Although some of the practical reasons for oral health's marginalization from general health have been described, it must not remain a professionally situated subcategory of health. Achieving health must be considered a multidisciplinary endeavor, a rich collective of theory, research and response involving many disciplines and many levels of the community. Ensuring that members of society are not subjects of undue burdens of poor health arising from oral disease and disability requires that we continue to engage and reflect carefully on the meaning and proper domain of oral health. Justifying what we ought to be doing in order to sort out legitimate needs and social responsibility in the provision of oral health care is the subject of the remaining chapters.

Notes

[1.] Preamble to the Constitution of the World Health Organization as adopted by the International Health Conference, New York, 19-22 June, 1946; signed on 22 July 1946 by the representatives of 61 States (Official Records of the World Health Organization, no.2, p. 100) and entered into force on 7 April 1948.

[2.] Vitiligo refers to an inconsequential pigmentation of the skin characterized by the formation of white patches.

[3.] Specifically, Engelhardt tracks the history of medical developments surrounding the "disease of masturbation" over the past two centuries to illustrate how therapy and conceptions of the disease have changed on the basis of changing values. "The disease of masturbation is an eloquent example of

the value-laden nature of science in general and of medicine in particular"
(Engelhardt 1999). The nineteenth century saw the acceptance of a model
of diagnosis and therapy where pathophysiological signs and symptoms of
masturbation arose from a number of possible etiologies including: unnatural
sexual overexcitation, associated guilt and anxiety, and response to a culture
that condemned the activity. Invasive physical therapies and interventions
were documented in the medical literature to have cured the myriad of
symptoms associated with the disease."The theoretical framework, though ...
was not value free (it was a disapproved activity) but structured by the values
and expectations of the times" (Engelhardt 1999). This is problematic for
Engelhardt who argues that because diseases are, in fact, socially constructed
phenomena, they are misplaced within the exclusive, physiological jurisdic-
tion of medicine. There have been vast changes in attitudes (societal and
medical) about the"disease" of masturbation (e.g., articles written about using
masturbation to overcome the disease of frigidity or orgasmic dysfunction)
that reflect changes in values from the nineteenth to the twentieth century.
"The variations are not due to mere fallacies of scientific method, but involve
a basic dependence of the logic of scientific discovery and explanation upon
prior evaluations of reality...Values influence the purpose and direction
of investigations and treatment... and play a role in the development of
explanatory models" (Engelhardt 1999).

Bibliography

Boorse C. Health as a Theoretical Concept. *Philosophy of Science* 1977, 44:
542-573

Boorse C. On the Distinction Between Disease and Illness. In Lindemann
Nelson J & Lindemann Nelson H (Eds.). *Meaning and Medicine: A Reader
in the Philosophy of Health Care*. New York: Routledge and Chapman Hall,
Inc., 1999; pp.16-27

Burke FJT & Wilson NHF. Measuring Oral Health: an Historical View and
Details of a Contemporary Oral Health Index. *International Dental Journal*
1995, 45: 358-370

Callahan D. *What Kind of Life?* New York: Simon and Schuster, Inc., 1990

Callahan D. The Who Definition of Health. In Teays W & Purdy LM (Eds.).
Bioethics, Justice and Health Care. Belmont CA: Wadsworth Publishing
Company, 2001; pp. 7-11

Canadian Dental Association. Definition of Oral Health among Items Endorsed
by Board of Governors. *Communique* 2001, March/April: 1-15

Canadian Dental Association. Code of Ethics. 1991. On-line at: http://www. cda-adc.ca/en/cda/about_cda/code_of_ethics/index.asp (access verified on 11/3/05)

Daniels N. Health Care Needs and Distributive Justice. In Lindemann Nelson J & Lindemann Nelson H (Eds.). *Meaning and Medicine: A Reader in the Philosophy of Health Care.* New York: Routledge and Chapman Hall, Inc., 1999; pp. 215-235

Dharamsi S & MacEntee M. Dentistry and Distributive Justice. *Social Science and Medicine* 2002, 55: 323-329

Engelhardt HT. The Disease of Masturbation: Values and the Concept of Disease. In Lindemann Nelson J & Lindemann Nelson H (Eds.). *Meaning and Medicine: A Reader in the Philosophy of Health Care.* New York: Routledge and Chapman Hall, Inc., 1999; pp. 5-15

Engelhardt HT. Human Well-being and Medicine. In Engelhardt HT Jr. & Callahan D (Eds.). *The Foundations of Ethics and Its Relationship to Science: Science Ethics and Medicine Volume I.* New York: The Hastings Center Institute of Society, Ethics and the Life Sciences, 1976; pp. 120-139

Locker D. Concepts of Oral Health, Disease and the Quality of Life. In Slade GD (Ed.). *Measuring Oral Health and Quality of Life.* Chapel Hill: University of North Carolina, Dental Ecology, 1997; pp. 12-23

Ozar DT. Value Categories in Clinical Dental Ethics. *Journal of the American Dental Association* 1988, 116: 365-368

Ozar DT & Sokol DJ. *Dental Ethics at Chairside: Professional Principles and Practical Applications (2nd ed.).* Washington: Georgetown University Press, 2002.

U.S. Dept. of Health and Human Services. *Oral Health in America: A Report of the Surgeon General.* Rockville, MD: USDHHS, NIDCR, NIH, 2000. Available on-line at http://www.surgeongeneral.gov/library/oralhealth/ (access verified on 11/3/05)

Yewe-Dyer M. The definition of oral health. *British Dental Journal* 1993, 174: 224-225

Shafik Dharamsi

Social Responsibility and Oral Health Disparities: A Constructivist Approach

Introduction

There is increasing evidence that oral health policies that fail to consider the social determinants of health are unlikely to have the desired impact at the level of population and public health (Hobdell et al. 2003). Clearly, health and health care are influenced by the interaction of social, economic and cultural factors (Blane et al. 1996; Link & Phelan 1995; Kawachi & Kennedy 1997; Auerbach & Krimgold 2001), all of which contribute to the oral health disparities identified in western society (Fiscella & Williams 2004; US Dept. of Health and Human Services 2000; Locker & Matear 2000; Edelstein 2002). For instance, although Canada and the USA have remarkably high life expectancies, educational attainments, and incomes (UNDP 2004), they also fair remarkably poorly on the Human Poverty Index (12th and 17th respectively) with more than one million children in Canada and 11 million children in the USA living in poverty (CCRC 2004; Douglas-Hall & Koball 2005). We know that disparities in health are influenced more readily by the income gap between rich and poor than by the simple number of people in poverty (Wilkinson 1996), and in both countries today the gap seems to be increasing. Consequently, when it comes to health, the more vulnerable segments of the population are not only socio-economically disadvantaged (Budetti et al. 1999; Smith 1999, MacEntee et al. 2001; WHO 2003), they also carry a disproportionately high burden of illness (Kennedy et al. 1996; Poulton et al. 2002; Federal, Provincial & Territorial Dental Directors, 2003).

As a result, there is a growing desire in society to provide equitable access to health care for all and to reduce health-related costs without compromising on quality. Unfortunately, dental care in most parts of the world is a health service that continues to remain accessible predominantly to the socio-economically advantaged members of society.

Canadians, for instance, have a health care system built on the principles of universality, comprehensiveness, public administration, portability and accessibility, but oral health care is not a part of this system (Federal, Provincial & Territorial Dental Directors, 2002). Canada does not have a national oral health strategy, or central monitoring of oral health in the country (Armstrong 2005). Yet, it is now widely acknowledged that "you cannot be healthy without oral health ... [it] is a critical component of health and must be included in the provision of health care and the design of community programs" (US Dept. of Health and Human Services 2000).

Over the past decade several stakeholders have raised a number of concerns, calling for a closer examination of the inequities that are provoked by a restricted dental health care system, as well as the factors that affect access to oral health care. It has certainly spurred a call for greater sensitivity to the social determinants of health, and perhaps more interestingly, the issues have also raised concerns around the ethic of social responsibility in dental practice and dental education (Boyd 1993; Woolfolk 1993; Gershen 1993; Formicola 1988; Haden et al. 2003).

However, social responsibility is a concept with many dimensions that have not been explored adequately within the context of dentistry and the needs of a profession struggling with the relationships of practicality, affordability and equity in the provision of oral health care for all. How is the idea of social responsibility considered within dentistry and how do its expression and understanding relate to the issues of access to dental care and oral health disparities?

Using the analytic construct of "discourse" (Mills 1997) this chapter explores the concept of social responsibility as it is discussed within a profession that is challenged increasingly by the realities of health disparities and the needs of disadvantaged populations. Discourses reflect prevailing ideologies, values, beliefs and the social practices that dominate; they have a profound influence on the social, political and economic structures of society, and on how individuals choose to function within them (Pratt & Nesbitt 2000). This chapter is based on a critical examination of the dental literature, editorials and letters in dental journals, keynote addresses at professional society meetings, as well as discussions with dental educators, clinicians, and politicians who were asked to speak freely about their sense of social responsibility and related issues that influence the practice of dentistry in western society (Dharamsi 2004). It examines the assumptions that underlie various views of social responsibility and the speculations on the sense of responsibility that operates currently within the dental profession toward disadvantaged populations. The analysis is based on the premise that no individual speaks entirely freely of their social and cultural context and affiliations (Kukla 2000). As a consequence, any construction of the concept of social responsibility is, in part, that of the individual, the profession, and the larger societal discourse.

The intent of this chapter is not to suggest a universal definition for social responsibility, but to describe ways this concept is considered and addressed within particular social contexts and social realities. Various constructions of social responsibility are presented. They are situated within the contexts of dentistry and dental education. The aim is to provoke critical reflection on the influences that shape the boundaries of what is acceptable and unacceptable within the community of professional dental practice, and to stimulate discussion and action toward eliminating oral health disparities and the challenges around equitable access to care.

Discourses of Social Responsibility

Social responsibility is context-dependent. Its meaning is culturally and historically specific. When applied to a context like professional practice, the concept becomes increasingly explicit. Recognizing the different ways social responsibility is constructed within the context of practice provides useful insight into what people see as reasonable and justifiable. For instance, the social responsibility to treat dental pain, regardless of compensation, is a responsibility that dentists say they hold sacrosanct; no one should be left in pain. This is a widely accepted code among dentists. It provides an agreed upon position for talking and thinking about social responsibility. However, it may be difficult for some to extend themselves beyond this code because the moral resolve to provide dental care for the vulnerable and less advantaged is influenced by the different ways we deal with the economic, educational, political and professional realities of the health care system, and how we position ourselves within it. We need to understand, therefore, what it is that influences how we experience these realities and how we decide to position ourselves accordingly.

Social Responsibility as an Economic Construct

References to dentistry as a commercial enterprise focus on the business side of providing dental services. There are those who are critical of it while others present it as an inevitable and necessary part of the dental health care system. The critics point to its hegemonic function in dentistry and resist what they consider an unacceptable construction of their professional identity and what it means to be a dentist and a professional within health care. They invoke issues of professionalism and rights to health care to support their position and criticisms. They are critical of the image of dentists as commercial entrepreneur, seen first as business-persons with a primary desire to economic success. They express a strong concern about a profession that they feel is absorbed by a corporate mentality, driven by profit. They hold firm to a professional identification more closely related to what they believe health care ought to be – accessible, universal and equitable. They say that the dental health care system as it is currently structured in many parts of the world is seen to give certain segments of the population an unfair advantage in accessing care. It is seen as the detrimental influence of the 'monetarization' of health care where the organization of health services is increasingly determined by economic priorities.

Yet others argue that it is naive to ignore the importance of fiscal responsibility and the economic realities within which health care is embedded. It is not about denying equity and accessibility, they say; it is about the realities of economics within a free-market system – a system that forms the bedrock upon which highly industrialized societies are based. Within this context, social responsibility is constructed in relation to economic factors that trust the market to be a fair arbiter for providing equal opportunity to all. The market is seen, therefore, as a vehicle for delivering health care efficiently. The notion of efficiency is based on the foundation of free enterprise, hard work and survival of the fittest. For the foundation to remain stable, its proponents argue, the market cannot be encumbered by non-market forces. As a result, proponents of this system tend to give priority to free enterprise over compulsory service to society. They see the market as a place for the development of individual capacity, self-determination and meritocracy. And although proponents of the market system do not deny the importance of issues of access and equity, they challenge the locus of responsibility for addressing these matters. They refer to welfare and other public mechanisms established through the taxes generated from market activities.

Conversely, those who notice the influence of social determinants on health, wealth and general well-being argue that the market indeed discriminates against those who are among the least advantaged in society and who find themselves marginalized from its benefits. The market, they argue, is constrained by vested interests and it can succumb to monopoly. They argue, therefore, that the market is an inappropriate vehicle for the delivery of health care, which they consider a fundamental social good, like education. A market oriented health care system is seen to introduce attitudes and actions that associate the patient with profit. Wealthier patients and those with insurance become preferred clientele.

For instance, posted on one of the information bulletin boards at a prominent dental school was an advertisement for a continuing education seminar by "one of the world's most successful and unusual Dentists of Australia" who conducts continuing education courses worldwide for dentist, teaching how to achieve a preferred clientele, and to work less and make more money. The brochure went on to state:

> Here's a dentist who was miserable and so, "fired" half his patients, locked his front door, took down all his signs, and only accepted new patients "By Referral." And now Paddi works 3 days a week, makes 3 times more money than the average dentist and has made happiness the focus of his practice! (…) Paddi has a negative accounts receivable and no bad debts – customers like to pay their bills! (…) This is what we all want in our practice. Paddi has an amazing story to tell and his philosophy of work will revolutionize the way you envision and operate your dental business (Lund, n.d.).

The message to all dentists, new and established alike is that they should all be striving to be like Dr. Lund – if you are not earning an "appropriate" level of income and you are miserable as a result, then fire your patients and get new "customers." Dr. Lund's approach is said to have "received high recognition from leaders both in and outside of dentistry…" His approach reinforces the dominant business discourse arising from the market paradigm. It influences how some dentists think about their practice and their profession. Some go as far as to argue that market influences promote primary objectives among many dentists to make an "obscene amount of money, to sit back and watch it role in…to come into work late and leave early." These dentists strive for a "different league," they are the "seven-series BMW guys":

> "…some make an obscene amount of money because they own several practices and they've been very good business people, as well as good dentists. They have several practices and they employ associate dentists working for the National Health Service and off they go…they just sit back and watch it role in! Now the dentist I worked for had two associates and he made probably 60-70 thousand pounds a year. Which is a very nice income level and he didn't bust his butt. He left at half four and he got in at ten. Now, private dentists make 120-200 thousand pounds a year. They are the seven-series BMW guys and they make huge amounts. They look toward North America and they see what we have here and they say, "well, we want a bit of this!" So you see, it's a move from very good income levels to obscene income levels" (Dharamsi 2004).

Dental marketing experts, for example, use the profit motive to have dentists rethink their professional worth. They capitalize on and perpetuate the pervading business culture and profit orientation. Within this discourse dentists are urged, with great emphasis, to consider raising their fees if they are to be seen as worthy professionals:

> "Many of you struggle with your fees. Many of you don't feel you are worth what you are charging. Many of you find it hard to justify raising your fees when it is suggested by me and others. The role that dentists play in our society is very important. Do you want some justification on raising your fees? Here is some information I got from my clinical director of the Master Dentist Program, Mike Miyasaki. I think it would be hard to find anyone who thinks basketball is more important to society than dentistry. So let's compare your fee to the best in basketball. Michael Jordan will make $10,000 a minute playing basketball, assuming he plays for 30 minutes each game. Also assuming he will make $40 million in endorsements (that's a conservative figure), he'll be making $178,100 a day, regardless of whether he's working or not. Taking his income and dividing it by 24 hours, he makes $7,420.83 an hour; every hour of the day. Again, whether he is working or not. While watching a movie, he makes $18,550. While playing golf, he makes $33,390, not including anything he wins betting. If he wants to buy a $90,000 luxury automobile, it will take him 12 hours of savings. In fact, he could go

to bed at 9:00 p.m. after spending every dime he had and still be able to afford it when the dealership opens at 9:00 a.m. the next morning. How long would it take you to save up for such a car? ... He will make more than twice as much as all of our past presidents for all of their terms... combined. The average dentist makes less than two tenths of one cent for every dollar he makes. I hope now you are thinking that maybe you don't get paid enough considering the difference in importance between a basketball player and a dentist. Do you want a little more help in realizing the insignificance of your income? Well think about this: Michael Jordan would have to save 100 per cent of his income for the next 270 years to have a net worth equivalent to that of Bill Gates" (Dickerson 1999).

Proponents of the market consider social responsibility an "expensive proposition." Others argue that as long as health care is situated in the market, it will be seen as a business first. This creates social pressures and a tension between the patient-first ethos of the healer and the survival-of-the-richest demands of private enterprise where profit is a fundamental end. Some argue that dentistry desperately needs a foundation in business ethics and that dentistry should "learn from its business confreres...and present a genuine corporate face of ethical unity in response to a demanding market" (Wiebe 2000). Introducing business ethics into the equation provides the tacit assurance that dentistry is first a commercial endeavor.

Although entrepreneurial thinking is a vital ingredient for the everyday running of a dental clinic, and some of the decisions taken by clinicians are clearly business oriented, Ozar (1985) concludes that it does not have to translate into a defining construct of dentistry. Yet, while dentists aim to maximize the oral health of their patients, the economic dimension of their strategies tends inevitably to exert its pragmatic influence. Those who see equitable access to health care as elemental and the health professions as guardians of that care, consider it unacceptable to place the providers' business interest over the patient's health – it is seen to compromise the fiduciary relationship between the profession and society, and this introduces a moral conflict that remains yet unresolved in professional practice.

Social Responsibility as a Professional Construct

Those who oppose the business discourse (either absolutely or in part) tend to invoke the virtues of being a health professional to defend their position. In turn, they use a professionalism discourse to counter the market-driven model of dental health care (Welie 2004a, 2004b, 2004c). Some believe that the concepts of social responsibility and professionalism are interdependent. Within this construct, to be regarded a profession, dentistry is seen as having certain standards or principles to uphold, regardless of the economic structures within which the dental health care system is embedded. The concept of professionalism, it is argued, has evolved to include the principled acceptance of certain obligations: a commitment to society to achieve a specified level of education, training and expertise, to agree to abide by stated principles and codes of conduct, and to place a high priority on society's welfare.

In this view, the image of a professional is one imbued with trust, and possessing expert knowledge not available to the laity. Professionals, therefore, are expected to use their knowledge and skill in the interest of the public good, for which they are granted a number of privileges: self-governance, autonomy and self-regulation. The knowledge professionals acquire through their specialized education and training may not be seen as proprietary or taken to be exclusive or discriminating in who receives care. Some worry therefore that dentistry fights hard to protect its privileges but fails to uphold its obligation to ensure that all members of society have access to their services. They see dentistry as a symbol of affluence and of the affluent. The implication is that the elite – that dentists too are seen to have become – shape, reproduce, and perpetuate a particular kind of social inclusion and exclusion around dentistry, defining what it means to be a dentist and to whom their services belong.

Although the dental profession, like most professions, is governed by a code of conduct and ethics within which members can be called upon to account for their decisions and actions, these codes tend not to insist on equitable access to care. Yet if the salient issues of equity and access are left largely to each individual dentist to determine, some dentist will decide they do not have to care for those who are vulnerable, and this conflicts with what others regard as inherent to the notion of professionalism.

While the underlying issue of professional privilege provides for some obvious and reasonable grounds for considering a social responsibility to meet the needs of the least advantaged, ultimately it all depends on where the subject of concern is situated – in the health of individual patients through individual dentists or the health of communities through a community of practitioners.

Social Responsibility as an Individual Choice Construct

A well-organized society is one where there is a healthy balance between individual pursuits and working to advance the common good. However, an emergent and dominant individualism in today's society is seen to affect interpretations of social responsibility. In this case, professionals are seen as having less commitment to their profession as a whole and more to themselves as beneficiaries of the profession to which they belong. It is thought to be a reflection of more and more people "bowling alone" (Putnam 2000). Prior to the advent of institutionalized social services communities functioned on a framework of reciprocity and concern for each other. Now this is seen as the government's responsibility and no longer part and parcel of one's civic attitude and practice.

Some argue, however, that the social net is woefully inadequate and that the dental profession ought to make a contribution to meet the shortfall. Social responsibility within this construct is vested in the concept of community, not individuals. Those who locate both the dentist and the patient in social communities see a collective responsibility for ensuring access to care, and the subject of community is the element of concern, not simply the individual. Others object that the ways in which large and complex societies are structured inevitably tend to create depersonalized tendencies among individuals and communities.

Various socializing factors also affect an orientation to social responsibility. Culture and family background as well as secondary socializing forces, such as education, have a powerful impact on world view and behavior. Education is thought to play a significant role in determining what constitutes acceptable professional practices and how dentists ought to interpret professional principles within the context of their communities (DeSchepper 1987). What students are taught and how they are taught is inextricably linked to particular orientations to social responsibility (Mouradian et al. 2003). If the delivery of dental care is to balance between the focus on the individual patient in the dental chair and a wider commitment to the oral health of society, then dental education should reflect that. However, the currency to graduate in most dental schools is not community service but to do well in a credit-based curriculum with an emphasis on the surgical art and science of dentistry. If students are overwhelmed by an educational milieu that favors technical and clinical competencies and overlooks education for civic duty, then social responsibility will remain peripheral to professional practice (Rubin 2004).

Moreover, the types of students who apply and are admitted into dental school also influence and are influenced by a particular discourse. The typical dental student comes from an upper or upper-middle class background and lives a privileged life; their socio-economic experiences are too far removed from the problems and issues facing disadvantaged segments of the population (Carlisle et al. 1998; Sinkford et al. 2001; Cavazos 2001). Many students who enter dental school appear to be rather individualistic and concerned primarily about a career that enables the earning of a good income and the achievement of a lofty social status. There is a sense also that the types of students attracted to dentistry are acutely aware of the way the profession is structured; and those with a strong orientation to social responsibility tend to choose professions other than dentistry to enable and nurture that ethic. Dentistry appears caught in a self-perpetuating cycle where the prevailing conduct of practice is driven by a corporate ethos and a discourse that attracts individualistic and materialistic oriented students who perpetuate the accompanying norms and standards within a system that is private and situated in the free market (Jamous & Peloille 1970; Frank 1999). This individualism is thought to predominate among the more privileged members of society who also hold a more dominant social place within it. As a result, the perceived outcome of the dominance is a pervasive hegemonic world-view that is accepted by the whole of society as natural and normal.

Theoretical Reflections on the Concept of Social Responsibility

The term "responsibility" emerges usually within a framework of action, inaction (as in failing to do something), intention and behavior. Responsibility involves personal agency, and it is something that is learned. It is a personal and acquired concept, with a definite dimension of choice – you can either accept or reject it.

Responsibility is concerned with intentions as well as behaviors, and it is linked to morality. I refer to morality as conduct examined and established within a society to understand and do what is right, while respecting the rights of others (Frankena 1962). Hence, being responsible entails moral and ethical behavior. Morality implies an ability and willingness to choose right over wrong. If being responsible is also a matter of moral principle, then fulfilling commitments due only to accountability or in anticipation of positive or negative consequences is insufficient. A responsible person is one who is responsible not solely out of self-interest, but because it is the right thing to do as a matter of principle and social standard independent of context or situation.

Responsibility is also influenced by social practice and the integrity of the individual within society. Consequently, the act of social responsibility, in contrast to the more general concept of responsibility, is influenced by the context of a person's social role, social position, and occupation. It is an act that goes beyond honesty, reliability, morality and honoring the rights of others. For example, the socially responsible person might leave the car at home and take the bicycle to work in an effort to improve the environment. Although not required by law, the bicycle rather than the car is used for the common good stemming from an ethic of social responsibility within a community. It also becomes a matter of choosing to contribute to the common good rather than being forced to do so.

Ideal notions of social responsibility will inevitably be absolutist, and incontestable. Ideal notions will not account for the messiness, complexities and dilemmas encountered and experienced in daily life. The conventional approach in the literature in responding to matters of equity and access is to situate them within the different theories on distributive justice and to pitch one against the other – libertarianism vs. egalitarianism vs. contractarianism, for example – in the hopes of arriving at a fruitful solution (Dharamsi & MacEntee, 2002). Unfortunately, theoretical conceptions of social responsibility do not always respond well to the discourses that develop and evolve contextually in relation to the micro and macro levels of economic, professional and political influences on health care. The notion of social responsibility is complex and to understand complex problems requires an understanding of the real world of practice. What goes unexamined when filtering such problems primarily through a theoretical lens is how discourses play a part in influencing how things work. There remain unresolved differences between what is considered a fair allocation of resources to public dental health care in particular, to provide a reasonable compensation to providers and an adequate range of services. We need practice-based evidence for evidence-based practice.

Toward a Cooperative Discourse

Clearly, there are fundamental practical, political, professional, policy, and educational implications of the different discourses of social responsibility in dentistry. Although it is not within the scope of this chapter to examine these, a brief mention will serve to orient us toward a cooperative discourse.

For instance, current social and related oral health policies and educational frameworks that seek to address health disparities are in need of fundamental reconceptualization – based not on welfarist ideology but on the mounting evidence of the influence of social determinants on health and the knowledge and power differentials in society that lead to inequities (Benzeval et al. 1995). A welfarist approach focuses on the negative consequences of illness requiring clinical treatment and significant resources. More fundamentally, however, it overlooks the affects of social organization (Syme 1996), and the mounting evidence of increasingly successful and empowering community-based initiatives (Petersen & Waddel 1998; Mittelmark, 1996; Dickson, Dunn-Pierce & Rosenbloom 1996). Moreover, the construct of the "social" within a welfarist model does not include non-dominant voices, thereby often excluding the perspectives of those who are most vulnerable. Constructive approaches require the engagement of a wide range of stakeholders (dentists, dental educators, those in the governance of dentistry, representatives of the public, those marginalized from care, and government officials and policymakers) to participate in open and honest dialogue and debate of the problems at hand. There must be a genuine willingness to understand and ultimately resolve the existing inequities. This requires a truthful cooperative discourse toward a consensus moral view among the different stakeholders (Habermas 1992). To arrive at a consensus requires an examination of the range of discourses that influence the potential and real impacts of various decisions and actions.

Implications for Dental Education

As dental schools across North America continue to work towards developing a socially responsive curriculum, there is an opportunity to examine the extent to which it influences the beginnings of the formation of a new professional identity in the next generation of doctors (Wotman et al. 2003). Bernstein's (1996) work on retrospective and prospective identities is helpful when examining professional identity formation. Retrospective identity is rooted in the past and affects the on-going formation of identity for the present and for the future. Hence, retrospective identity formation tends to advance the status quo. Prospective identity, on the other hand, is oriented towards the future, on the basis of which there is a concerted effort to shape what ought to be. In effect, the idea of prospective identities is an attempt to change the basis for collective recognition and relationships. Prospective identities are an outcome of new social movements, and the creation of a new and different discourse. In the case of dentistry, it suggests a new and different way of engaging with economic, professional and political realities to enable the development of new ways of looking at the dental profession and its place in society. Curricular reform efforts should try to achieve what Beane and Apple (1995) see as an integral part of democratic schools that seek progressive change:

• The open flow of ideas, regardless of their popularity, that enables people to be as fully informed as possible

• Faith in the individual and collective capacity of people to create possibilities for resolving problems

• The use of critical reflection and analysis to evaluate ideas, problems and policies

• Concern for the welfare of others, equity and "the common good"

• Concern for the dignity and rights of individuals and minorities

• An understanding that democracy is not so much an "ideal" to be pursued as an "idealized" set of values that we must live and that must guide our life as people

• The organization of social institutions to promote and extend the democratic way of life

How we educate the next generation of health care workers will determine the potential impact health and human service endeavors will have in addressing health disparities. Educators are challenged to be creative and innovative, to develop, implement and evaluate experiential community-based educational approaches that provide students the opportunity to engage in transformative educative experiences that can facilitate a prospective professional identity formation, leading ultimately to a new and different community of practitioners (Mezirow 1990; Nemerowicz & Rosi 1997; Hobdell et al. 2002; Strauss et al. 2003). Educators in such schools are enabled to examine critically the past and to prepare for the future to develop the capacity of their students to address the social determinants of health, to respond to health disparities and to care for vulnerable segments of the population. Education, as a result, creates a state of never being able to see and act in the world in the same way. Students are enabled to develop their skills and capacity as advocates, to be community responsive, to examine what is unspoken and taken-for-granted, and how the tacit can create inequities and injustices within any particular system (Oandasan et al. 2003). They begin to adopt a counter-cultural discourse (Nash 1996); they begin an intense examination of how existing views and actions either perpetuate inequity or promote justice; and they begin to challenge and change prevailing economic, professional and political norms and attitudes with the aim of moving toward a more socially responsible health care environment.

Closing Remarks

This chapter can serve as a possible point of departure for addressing how different stakeholders might approach and reconsider the role and responsibilities of individual dentists, of the profession at large, of educators, and of society and governments relative to the different perspectives of social responsibility in relation to health disparities. Health professionals generally seem to have a sense of what the issues are and they know what they want: "we want, as participants in institutional culture, to be able to notice our moral problems and to cope with them with sensitivity and integrity and to keep our health care institutions responsive to their moral goals" (Jameton 1999). This chapter provides a beginning for examining further how different stakeholders can be more sensitive to the discourses that inform what is aspired to and what is actually practiced. Discourses are not just "words" but a body of ideas, concepts and beliefs established as knowledge and what is accepted and practiced. Discourses are ways of thinking and deciding about what is right, what is reasonable and what might be considered normal. They provide subconscious justifications for how we reason and act. In effect, the different discursive constructions of social responsibility for addressing health disparities provide an insight into what might determine the dental profession's response; and it is these same discourses that will influence the social, political and educational interventions that seek to address disparities and promote equity for those marginalized from care.

Acknowledgment

The author wishes to express his appreciation for the advice of Dr. Michael MacEntee and Dr. Dan Pratt in the preparation of this chapter.

Bibliography

Armstrong RR. Access and Care: Towards a National Oral Health Strategy – Report of the Symposium. *Journal of the Canadian Dental Association* 2005, 71(1): 19-22

Auerbach JA & Krimgold BK (Eds.). *Income, Socioeconomic Status and Health: Exploring the Relationships.* Washington, DC: National Policy Association, 2001

Beane J & Apple M. The Case for Democratic Schools. In Apple M & Beane J (Eds.). *Democratic Schools.* Alexandria, VA: ASCD, 1995

Benzeval M, Judge K & Whitehead M (Eds.). *Tackling Inequalities in Health: an Agenda for Action.* London: Kings Fund, 1995

Bernstein B. *Pedagogy, Symbolic Control and Identity.* London: Taylor and Francis, 1996

Blane D, Brunner E & Wilkinson R. *Health and Social Organization: Towards a Health Policy for the 21st Century.* London: Routledge, 1996

Boyd MA. Curriculum Focus: Traditional Dental Education Confronts the New Biology and Social Responsibility. *Journal of Dental Education* 1993, 57: 340-342

Budetti J, Duchon L, Schoen C & Shikles, J. *Can't Afford to Get Sick: a Reality for Millions of Working Americans. Report from the Commonwealth Fund 1999 National Survey of Workers' Health Insurance.* Commonwealth Fund 1999. Retrieved August 20, 2005 from http://www.abtassoc.com/reports/commfund.pdf (access verified on 11/3/05)

Canadian Children's Rights Council. *One Million Too Many: Implementing Solutions to Child Poverty in Canada. 2004 Report Card on Child Poverty in Canada.* Canadian Children's Rights Council 2004. Retrieved February 9, 2005, from (access verified on 11/3/05)

Carlisle D, Gardner J & Liu H. The Entry of Underrepresented Minority Students into U.S. Medical Schools: an Evaluation of Recent Trends. *American Journal of Public Health* 1998, 88(9): 1314-1318

Cavazos L. Strategies for Enhancing the Diversity of the Oral Health Profession. *Journal of Dental Education* 2001, 65:269-272

DePaola DP. Beyond the University: Leadership for the Common good. In: *75th Anniversary Summit Conference Discussion Papers and Proceedings.* American Association of Dental Schools, October 12-13, 1998. Available on-line at http://www.adea.org/DEPR/Summit/depaola.pdf (access verified on 3/11/05)

DeSchepper EJ. The hidden curriculum in dental education. *Journal of Dental Education* 1987, 51(10): 575-577

Dharamsi S. *Discursive Constructions of Social Responsibility.* (Doctoral dissertation, University of British Columbia). Ottawa: National Library of Canada/Bibliothèque Nationale du Canada, 2004

Dharamsi S & MacEntee MI. Dentistry and Distributive Justice. *Social Science & Medicine* 2002, 55: 323-329

Dickerson WG. Will Raising Your Fees Ruin Your Business? *Oral Health* 1999, 89(2): 21

Dickson M, Dunn-Pierce T & Rosenbloom J. Pasantia: A Process for Engaging Communities in Dialogue. *Canadian Journal of Community Dentistry* 1996, 11(1): 12-15

Douglas-Hall A & Koball H. *Basic Facts about Low-income Children in the United States. National Center for Children in Poverty.* Columbia University, Mailman School of Public Health, 2005. Retrieved February 22, 2005 from http://www.nccp.org/ (access verified on 11/3/05)

Edelstein BL. Disparities in Oral Health and Access to Care: Findings of National Surveys. *Ambulatory Pediatrics* 2002, 2(2 Suppl): 141-147

Federal, Provincial and Territorial Dental Directors. *A Canadian Oral Health Strategy: Report of the Federal, Provincial and Territorial Dental Directors.* February 2003. Retrieved February 9, 2005 from http://www.fptdd.ca/COHS.html (access verified on 11/3/05)

Federal, Provincial and Territorial Dental Directors. *Oral Health: Its Place in a Sustainable Health Care System for Canadians: A Submission to The Commission on the Future of Health Care in Canada by the Federal/Provincial/Territorial Dental Directors.* January, 2002. Retrieved February 9, 2005 from www.caphd-acsdp.org/fptddsub.pdf (access verified on 11/3/05)

Fiscella K & Williams DR. Health Disparities Based on Socioeconomic Inequities: Implications for Urban Health Care. *Academic Medicine* 2004, 79: 1139-1147

Formicola AJ. "Service-first" Philosophy. *Journal of Dental Education* 1988, 52: 509-512

Frank HR. *Luxury Fever: Money and Happiness in an Age of Excess*. Princeton: Princeton University Press, 1999

Frankena WK. The Concept of Social Justice. In Brandt R (Ed.): *Social Justice*. Englewood Cliffs, New Jersey: Prentice Hall, 1962; pp. 1-29

Gershen JA. Response to the Social Responsibility Model: The Convergence of Curriculum and Health Policy. *Journal of Dental Education* 1993, 57: 350-352

Habermas J. *Moral Consciousness and Communicative Action*. Cambridge: Polity Press, 1992

Haden NK, Catalanotto FA, Alexander CJ, et al. Improving the Oral Health Status of All Americans: Roles and Responsibilities of Academic Dental Institutions: The Report of the ADEA President's Commission. *Journal of Dental Education*. 2003, 67: 563-583

Hobdell, M, Oliveira, ER, Bautista, R, Myburgh, NG, Lalloo, RS, Narendran, S & Johnson, NW. Oral Diseases and Socio-economic Status (SES). *British Dental Journal* 2003, 194(2): 91-96

Hobdell M, Sinkford J, Alexander C, et al. Ethics, Equity and Global Responsibilities in Oral Health and Disease. *European Journal of Dental Education* 2002, 6(Suppl 3): 167-78

Jameton, A Culture, Morality, and Ethics. *Critical Care Nursing Clinics of North America* 1990, 2: 443-451

Jamous H & Peloille B. Professions and Self-Perpetuating Systems. In Jackson JA (Ed.). *Professions and Professionalisation*. London: Cambridge University Press, 1970

Kawachi I & Kennedy BP. Socioeconomic Determinants of Health: Health and Social Cohesion: Why Care About Income Inequality? *British Medical Journal* 1997, 314: 1037-1040

Kennedy BP, Kawachi I & Prothrow-Stith D. Income Distribution and Mortality: Cross-Sectional Ecological Study of the Robin-hood Index in the United States. *British Medical Journal* 1996, 312: 1004-1007

King TB & Gibson G. Oral Health Needs and Access to Dental Care of Homeless Adults in the United States: a Review. *Special Care Dentistry* 2003, 23(4): 143-147

Kukla A. *Social Constructivism and the Philosophy of Science*. Routledge, New York, 2000

Link BG & Phelan J. Social Conditions as Fundamental Causes of Disease. *Journal of Health and Social Behavior* 1995, Extra issue: 80-94

Locker D & Matear D. *Oral Disorders, Systemic Health, Well-being and Quality of Life. A Summary of Recent Research Evidence.* (Health Measurement and Epidemiology Report No. 17). Community Dental Health Services Research Unit, Faculty of Dentistry, University of Toronto, 2000

Lund P. *Happiness & Profits.* Retrieved March 15, 2005, from http://www.solutionspress.com.au/content/standard.asp?name=DrPaddiLund_HappinessAndProfits (access verified on 11/3/05)

MacEntee M, Harrison R & Wyatt C. *Strategies to Enhance the Oral Health of British Columbians, Specifically Aboriginal Peoples, Tobacco-users, and Those of Low Socioeconomic Background. Report Prepared for the Ministry of Health,* Government of British Columbia, March 2001

Mezirow J. *Fostering Critical Reflection in Adulthood: a Guide to Transformative and Emancipatory Learning.* San Francisco: Jossey Bass, 1990

Michael M, Andrew H, Oliver F, Whitney A, et al. Poverty and Ill Health: Physicians Can, and Should, Make a Difference. *Annals of Internal Medicine* 1998, 129(9): 726-733

Mills S. *Discourse.* London: Routledge, 1997

Mittelmark M. Centrally Initiated Health Promotion: Getting on the Agenda of a Community And Transforming a Project to Local Ownership. *Internet Journal of Health Promotion,* 1996. URL: http://www.monash.edu.au/health/IJHP/1996/6

Mofidi M, Rozier G & King, RS. Problems with Access to Dental Care for Medicaid-insured Children: What Caregivers Think. *American Journal of Public Health* 2002, 92(1): 53-58

Mouradian W, Berg J & Somerman M. The Role of Cultural Competency in Health Disparities: Training of Primary Care Medical Practitioners in Children's Oral Health. *Journal of Dental Education* 2003, 67:860-868

Nash DA. It's Time to Launch a Counter-Cultural Movement. *Journal of Dental Education* 1996, 60: 455-457

Nathanson V. Humanitarian Action: The Duty of All Doctors. *British Medical Journal* 1997, 315: 1389-1390

Nemerowicz G & Rosi E. *Education for Leadership and Social Responsibility.* London: The Falmer Press, 1997

Oandasan IF & Barker KK. Educating For Advocacy: Exploring the Source and Substance of Community-responsive Physicians. *Academic Medicine* 2003, 78(10 Suppl):S16-19

Ozar DT. Three Models of Professionalism and Professional Obligation in Dentistry. *Journal of the American Dental Association* 1985, 110(2): 173-177

Petersen A & Waddel C. *Health Matters: A Sociology of Illness, Prevention and Care.* Buckingham: Open University Press, 1998

Poulton R, Caspi A, Milne BJ et al. Association Between Children's Experience of Socioeconomic Disadvantage and Adult Health: a Life-course Study. *Lancet* 2002, 360: 1640-1645

Pratt DD & Nesbit T. Discourses and Cultures of Teaching. In: Hayes E & Wilson A (Eds.). *Handbook of Adult and Continuing Education.* San Francisco: Jossey-Bass, 2000

Putnam RD. Bowling Alone: The Collapse and Revival of American Community. New York: Simon & Schuster, 2000

Rubin RW. Developing Cultural Competence and Social Responsibility in Preclinical Dental Students. *Journal of Dental Education* 2004, 68(4): 460-67

Sinkford J, Harrison S & Valachovic R. Underrepresented Minority Enrollment in U.S. Dental Schools – The Challenge. *Journal of Dental Education* 2001, 65(6): 564-570

Smith JP. Healthy Bodies and Thick Wallets: The Dual Relation Between Health and Economic Status. *The Journal of Economic Perspectives* 1999, 13(2): 145-166

Strauss R, Mofidi M, Sandler ES et al. Reflective Learning In Community-Based Dental Education. *Journal of Dental Education* 2003, 67(11): 1234-1242

Syme SL. To Prevent Disease: The Need For A New Approach. In Blane D, Brunner E & Wilkinson R. (Eds.). *Health and Social Organization: Towards a Health Policy for the 21st Century.* London: Routlage, 1996

United Nation Development Program's Human Development Index. 2004. Retrieved February 16, 2005, from http://hdr.undp.org/reports/global/2004/pdf/hdr04_HDI.pdf (access verified on 11/3/05)

U.S. Dept. of Health and Human Services. *Oral Health in America: A Report of the Surgeon General.* Rockville, MD: USDHHS, NIDCR, NIH, 2000. Available on-line at http://www.surgeongeneral.gov/library/oralhealth/ (access verified on 11/3/05)

Welie JVM. Is Dentistry a Profession? Part 1. Professionalism Defined. *Journal of the Canadian Dental Association* 2004a, 70(8): 529-32

Welie JVM. Is Dentistry a Profession? Part 2. The Hallmarks of Professionalism. *Journal of the Canadian Dental Association* 2004b, 70(9): 599-602

Welie JVM. Is Dentistry a Profession? Part 3. Future Challenges. *Journal of the Canadian Dental Association* 2004c,70(10): 675-678

Wiebe RJ. The New Business Ethics. *Journal of the Canadian Dental Association* 2000, 66: 248-249

Wilkinson RG. *Unhealthy Societies: The Affliction of Inequality.* London: Routledge, 1996

Woolfolk MW. The Social Responsibility Model. *Journal of Dental Education* 1993, 57: 346-349

World Health Organization. *The World Oral Health Report 2003: Continuous Improvement of Oral Health in the 21st Century – the Approach of the Who*

Global Oral Health Programme. WHO: 2003. Retrieved February 12, 2005, from http://www.who.int/oral_health/publications/report03/en/ (access verified on 11/3/05)

Wotman S, Lalumandier J, Canion S & Zakariasen K. Reexamining Educational Philosophy: the Issue of Professional Responsibility, "Cleveland First". *Journal of Dental Education* 2003, 67(4): 406-411

Gerald R. Winslow

Just Dentistry and the Margins of Society

Introduction

The United States Surgeon General's report, *Oral Health Care in America*, probably surprised none of its readers when it offered this assessment of our nation's oral health condition: "What amounts to a 'silent epidemic' of oral diseases is affecting our most vulnerable citizens – poor children, the elderly, and many members of racial and ethnic minority groups" (US Dept. of Health and Human Services 2000, p. 1). Without question, oral health-care professionals now have the skill and technology to provide remarkably successful preventive measures and restorative treatments. By the standards of earlier times, and in comparison with much of the rest of the world, contemporary American oral health care is an astonishing triumph. But for millions of Americans who exist at the margins of society's privileges, the accomplishments of today's dental care have little or no effect.

As one who regularly teaches ethics courses to dental students, I have this question: What should students of the oral health-care professions be taught about social justice and access to equitable oral health care? Related to this question are others. Are there sufficient ethical resources in our society, and more specifically within the oral health professions, to serve as the basis for establishing a commitment to care for those on society's margins as a matter of fairness? Is the language of justice the appropriate idiom to awaken in new members of the dental professions a sense of responsibility to serve those who face the greatest obstacles to adequate oral health care? By long tradition, restorative dentistry has given careful attention to what are called "margins." The question I am asking is whether we can find, in our shared language of justice, the necessary resources to enhance dentistry's common commitments to some different margins – the edges of society's favor where millions of our fellow citizens live their lives.

Now, my thesis: We should teach students that there is an ethical obligation, founded on social justice, to work cooperatively with organized oral health care so that all members of society have equitable access to basic oral health care. This vision of social justice should feature strategic concern for the most vulnerable members of society. I have focused deliberately on the education of students because the vision of social justice set forth here is so far from current reality in American society that it can only be understood in terms of a hoped-for future. This future will, to some significant extent, be in the hands of our students, and eventually their students. Those of us who have the honor of teaching aspiring students of the dental professions need to find the most effective approaches to fostering commitment to social justice – the inclination to help build a society that is fair in its provision of oral health care. In this task, we should draw as broadly as possible from the ethical resources of our culture.

The expression "social justice," as I am using it, refers to the convictions of a society about what it owes its constituent members and, in turn, the responsibilities those members have to the whole society. Many of the important questions of justice are interpersonal. They have to do with the way individuals relate to each other and whether these relationships are characterized by what we often call fairness. But questions of social justice have to do with the way social institutions, such as health care, distribute both benefits and burdens throughout society. The way we balance such values as liberty, utility, equality, and efficiency sets the pattern of justice in our society.

No doubt, the diverse visions of social justice we bring to such questions are shaped significantly by our varied biographies. I am no exception. I was reared in a family with modest means and six children. We had no health-care insurance, nor did most of our fellow citizens at that time. In fact, when I was born in the 1940s, less than ten percent of Americans had health-care insurance. This began to change rapidly during my childhood so that about fifty percent of Americans had health insurance when I was in elementary school, and over eighty percent had some form of health insurance by the time of my early adulthood. But despite this remarkable rise in the percentage of Americans with health-care insurance, dental care was typically not included. At present, nearly three times as many Americans lack any insurance for oral health care as have no general health-care insurance (United States Surgeon General, 2000). For my family of origin, dental care was considered optional unless a family member had a toothache. Even then, we purchased only as much care as we could afford, which turned out to be very little and of dubious quality. While I now have generous dental insurance coverage, my memories of living with severe toothaches, and even an abscess, are still vivid. So I am troubled by the knowledge that millions of children in our society receive no regular dental care. They suffer from perfectly preventable dental diseases that diminish the quality of their lives now, and damage their prospects for future health. I believe we could do better, and should aspire to do so.

Challenges

Attempts to include oral health needs in the package of basic health-care coverage to which all fellow citizens should be entitled are likely to face difficulties. Any honest appraisal of currently held cultural convictions will turn up several obstacles to ensuring access to oral health care as a matter of social justice. A list of the most obvious of these barriers includes the following:

1. *Missing Vision.* Our society is marked by the absence of a widely shared vision of social justice for health care. Unlike the rest of the industrialized world, we continue to tolerate the fact that tens of millions of our fellow citizens have no health-care insurance coverage. Our collective conscience seems mostly unfazed when witnessing the tattered patchwork of social safety nets we have created for health care. The closest we have come to a national health plan is something called the Emergency Medical Treatment and Active Labor Act, which ensures that all citizens who arrive at a hospital emergency room must be assessed and provided with basic emergency care regardless of their insurance coverage or ability to pay (EMTALA, 1986). The majority of our populace seems satisfied with this arrangement of using hospital emergency departments for last-resort provision of health care, despite the inefficiency and excessive costs this represents.

2. *Dispensable Oral Health.* Oral health care, because of the mistaken but persistent belief that it is less essential and thus more optional, generally fares even more poorly than the rest of basic health care when it comes to equitable access. Despite impressive evidence that oral health is foundational for much of the rest of health and that dental disease can lead to many other health problems, an irrational segregation of oral health from basic health-care coverage remains the norm. For example, explaining why there must not be a "right" to health care, Baumrin

(2002, p. 81), sets forth three prioritized lists of possible health-care services. He argues that attempting to provide the general populace with even the services on his second list "would outstrip the resources of the best-intentioned, best-endowed nation....." And dental care does not appear until his third, least essential list, along with "well care" and "nutrition."

Lamenting this tendency to locate oral (and mental) health at the low end of health-care priorities, Teitleman (2002, p. 256) wonders about the availability of compassion in our society. He finds this peculiarly puzzling in the case of oral health because, unlike most other diseases, sooner or later all of us will have trouble with teeth or gums. Still, as Teitleman (2002, p. 257) observes: "At the dental end of the spectrum, moral pressure to provide universal access to care is nonexistent because dental disease does not have outcomes that touch us deeply." Maybe not, but any person with an aching tooth and no access to dental care might wonder why not.

3. *Market Freedom.* Commitment to a kind of libertarian ethic of the free market for health care is especially pervasive in dentistry. The cultural icon of the ruggedly individualistic entrepreneur selling dentistry on the open market is widely admired. For most of my dental students, some version of this ideal is highly influential. It is generally coupled with a fear of losing professional autonomy to some faceless bureaucracy. And it is often accompanied by the conviction that oral health-care professionals should be as free to market the commodity of their services as any other person in business. On this view, no one should be forced to purchase dental care, and no one should be forced to provide it for free or at a rate the professional finds unacceptably low. What is more, no one should have income confiscated through taxes in order to pay for others' care. In other words, people deserve whatever dental care they can pay for at the going market rates. Any other system is perceived as a threat to liberty.

4. *Potentially Unbounded Costs.* The reality that most oral health-care needs can be treated in a variety of ways and that these represent widely different costs creates a serious challenge for determining what would be included in "basic" dental care. Millions of people have read the now famous (some would say infamous) article in the 1997 *Reader's Digest* describing the incredible divergence of diagnoses and treatment plans the author received from various dentists around the country (Ecenbarger, 1997). One commonly offered explanation given by dentists is

that they are free to offer dental treatments that may be more or less extensive, and thus expensive, than would be offered by other dentists, and patients are free to accept or reject these different treatment plans. This diversity, when coupled with the dental profession's reluctance to establish standards of care, makes it difficult to ascertain what care should be considered essential and creates anxiety about how costs for dental care could be adequately controlled.

5. *Unfairness to the Unwary.* Many of my dental students express concern that their practice might become known as the only place where charity care is readily available. The fear is that the path to their office will become well worn by the traffic of those who are least able to pay. This, it is said, would be unfair not merely to the dentists involved but also to their employees and families.

Thoughtful readers could, at this point, easily lengthen this list of challenges to any proposal that basic oral health care should be made available to all citizens as a matter of social justice. The purpose of listing some major examples of such hurdles is simply to acknowledge, from the outset, that a just system of oral health care will only be established when enough members of our society are willing to meet these challenges. For this to happen, the leadership of organized dentistry will be essential. And the future leaders of the oral health professions are attending our classes now.

Justice and Oral Health Care

Graduates from educational programs in oral health care now enter a profession that has already expressed a commitment to justice. The American Dental Association's (ADA) *Principles of Ethics and Code of Professional Conduct* (2005, pp. 5 and 6) includes justice as its fourth principle: "The dentist has a duty to treat people fairly." This section of the ADA code is brief and includes such diverse elements as "justifiable criticism" of other dentists, the provision by dentists of expert legal testimony, and the prohibition of rebates and split fees. Nevertheless, there are hints of a commitment to basic social justice here and elsewhere in the ADA's code. For example, the code avers: "In its broadest sense, this principle [of justice] expresses the concept that the dental profession should actively seek allies throughout society on specific activities that will help improve access to care for all." The statement, with its reference to seeking allies, may seem somewhat oblique. But the commitment to improve access to needed oral health care "for all" is significant.

Similarly, but rather more boldly, the American Dental Hygienists' Association (ADHA, 2001) has officially affirmed that "oral health care – a fundamental component of total health care – is the right of all people." The ADHA's *Code of Ethics*, under the heading of "Justice and Fairness," adds: "We value justice and support the fair and equitable distribution of healthcare resources. We believe all people should have access to high-quality, affordable oral healthcare" (ADHA, 1995). Statements like this indicate that the announced ethical virtues of organized dentistry include a commitment to help create a system of oral health care that provides fair access to all citizens.

There is also a small but interesting scholarly literature developing on social justice and oral health care. Dharamsi and MacEntee (2002, p. 323) correctly observe that "there is remarkably little reference in the literature to the theories of distributive justice that might offer guidance on how an equitable oral health service could be achieved." But their essay has helped to change this. After describing libertarian, egalitarian, and contractarian theories of justice, they conclude, "the greatest rewards for society can be derived from an egalitarian perspective on prevention supplemented by a social contract for curative care that will render maximum benefit to the least advantaged (p. 327)." More recently, McNally (2003) has reflected helpfully on the relationship between theories of justice and oral health care for the elderly. Building to some extent on the influential work of Norman Daniels (1985), McNally concludes that a commitment to social justice would lead to more equitable care for the oral health needs of elderly patients.

In their reflections on justice and health care, these authors and others like them, including myself (Winslow 1982), typically compare available theories of justice in an attempt to find an approach that is both rationally appealing and practically appropriate to the distinctive goods that health care has to offer. The hope is to find a comprehensive account of justice for health care that will be rationally compelling to fair-minded members of our society. In this quest, most of the recent works on justice and oral health care reflect the significant influence of Norman Daniels. For over twenty years, Daniels has applied the seminal thinking of John Rawls' contractarian theory of justice to health care. Since the appearance of Daniels' book, *Just Health Care* (1985), he has produced a steady stream of articles refining his basic thesis for establishing a system of health care that we should count as just. Recently, he has produced a valuable summary of this work (Daniels, 2002).

From the beginning, Daniels has asked why health care should be considered different from many other social goods that we are content to have markets distribute without regard for the end results of the distribution. Why should health care be placed in a category different from, say, electronic goods or tickets to concerts? His answer is that health care, at least at some basic level, is essential to preserving the functions that are considered normal for members of our species. And being able to carry out these functions is necessary for members of society in order for them to have fair equality of opportunity. In Daniels' words (2002, p. 7), "by keeping people close to normal functioning, health care preserves for people the ability to participate in the political, social, and economic life of their society." Preserving this "normal opportunity range" is the crucial reason why health care should be made available to all citizens. Daniels deliberately rejects the notion that health care's morally special status is because of its importance to human happiness. People may be happy or unhappy whether relatively well or not. What is needed, he argues, is a "more objective" assessment of how preventable or curable illness might restrict the opportunities of a person to enter into the fullest possible range of opportunities in society.

Behind Daniels' work on justice and health care, and informing this work at nearly every turn is the analysis of justice presented by John Rawls, who, even recently, was described as "the most distinguished political philosopher of our time" (Stout, 2004, p. 64). In Rawls' masterwork, *A Theory of Justice* (1971), the reader is invited to imagine a situation in which hypothetical members of society come together to formulate the principles of justice that will govern their common life. Rawls stipulates that these original contractors must be equal, reasonable, and self-interested. They understand that they will live in the society they are designing, but they do not know which positions in society they will occupy – they are in Rawls's terms behind a "veil of ignorance" regarding their own identifying information, including their eventual stations in life. In this so-called "original position," Rawls contends that rational participants would establish two basic rules. First, they would insist that all members of society be accorded "an equal right to the most extensive basic liberty compatible with similar liberty for others" (Rawls, 1971, p. 60). Second, the rational contractors would insist that social or economic inequalities work to the benefit of all members of society, and that favored positions in society be open to all. As Rawls elaborates these principles, they can most easily be thought of as three intertwined but distinct norms. The first calls for equal liberty rights. The second becomes Rawls' now famous "maximum" rule, which prescribes that social and economic inequalities can only be justified if they "maximize, or at least all contribute to, the long-term expectations of the least fortunate group in society" (Rawls, 1971, p. 151). The third mandates that there be fair equality of opportunity. Rawls thus summarizes his "general conception" of justice (1971, p. 303): "All social primary goods – liberty and opportunity, income and wealth, and the bases of self-respect – are to be distributed equally unless an unequal distribution of any or all of these goods is to the advantage of the least favored."

For Norman Daniels, the most salient part of this conception of justice, when it comes to the distribution of health care, is the preservation of normal human functioning for the sake of preserving reasonably fair equality of opportunity.

I find Daniels' account of just health care convincing. And it is obvious that it applies as fully to oral health care as to any other essential part of health care. The child who is deprived of adequate oral health care and reaches maturity with seriously compromised oral health is not likely to experience fair equality of opportunity. The adult who is unable to secure needed restorative dentistry may find important opportunities closed for that reason. In a society with our level of wealth, it is inconceivable to me that we should accept our current oral health-care disparities as fair. Certainly, our present inequalities would not be acceptable to rational participants forming a just social contract if they knew that they might be among those without access to essential oral health care.

It would be naïve, of course, to imagine that the liberal, contractarian vision of justice as fairness, represented in the works of Rawls, Daniels, and others, would be convincing to all members of our pluralistic society. I believe that this way of understanding justice is best understood as a means of vivifying our imaginations. By thinking in terms of the original position where reasonable contractors design a cooperative society characterized by justice, we are better able to imagine what justice requires if all members of society are to be respected fairly. However, this approach to justice can hardly tell us why all members of society should be given equal consideration. For this we would need to explore the deeper roots of justice in our culture.

Fortunately, we are not dependent on only one way of construing justice. Our cultural resources for thinking about justice are rich and deep. For example, Robert Bellah (1985, pp. 28-31) and his colleagues, in *Habits of the Heart*, suggest that our vision of a virtuous society is shaped by both the "republican" and the "biblical" traditions. One cultural stream gives us the tradition of shared citizenship in a republic that is governed by laws. Bellah's exemplar is Thomas Jefferson. But we might also think of Aristotle, who gives us the first detailed analysis of justice in our culture, and who teaches us that distributive justice formally requires similar treatment for those who are similar in morally relevant ways. For Aristotle, people should get what they deserve, and neither less nor more. His formulation of a proportional approach to distributive justice has remained influential in our culture for over two millennia.

Another, even older, cultural stream gives us the tradition of justice as a requirement of the Creator who has endowed all persons with a dignity that is more enduring than our assessment of their value to society. Bellah's exemplar is the Puritan leader John Winthrop who led in the establishment of the 17th century Plymouth community on Cape Cod. But we might also think of Amos, that Hebrew prophet of the eighth-century BCE, who cried out against those who "trample on the heads of the poor as upon the dust of the ground and deny justice to the oppressed" (Amos 2:7). For Amos, and his fellow Hebrew prophets, justice required strategic attention to the needs of the vulnerable not because they are more important, but because they are nearly always the ones in any society who are least likely to get fair treatment.

The combination of these two cultural streams, the philosophical and the prophetic, provides the deepest cultural roots for our shared sense of justice. I believe their pervasive influence helps to explain, in part, the cultural resonance of Rawls' contractarian theory of justice, with its provision not only for the formal principles of equal consideration and fair processes but also its emphasis on improving the well-being of those who are least advantaged in society.

The point of this observation is not to elide the interesting and significant differences of varying theories of justice as they coexist in our culture. Nor do I wish to suggest that religious and philosophical understandings of social justice can be readily harmonized. In her analysis of six leading philosophical and religious theories of justice, Lebacqz (1986) argues that such theories are like unmatched fragments that should be brought into contact with each other, however uneasily, in order to provide a more complete understanding of what we now mean by justice in our culture. The value of this approach is that it acknowledges an undeniable fact about the ethical condition of our pluralistic society: we will not find it possible to settle on only one philosophical or religious account of social justice. Nor need we do so. It is possible to proceed toward a more comprehensive and coherent account of social justice without insisting on a perfectly unified version. This can be done in a democratic republic like ours through a process of dialogue among the various accounts of social justice in order to discover the widest possible convergence. What this approach sacrifices in neatness it gains in the creation of adequate social consensus.

If we take the ethical aspirations of the oral health-care professions as evidence for such consensus, we should not despair. As we have already seen, organizations like the ADHA and the ADA have espoused, as a matter of justice, the goal of making oral health care accessible to all citizens. They also renounce unfair discrimination. The ADA's code (2005, p. 5), for example, expresses the commitment that "the dentist's primary obligations include dealing with people justly and delivering dental care without prejudice." The chasm we sense between these aspirations and the reality of oral health-care disparities is not primarily the result of failure to converge on the ideals of justice. Rather, it is a profound failure to achieve the goals of fair access that the oral health-care professions have promised to champion.

How do we account for this failure? Must we conclude that our society simply lacks both the compassion and the sense of social justice required to move us more effectively toward equitable access to needed oral health care? Are we justified in the cynical conclusion that the oral health professions, along with the rest of society, have merely been posturing with platitudes that few had any intention of following? I do not believe this. While the challenges to providing more fairly accessible oral health care, enumerated above, are real and difficult, they are not insurmountable. As one who teaches students of the oral health professions, and in my case one who professes ethics, I must retain hope that we can do better and that education can have a significant influence for social justice.

Education for Justice

In the well-known opening line of one of Plato's dialogues, Meno questions Socrates: "Can you tell me Socrates, whether virtue is acquired by teaching or by practice; or if neither by teaching nor practice, then whether it comes to man by nature, or in what other way?" Teachers of ethics have been pondering this question ever since. Recently, Charles Bertolami (2004) sparked a debate among dental educators over this matter with his essay claiming that ethics education for dental students has marginal, if any, desired impact. Bertolami's assessment is that ethics courses are boring and do little to provide the kind of personal introspection that would be needed for genuine changes in students' attitudes and behaviors. The flurry of responses elicited from ethics professors, administrators, and dental students indicates that Meno's question for Socrates is still entirely alive (e.g., Koerber, et al., 2004; Jenson, 2005).

In this recent debate, it was disappointing to see so little attention given to the careful work of scholars who have studied the way professional education affects moral development. For example, Muriel Bebeau has devoted decades to meticulous research, much of it with dental students, aimed at uncovering how professional students develop in their moral judgment and behavior (e.g., Bebeau, 2002). It is not my purpose here to summarize such work. But, having spent decades seeking to teach ethics to students of the health-care professions, I want to offer some reflections on salient elements of education for social justice. And since I earlier described five challenges to the flourishing of greater justice for oral health care, I will briefly mention five pedagogical strategies that I have reason to believe will help to meet these challenges.

1. *Raising consciousness.* Most of my dental students have not read the Surgeon General's *Oral Health Care in America*. They are largely unaware of the extent of unmet dental needs in our society and the way the burden of those needs falls unfairly on the most vulnerable. This is not entirely because all or most of these students come from the socially privileged sectors of society. It has much to do what the Surgeon General called the "silent epidemic." The oral health-care needs of the frail elderly and the mentally handicapped, for example, are largely hidden from view. One of the tasks of ethics education is to provide accurate information about such oral health-care disparities. As Bebeau (1993 and 2002) has shown, professional students cannot progress in their

moral development if central issues of ethics are not even detected by their ethical radar. Raising consciousness by sharing accurate information is only a first and, by itself, inadequate step. But even though we must grant that such information is not sufficient, the lack of it is often enough to leave us blinded to the injustices of our time.

2. *Engaging in service.* The school of dentistry that I know best has instituted a requirement that all students become involved in what is now widely called "service-learning." By participating in a variety of outreach programs for those who are least likely to get adequate dental care both in the local community and abroad, students come into first-hand contact with the reality of unmet dental needs. Through the work of clinics for the indigent, students also become acquainted personally with the stories of those who are in need. More research on how this affects students' knowledge and attitudes would be helpful. But listening to students describe their opportunities for service, I have the impression that direct involvement in the care of the vulnerable is a powerful antidote for the complacency that so often cuts the nerve of social justice. The belief that nothing can be done to move our society toward greater equity is refuted by every moment that care is provided to a person who would never have received it without a deliberate effort to reach out. Such charitable care does not take the place of a system of social institutions that are fair. But I believe there is evidence that it does open the hearts and minds of students to the need for a better system.

3. *Telling better stories.* When I first started teaching dental ethics, I was surprised by the dearth of well-told stories about past or present heroes of oral health care. Medicine can tell stories from Hippocrates and Maimonides to Osler and Salk. Nursing has its Nightingale and Lavina Dock. But who, I wondered, were the comparable exemplars in the story of dentistry? When and how well do we tell their stories? There is a reason for wondering about this. Publication of professional codes of ethics is important for the identity of any profession and for sealing the social compact that gives a profession its stamp of trustworthiness in society. Such codes are the publicly announced ethic of the profession. But they seldom, if ever, inspire the grander virtues that characterize the lives of those members of a profession we most admire. For this we need vivid stories of those who have gone beyond the minimal requirements that typify codified ethics. In telling such stories, a profession helps its new members envision the embodiment

of what moral excellence means. I concluded that dentistry needed more good stories. Fortunately, a recent work has taken a major step toward meeting this need. In their new book, *Dentists Who Care*, Rule and Bebeau (2005) recount "inspiring stories of professional commitment." This valuable resource, if it is used in dental education, can help to awaken in students an awareness of the lives of those who, by their example, stir others to make positive differences for social justice.

4. *Unveiling creative options.* One of the benefits of better stories is the way in which students may become aware of creative systems for meeting the needs of persons lacking adequate care without unfairly burdening a particular oral health-care professional. While a strong case can be made for more effective involvement of federal and state governments, it is important for students to know that social justice can also be pursued through the creative efforts of local communities and voluntary organizations. In our culture, such programs often prepare the way for more comprehensive social programs by revealing what works and what does not.

Take for example the efforts of Dientes Community Dental Care in Santa Cruz County, California. This organization takes as its mission "creating lasting oral health for the underserved children and adults" of their community and of neighboring communities (Dientes, 2005). It schedules more than eight thousand dental appointments annually for patients who cannot afford the cost of private care. And it provides the full range of oral health care, including both urgent care and extensive restorative dentistry. When able to do so, patients pay for their care, but the charges are typically about one-half those of private dentistry. Care is provided by a mix of paid and volunteer oral health-care professionals. In this way, children, seniors, homeless persons, and others with low or no income are provided the opportunity to receive needed care.

While such programs cannot substitute fully for a comprehensive plan for the health care of our society's citizens, they can help show the way. Social justice and charity care are not the same thing. But the Dientes clinic is not simply about charity care. Dientes takes full advantage of the patchwork of resources available for impoverished patients in an attempt to create a more coherent point of entry for their dental care. In doing so, it helps bring a greater measure of social justice to the communities it serves. And it proves that the pursuit of social justice does not rely solely on national initiatives.

Nor do all programs that have national impact rely on the federal government. A stellar example is the National Foundation of Dentistry for the Handicapped (2005). The NFDH's program, Donated Dental Services (DDS) has organized care for nearly fifty thousand persons in thirty-four states. The organization screens patients for eligibility based on need and then coordinates the care, including such needs as transportation and communication. Between now and the day our society decides to provide all members with basic health care, organizations like NFDH labor valiantly to meet the needs of those least able to care for themselves. And, in so doing, we may hope to be reminded of the great need for a more comprehensive system of just health care.

5. *Acknowledging limits.* Human beings can invent more things than they can pay for. This is as true of new, and often expensive, health-care technology as for any other sector of our economy. But our culture is peculiarly resistant to this truth. We often seem to prefer the belief that any useful health-care technology should be made widely, though obviously not universally, available to those in need, no matter how costly or marginal the benefits. If social justice requires that all members of society receive the same health care that the wealthiest members can afford to purchase, then pursuit of this goal is a formula for national bankruptcy. But most thoughtful, fair-minded observers of our health-care system have concluded that what justice requires is not everything that can be invented, but the basic care that is needed to function as fully as reasonably possible in the life of society. Over twenty years ago, for example, the President's Commission for the Study of Ethical Problems in Medicine (1983) concluded that fairness in health care did not require absolute equality, since individual needs are variable and social resources are limited. Rather, the Commission defined an equitable system as that which provides an "adequate level of health care." And this level was described as "enough care to achieve sufficient welfare, opportunity, information, and evidence of interpersonal concern to facilitate a reasonably full and satisfying life" (President's Commission, 1983, p. 20).

The point is that we should focus our concern on the floor of health care beneath which no member of society should be required to fall rather than the ceiling of health care above which members of society would be forbidden to purchase more. The ceiling approach appears to have worked poorly in most places where it has been tried because those who are financially able typically find ways to buy the care they want. Settling on what the essential floor should be is one of the more challenging tasks for any just system of health care. As Norman Daniels (2002, pp. 16-18) has suggested, the best we can do is to establish fair social processes for settling on what comprises basic care owed to all. If the decisional process is fair and reasonable, then I am convinced basic oral health care will be included on the list of essential care.

Conclusion

We can and should teach students of the oral health-care professions that there is an ethical obligation, founded on social justice, to advance toward a health-care system that provides all members of society equitable access to basic oral health care. Our current system that leaves millions of our most vulnerable neighbors in need of care is not just unfortunate. It is unfair. We who teach do well to consider the effect of our work in bringing our students and our society to a clearer, more compelling vision of social justice.

Bibliography

American Dental Association (ADA). *Principles of Ethics and Code of Professional Conduct*, revised to January, 2005. Available online at www.ada.org

American Dental Hygienists' Association (ADHA). *Code of Ethics for Dental Hygienists*. 1995. Available online at www.adha.org/aboutadha/codeofethics.htm

American Dental Hygienists' Association (ADHA). Access To Care Position Paper. 2001 Available online at www.adha.org

Baumrin B. Why There Is No Right to Health Care. In Rhodes, R et al. (Eds.): *Medicine and Social Justice: Essays on the Distribution of Health Care*. Oxford: Oxford University Press, 2002; pp. 78-83

Bebeau M. Designing an Outcome-based Ethics Curriculum for Professional Education: Strategies and Evidence of Effectiveness. *Journal of Moral Education* 1993, 22: 313-326

Bebeau M. The Defining Issues Test And The Four Component Model: Contributions to Professional Education. *Journal of Moral Education* 2002, 31: 271-295

Bellah R et al. *Habits of the Heart*. New York: Harper & Row, 1985

Bertolami C. Why Our Ethics Curricula Don't Work. *Journal of Dental Education* 2004, 68: 414-425

Daniels N. *Just Health Care.* New York: Cambridge University Press, 1985

Daniels N. Justice, Health, and Health Care. In Rhodes R et al. (Eds.). *Medicine and Social Justice: Essays on the Distribution of Health Care.* Oxford: Oxford University Press, 2002; pp. 6-23

Dientes Community Dental Care (2005). Information available online at www.dientes.org

Ecenbarger W. (February 1997) How Honest Are Dentists? *Readers Digest* 50-56

EMTALA: The Emergency Medical Treatment and Active Labor Act. (1986) Codified at 42 USC 1395dd, part of the U.S. Code

Koerber A et al. Enhancing Ethical Behavior: Views of Students, Administrators, and Faculty. *Journal of Dental Education* 2005, 69: 213-224

Jenson L. Why Our Ethics Curricula Do Work. *Journal of Dental Education* 2005, 69: 225-228

Lebacqz K. *Six Theories of Justice: Perspectives from Philosophical and Theological Ethics.* Minneapolis: Augsburg Publishing House, 1986

McNally M. Rights Access and Justice in Oral Health Care. *Journal of the American College of Dentists* 2003, 70: 56-60

National Foundation of Dentistry for the Handicapped (2005). Information available online at www.nfdh.org

Rawls J *A Theory of Justice.* Cambridge, MA: Harvard University Press, 1971

Rule J & Bebeau M. *Dentists Who Care: Inspiring Stories of Professional Commitment.* Chicago: Quintessence Publishing, 2005

Stout J. *Democracy and Tradition.* Princeton: Princeton University Press, 2004

Teitleman M. The Medical, the Mental, and the Dental: Vicissitudes of Stigma and Compassion. In Rhodes R et al. (Eds.). *Medicine and Social Justice: Essays on the Distribution of Health Care.* Oxford: Oxford University Press, 2002; pp. 248-258

U.S. Dept. of Health and Human Services. *Oral Health in America: A Report of the Surgeon General.* Rockville, MD: USDHHS, NIDCR, NIH, 2000. Available on-line at http://www.surgeongeneral.gov/library/oralhealth/ (access verified on 11/3/05)

Winslow G. *Triage and Justice.* Berkeley: University of California Press, 1982

Jos V.M. Welie & James T. Rule

Overcoming Isolationism.
Moral Competencies, Virtues and the Importance of Connectedness

Disparities as a Symptom of Dentistry's Isolationism

The assumption underlying this chapter, in fact this whole book, is that oral health disparities are not only unfortunate but also unfair. This is as true for highly developed and wealthy countries such as the United States as it is for developing countries. As evidenced by the many reports that have been written of late by individuals as well as by dental associations and organizations, this assumption is shared widely within the profession of dentistry. But that is about as far as the agreement appears to go. As soon as the question is raised how to create a fairer oral health care system, a series of new questions immediately arises: "What kind of justice?" "Whose justice?" "As an individual dental professional am I obligated to care in some way for the underserved, or is it acceptable to leave such care to charitable efforts or a governmental clinic?" "If I am obligated, how, and how much?" "Why should I be obligated to participate in governmental service programs such as Medicaid?"

While the general concept of justice in oral health care sounds extraordinarily desirable, its devil is in the details. It seems easy to agree that we all should be fair – the fundamental implication of justice – and that we all should receive what we are due. However, it is extraordinarily difficult to agree on who gets what, mainly because we disagree on what circumstances in life are morally relevant. How relevant, for example, are the needs of patients? How much should their ability to pay matter? To what extent does the dentist's personal autonomy outrank the needs of his or her patients? Does it matter whether patients' clinical conditions or personal circumstances are their own fault? In considering such questions, it is difficult to imagine a concept more controversial than the principle of justice (see also Rule & Bebeau 2005, p. 190).

Indeed, the other chapters in the first part of this book underscore the diversity of views on fairness and justice in health care. Theories proposed and advocated range from game theory to free-market libertarian approaches, and from egalitarian theories based on the concept of access to basic oral health care for everyone to models inspired by the Judeo-Christian notion that the most vulnerable and marginalized have the greatest claim on available health care resources. In short, we appear easily able to agree about what is unjust, but have great difficulty agreeing what is just.

Oral health disparities have many different causative factors, some of which go far beyond the scope of the profession. But individual dentists and the profession as a whole *are* part of the problem and *do* share in the responsibility to fix it. We submit that the reason for dentistry's relative ineffectiveness in reducing oral health disparities – relative, that is, to other health professions – is not due to the lack of a generally agreed-upon theory of justice in oral health care. Hence the development of such a theory – if one can ever be developed – is not likely to solve the problem. Rather, we argue that the root cause lies at a deeper level, namely isolationism. As the American Dental Education Association (ADEA) has pointed out: "Reduced access to oral health care is one of the prices of professional isolation that has too often characterized dentistry" (Haden et al. 2003, p. 13). For indeed, there are other dire consequences of dentistry's isolationist tendency, such as the low interest among dentists in an academic career; a widespread aversion of policies and protocols even though the individual dentist is no longer able to stay abreast of the rapid scientific and technological advances; and the continued hesitance to engage in peer review in spite of the rising need for professional self-regulation.

Dentistry has a long history of disconnectedness. Throughout its history, dentistry has been practiced largely in separation from other branches of medicine. Whereas the traditional medical disciplines of internal medicine, surgery and obstetrics gradually merged, dentistry remained a separate discipline. Prior to the very recent emergence of podiatry and optometry, teeth were the only part of the body that always retained its own group of healers. All other body parts, organs and organ systems were treated by medically trained healers. This isolation of the teeth from the rest of the body has had far-reaching consequences. Dental education is largely apart from medical education. Dentists and physicians have separate licensing boards and regulations. Dental and medical insurances are organized separately, and in many countries dental care is not part of publicly supported health care financing systems (e.g., the Medicare system in the US which makes health care available to the elderly does not cover dental care). And patients have to seek (and pay) a separate set of care givers for their oral health care. Moreover, the ADEA points out that dentistry's "isolation gives the impression to other health professionals, policymakers, and the public that oral health is not as important as general health" (Haden et al. 2003, p. 13). It may even be the case that many dentists themselves are less appreciative of the importance of oral health compared to medical care and perhaps consider themselves as less important than physicians.

In addition, there are structural forces at work in dentistry that foster patterns of isolation. The large majority of physicians, even those with private outpatient practices, tend to work closely with other physicians in clinics and hospitals. They tend to cooperate with a diverse cadre of other professionals such as nurses, physical therapists, clinical psychologists, and social workers. Dentists, on the other hand, generally work alone, or in relatively small practices that include a few additional hygienists and dental assistants. And they clearly like it that way as is evidenced by the persistence of this practice model. Dentists like to be their own boss, run their own offices, and practice dentistry *their* way. They tend to be suspicious of protocols and utilization reviews, practice standards, professional regulations, and governmental control. This focus on their own privacy may impact negatively on their inclinations and attempts to deal with broader issues, even such important ones as the staggering disparities in oral health. Hence the tendency of dentists and the profession at large to look outside of dentistry for solutions to oral health disparities – to state and local government, to insurance companies, to patients themselves.

If isolation is the problem – or at least a significant part of the problem – the obvious solution is to foster its opposite. What is needed, in the words of Hershey (then vice-chancellor for health affairs at the University of North Carolina at Chapel Hill as well as a dental school faculty member and practicing dentist), is "a willingness to be connected – a willingness to go beyond the isolation of narrowly interpreting one's professional role in order to be connected to the concerns of other individuals and to the overall well-being of society" (1994, p. 33). Or in the words of DePaolo (then President and Dean of Baylor College of Dentistry): "It is ... imperative that students in all education settings, including dental education, be taught in a manner where they are connected to the world and the *quality of connectedness* is ingrained in the very culture of the institution" (1994, p. 39-40; emphasis in the original).

Hershey and DePaolo coined the term "connected." The literature is actually replete with different terms that try to capture this sense of "connectedness" such as "belonging," "civil engagement," "community spirit," "community mindedness," "public conscience," "social responsibility," and even "cultural competence"[1]. We submit that if dentists acquire a much more robust sense of connectedness, that will be an important step in the reduction of oral health disparities. In addition it will render them more inclined, comfortable, and capable "of meeting the nation's need for oral health professionals engaged in the practice of clinical oral health care, public health practice, biomedical and health services research, education and administration; and oral health professions who can contribute to the fields of ethics, law, public policy, government, business, and journalism" (DePaolo & Slavkin 2004, p. 1143).

Four Realms of Connectedness

Even if organized dentistry has a long history of contributing to the isolation of its members, and even if individual dentists willingly seek some degree of isolation, most dentists are increasingly cognizant that good oral health care demands connectedness. The days in which the dentist could paternalistically decide what patients need without involving them in the decision are long gone. Patients must honestly inform their dentists about their needs, symptoms, habits, fears, and expectations, and in turn must be fully informed by their dentists about their diagnosis, prognosis and treatment options. Dentists must diligently foster their patients' trust by maintaining confidentiality, allowing them full access to their records, and abstaining from any behaviors that could jeopardize patient trust. Although patients cannot demand treatment but have to respect the professional autonomy of the dentists, so dentists must respect their patients' autonomy and always obtain consent before initiating treatment.

These examples all underscore the importance of connectedness between dentist and patient. There is widespread acknowledgment today that a strong fiduciary relationship, in which the patient is a full partner in the therapeutic process, is essential for successful outcomes. But this understanding of connectedness is limited to the sphere of dentists and their "own" patients. The kind of connectedness that Hershey and DePaolo advocate goes beyond the dental office. Besides a commitment to their patients, connectedness can be broken down into three additional realms: the profession that they choose to be part of; the community in which they practice; and the society at large with which the profession has an implicit contract.

Nothing in this is earth-shattering or new. These three additional realms are already acknowledged even if not as explicitly and robustly as they should be. Consider, for example, the issue of *professional* commitment. The very definition of "profession" is intrinsically a social concept. "Many individual expert service providers are committed to serve others and may have even promised to do so publicly. But the social phenomenon of a profession always refers to a collective. It does not make sense for anyone to claim the status of a professional if there is no profession to which one belongs. Indeed, society's trust in professionals is not vested in the individual service providers but in the profession at large" (Welie 2004, p. 599).

Furthermore, many dentists already assume leadership roles in their *communities* and apply their specific expertise and skills for the betterment of those communities. Their engagement ranges from health education projects in schools to the provision of oral health care for the homeless, and from lobbying for water fluoridation to serving in elective office.

And many dentists likewise exhibit deep concern for the well-being of *society at large* and the importance of cooperating with other players in society. Public health dentistry nowadays is an acknowledged specialty and indeed a concern of every dentist. The American Dental Association (ADA)'s code of ethics specifically states that "dentists have an obligation to use their skills, knowledge and experience for the improvement of the dental health of the public" (§3A). Moreover, "the dentists' primary obligation is service to the patient *and* the public-at-large" (§3; italics added). More recently, environmental protection has come to the foreground. As Mandel points out, "dental practice today involves a growing list of safety concerns that are important areas for discussion – as well as oral health research – and include infection control, radiation safety, mercury hygiene, amalgam and silver halide disposal, waterline biofilms, and nitrous oxide leakage and its reproductive effects" (1997, p. 134). Access to oral health care is yet another issue of concern. The Code of

Ethics of the ADA acknowledges that dentists must "actively seek allies throughout society on specific activities that will help improve access to care for all" (§4).

If we grant that dentistry must overcome its historical tendency towards isolationism; if we grant that dentists must develop a more robust sense of connectedness not only to their own patients, but also to the profession of which they have chosen to be part, to the community in which they will be practicing, and to the society at large with which the profession has an implicit contract; then we must also train future dentists to do so.

In our chapter on dental education included in the third part of this book, we will provide some practical suggestions for dental schools to consider. Here, we are concerned with the particular competencies that are needed in order to become and remain connected in all four realms. For it is certainly a challenge, the successful execution of which requires much more than an altruistic bent or good will. It requires knowledge, experience, motivation and practical skills. In short, it involves specific competencies of a moral nature.

Technical Competencies vs. Moral Competencies

Modern curricula are organized around specific sets of "competencies" that dental students are supposed to acquire in the course of their years in dental school. The educational competencies mandated by the US Commission on Dental Accreditation (ADA-CODA) cover a wide array of actions. Dental students must understand, apply principles, manage, evaluate, recognize, and perform intellectual and technical skills as they provide care. Often they involve prescribed ways of executing complex interventions that demand high levels of theoretical expertise and the manipulation of instruments, materials and even the bodies of other human beings. As essential as these technical competencies (from the Greek *techne* meaning craft, proficiency or practice) are to the provision of adequate care, they do not present the entire picture of what is expected of dental professionals.

Consider the earlier example about informing patients. There is a technical aspect to this task. A dentist is technically competent to inform a patient if she is capable of giving the patient adequate insight into his condition and the therapeutic options that are available. This technical competency involves linguistic skills (e.g., clarity of speech; translation of technical jargon), psychological skills (e.g., recognition of the patient's intellectual level; managing patient fears), and inter-cultural skills (e.g., familiarity with culturally defined social patterns; foreign language skills). But the core competency involved in informing patients is not technical but moral. It is about establishing a relationship of mutual respect and trust; motivating the patient to become an active partner in the healing process; respecting the patient's autonomy to make decisions about her own oral health care. In short, moral competencies are aimed at the protection of important values.

Technical and moral competencies are complementary. In order to be a truly "good" dentist, one must have acquired both types. But there is also a crucial difference between them. A dentist is technically competent to do X, if the dentist can perform task X successfully. In general, to prove that she is competent, the dentist has to actually do X successfully. However, the dentist does not have to continue doing X or even want to do X in order to be competent to do X. The only requirement is that, if challenged, she can prove that she (still) can do X successfully. In this regard, the technical competencies of dentists do not differ markedly from the technical competencies of other practitioners. A concert pianist is competent if he can play Rachmaninov when challenged to do so; he has not actually to play this or any other piano music in order to be competent. But moral competencies assume that the practitioner not only is able to successfully complete the underlying task, but is willing to do so and, when faced with the task, actually does do so.

It is makes perfect sense to say that Dr. Janet Jones is technically competent to inform her patients (i.e., that Dr. Jones is an informative dentist), but she frequently does not do so (e.g., because she has too many patients and tends to have too little time to inform patients well; or maybe because he just does not think it's that important). But it does not makes sense to say that Dr. Jones is morally competent to inform patients (i.e., that Dr. Jones is an honest dentist), but frequently withholds information or even lies to patients. A dentist is honest if and only if (s)he is eager to inform patients truthfully and actually strives to do so. Moral competencies are attitudinal and habitual.

Indeed, the Latin word "moralis," and likewise the Greek word "ethikos" mean "habitual." The French mathematician and philosopher Blaise Pascal (1623-1662) spoke about the "habits of the heart." But the synonym of moral competency that is probably best known – at least among ethicists – is the term "virtue." The German ethicist Dietmar Mieth literally translates virtue (Tugend) as "practical competence" (Handlungscompetenz) (1984, p. 61).

In fact, virtue ethics is the oldest ethical theory. Nowadays, ethical theory is dominated by principles, rights and duties, by maxims, rules and imperatives. Codes of ethics abound, as do decision making models that seek to apply these general norms to specific cases. But all of these perspectives are actually rather modern inventions. From Socrates to Aristotle, and from Aquinas to Pascal, ethics was foremost thought of in terms of virtues. The key question was never "what is the right thing to do in situation Z?" But "how to live a good life, how to be a good person, a good citizen, a good statesman, a good dentist." And – in the parlance of modern dental education – "what are the specific competencies required to achieve those ends?"

Virtue Ethics as a Background for Moral Competencies

As background for further discussion of moral competencies, additional comments on virtue ethics are necessary. Given its long history, there is a rich literature on the subject, and many overlapping catalogues of virtues have been proposed, each reflecting the particular socioeconomic and historical era in which they were developed. The most famous catalogue consists of the four "cardinal virtues." It can be traced back to Plato's *Symposium* in which one of the speakers organizes his speech in praise of love around these four virtues: prudence, justice, fortitude, and temperance. The great medieval theologian, Thomas Aquinas, discussed them at great length. In the mid-20th century, Joseph Pieper tried to recast these classic virtues for a more modern era.

Prudence. Pieper paraphrased "prudence" as "perfected practical reason" or "situation conscience" (1965, p.11). The medical ethicists Pellegrino and Thomasma essentially agree and characterize it as "the capacity for moral insight...." (1993, p.84). Its practicality serves as a link between "the intellectual virtues – those that dispose to truth (science, art, intuitive and theoretical wisdom, etc.) – and those that dispose to good character (temperance, courage, justice, generosity, etc.)" (p. 84). As such it serves as an orientating "guide to the right way of acting with respect to all the virtues" (p. 85). It helps us see what is truth and how to evaluate actions from a moral perspective. Its opposites are thoughtlessness and indecisiveness, but also cunning and covetousness (Pieper 1965, p. 19, 21). Prudence "is not only the quintessence of ethical maturity, but in so being is also the quintessence of moral freedom" (p. 31).

Justice. Pieper translates "justice" into the ability to give each person what is his or her due (1965, p. 44); not because that person is loved – he may be a complete stranger – but because he has a righteous claim on us (p. 54). He differentiates among three kinds of justice that are relevant to our purposes: *commutative*, denoting exchanges between persons; *legal*, referring to the relationships of individuals towards society at large; and *distributive*, indicating relationships of society towards individuals.

Fortitude. Fortitude is courage or bravery. It comes third because not all bravery is good. One can be brave in fighting for the wrong cause. So only the person who is prudent and just can be genuinely brave (Pieper 1965, p. 122-123). Pieper reminds us that courage presupposes vulnerability. One can only be brave if one can be hurt or suffer. Thus courage entails endurance and readiness to face the challenge and endurance. It is indeed a difficult virtue to fulfill in the current milieu of interactions with government, third-party, and community requirements (Pellegrino & Thomasma 1993, p. 112).

Temperance. All three foregoing virtues focus outwardly: prudence looks at reality; justice is concerned with our fellow human beings; and fortitude in essence is self-forgetfulness. But the fourth cardinal virtue, temperance, aims at self-preservation. "The purpose and goal of *temperantia* is man's inner order, from which alone this 'serenity of spirit' can flow forth" (Pieper 1965, p. 147). Nowadays, we may have little affinity with the traditional examples, such as chastity, virginity and fasting. But as Mieth has commented, the essence of this virtue is the difference between heteronomy (i.e., being restricted by temptations, obsessions and external pressures), and autonomy (i.e., self-determination). Understood as the competence to live a genuinely autonomous life, the old virtue of temperance gains new appeal (Mieth 1984, 34-35).

As mentioned, the four cardinal virtues are the most famous, but nevertheless only one set among many. For example, early Christian authors added the three theological virtues of faith, hope and charity. Medieval chivalrous culture proclaimed four primary – but different – knightly virtues: moderation, faithfulness, leniency, and honor (Mieth 184, p. 36). With the rise of the middle class in early modernity, yet other virtues were praised. The French revolutionaries hailed liberty,

equality, and fraternity. Benjamin Franklin produced a much longer list:
1. temperance; 2. silence; 3. order; 4. resolution; 5. frugality; 6. industry;
7. sincerity; 8. justice; 9. moderation; 10. cleanliness; 11.tranquillity;
12. chastity; and 13. humility.

We can further expand the list by adding classifications of virtues
developed in non-western philosophy. Confucian culture offers an
excellent example. It has as its primary influence an ethics of virtue, of
which the most important virtue is "Jen" (Bretzke 1995). Jen is difficult
to translate. Terms used include humanity, humanness, humanitarian-
ism, goodness, benevolence, and love (p. 9). The second most important
virtue is Li (or propriety). Its essence is the "observance of the proper
ritual behavior ... with a proper attitude or intention of sincerity" (p.
12). The two virtues, combined with chih (wisdom), i (righteousness),
and hsin (sincerity) make up the "five constant virtues." Other important Confucian virtues include filial piety, integrity, trustworthiness,
self-respect, magnanimity, and earnestness.

As the forgoing examples make clear, virtues guide our relationships
to other human beings and society at large. In that regard, they do
not differ from rights, duties, principles, rules, and laws. But virtues
differ from all of these other ethical concepts in that virtuous behavior
always also benefits the person him- or herself. Consider the following
example. In recent years, a series of new rules and regulations have been
promulgated by the US federal government on patient confidentiality and privacy protection (HIPAA) [2]. For the sake of patients, all
dentists and other health care providers are obligated to abide by these
rules. By doing so, dentists do not really experience personal gain. In
fact, many dentists are annoyed by these rules because they increase
paperwork, legal risks, and overhead costs. There are probably many
dentists who every now and then sigh: "I try to abide by those HIPAA
rules but I hate them nonetheless." Contrast these rules with the virtue
of trustworthiness. The dentist who strives to be trustworthy not only
benefits his or her patients but is also a better dentist for it, indeed a
better person. It would not make sense for a dentist to say: "I try to be
a trustworthy person, but I hate doing so." It may not always be easy to
be a trustworthy dentist, an honest dental assistant, a compassionate
hygienist. But the caregiver who manages to be virtuous is always a better
person for it. Indeed, (s)he is a "happier" person in the Aristotelian sense
of a "succeeded" person, the person who has become what (s)he wanted
to be.

Thus, virtue ethics is always intrinsically connected to the successful fulfillment of one's aspirations to become a certain kind of person. Although virtue ethicists tend to focus on human happiness in general, we have already encountered examples of more specific approaches: chivalrous virtues, civil virtues, and theological virtues. These catalogues of virtues presume an understanding of what it means to be a successful knight, a successful citizen, a successful Christian respectively. Likewise, any catalogue of virtues for dentists assumes an understanding of what it means to be a successful dentist, a good dentist. We cannot simply "apply" general ethical notions to the specific practice of dentistry if we seek to develop a virtue ethics approach. Virtue ethics is never "applied ethics" but always a reflection of the definition of the practice itself.

Virtue Ethics versus Duty-Based Ethics

Virtue ethics is not the most prevalent approach to health care ethics. Traditionally, health care ethics was a form of deontology or duty-based ethics. Health care providers were assumed to have certain duties, spelled out in codes of ethics or oaths that those entering the profession were expected to pledge. In many romance languages "medical ethics" is still called "medical deontology" (e.g., "deontologia medica" in Italian and Spanish, and "déontologie médicale" in French).

This is not the place to elaborate on the theoretical differences between duty-based ethics and virtue ethics. But one illustrative example may be helpful. Consider the difference between beneficence and benevolence. "Beneficence" literally means "to act for the (patient's) good." The American College of Dentists (ACD) considers beneficence one of nine "core values" and defines it as "the obligation to benefit others or to seek their good" (ACD Core Values). The American Dental Association's Code of Ethics likewise states that "professionals have a duty to act for the benefit of others. Under this principle, the dentist's primary obligation is service to the patient and the public-at-large." These definitions make clear that beneficence is more than a technical competency. Knowing how to act for the good of the patient is not enough. Both the ACD and ADA clearly expect dentists to *actually do* good things for patients. However, there is no indication that dentists should also *want* to do good things for patients. This is consistent with classic duty-based ethics (or deontology): The only thing that matters is *that* you act in accordance with duties, not *why*. Deontology focuses on the formal justification of duties and laws. In contrast, virtue ethics focuses on what kind of a person we want to become, what kind of world we should strive for. In addition to "bene-ficence" (doing good), virtue ethics would insist on "bene-volence" (wanting the (patient's) good).

Virtue Ethics versus Principlism

We have seen that health care ethics traditionally was thought of as duty-based ethics. More recently American bioethicists Beauchamp and Childress wrote their seminal work, *Principles of Biomedical Ethics*, first published in 1979, now in its 5th edition. Ever since, principlism has been the dominant theory in health care ethics. Even the ADA in the mid 1990s deemed it opportune to reorganize its code of ethics according to four principles of bioethics proposed by Beauchamp and Childress (autonomy, nonmaleficence, beneficence, and justice), but adding a fifth principle (veracity).

Beauchamp and Childress define principles as norms or (in the case of beneficence and justice) clusters of norms. But unlike rules, principles are less detailed and thus leave more room for judgment in specific cases. The authors acknowledge that a principlist approach to bioethics does not exclude virtues. Indeed, they consider virtues complementary and in later editions have devoted a whole chapter to "Virtues and Ideals in Professional Practice." But it is the principles that enable analysis and justification of acts and policies in health care (Chapter 8).

As mentioned, the ADA appears to have adopted principlism. However, upon closer reading of its Code of Ethics, it becomes clear that the ADA does not interpret principles strictly as justificatory norms, but rather as "the aspirational goals of the profession" (Code of Ethics, Introduction). Consider the description veracity: "This principle expresses the concept that professionals have a duty to be honest and trustworthy in their dealings with people. Under this principle, the dentist's primary obligations include respecting the position of trust inherent in the dentist-patient relationship, communicating truthfully and without deception, and maintaining intellectual integrity." (Section 5). Although the Code uses jargon that is typical of deontological or duty-based ethical theories – "... professionals have a duty to be..." – the examples reference what traditionally have always been understood as virtues: honesty, trustworthiness, and integrity.

Dentistry and Virtues

Other authors writing on dental ethics have more explicitly embraced virtue ethics. The ACD defines ethics as "the moral principles or virtues that govern the character and conduct of an individual or group" (Ethics Handbook). The College proposes the same five principles as does the ADA, but calls them "core values." It then adds compassion, integrity, tolerance, and professionalism. The first three are classic virtues, but even professionalism is a matter of commitment to the profession and to service of the public according to the ACD. Still more to the point is Rubin's adopting the Confucian virtues of compassion (humanity, kindness), righteousness (selfless, doing for one's own sake), propriety (respect, correctness in dealing with others), and wisdom (knowledge) to evaluate the impact of the outreach programs at the University of Pittsburgh School of Dental Medicine (Rubin 2004; 462).

One of us (JTR) recently co-authored with Muriel Bebeau a book entitled *Dentists Who Care: Inspiring Stories of Professional Commitment* (Rule & Bebeau 2005). Although Rule and Bebeau do not themselves classify their book as an exercise in virtue ethics, there is no question that the dentists described in the book are prime examples of "good dentists," of what ethically it means to "succeed" as a dentist.

In the subsequent section, we provide a "catalogue" of virtues for the practice of dentistry. We have organized the various virtues into three categories by their respective focus: (i) the relationship of the dentist to him- or herself; (ii) the relationship between dentist and patient; and (iii) the relationship to the profession, community and society. This breakdown is somewhat artificial in two regards. First, virtues always impact both others and the person him- or herself, as we have already seen. Second, most virtues are in some way interconnected with other virtues and are often interdependent. For example, a dentist's competence for justice may lead him/her to strive for better oral health care for illegal immigrants. But this is a controversial position to embrace and one that runs counter to established laws, thus requiring one more competence: fortitude or moral guts.

Moral Competencies Concerning the Relationship of the Dentist to Him –or Herself

In this first category of moral competencies we list those that pertain to the self: finding oneself, accepting oneself, and sustaining oneself. We live in an era that emphasizes individual freedom, independence, and self-determination. Thus, it is ever the more important that people also develop the moral competencies to determine their own selfhood successfully. For if people lack such competencies, pluralism can easily lead to subjectivism in which all values are a matter of personal taste. Individual freedom, independence, self-determination become hollow ideals if "anything goes."

Notwithstanding dentistry's tendency towards isolationism, few members of the profession would defend an "anything goes" attitude. Yet there are many demands and pressures that can threaten one's sense of self. The economic challenges of running a private practice intersect with the professional challenges of relieving the needs of patients. The dentist wields many powers over potentially vulnerable patients. There are multiple temptations as well, ranging from narcotics to insurance fraud. And a dentist is never merely a dentist, but always also a spouse or partner, father or brother, mother or daughter, neighbor and friend, colleague or teacher. Thus it is not easy to find, accept and sustain oneself throughout one's career as a dentist. It requires certain moral competencies. Without any claim to exhaustiveness, we discuss three of these competencies: integrity, tolerance, and temperance.

Integrity. Probably the best known and most discussed moral competency in modern dental practice is integrity. Literally, integrity means wholeness. A person of integrity has the ability persistently to maintain a certain degree of moral coherence – an integration of personal hopes and beliefs, values, and emotions – that is internally balanced and able to withstand immoral pressures from the outside. Indeed, integrity can also be translated as untouchability. A police officer with integrity is "untouchable" – as in the 1987 film by director De Palma about Federal Agent Eliot Ness and his small team of officers taking on gangster Al Capone. It was impossible for Capone to "break" Eliot Ness by driving a wedge between his moral convictions and his actual behavior. Ness's values could not be "corrupted."

Although it is difficult to specify what integrity means in daily life, the opposites are very clear. Hypocrisy, insincerity, bad faith, and self-deception are all examples of a failure to exhibit sincerity. Such moral incompetencies develop most easily when a person has not acquired a robust set of moral convictions or has been exposed too long to too many morally taxing challenges.

Tolerance. Tolerance is generally seen as a necessary condition for democratic and pluralist societies to survive. In order for individual freedom to flourish, each one of us has to tolerate others and let them do "their thing." Why then do we list this virtue in the first category of moral competencies that concern selfhood instead of in one of the subsequent categories that focus on relationships with others?

Tolerance in the sense of "letting others do their thing" is not really about relationships with others. After all, the very point is to leave others alone, to *not* get involved in their lives. Why then is it difficult to be tolerant of others? Why is tolerance a moral competence? It is because we ourselves have difficulty accepting otherness, accepting that the world, others, and even our own selves resist and defy our manipulations. Finding and sustaining oneself is as much a matter of striving and exerting as it is of letting-be and even letting-go. Without the ability to accept, to tolerate oneself, one's neighbors, and the world at large, one can easily get caught in a Sisyphysian struggle, a mission impossible. Alternately, apathy may take hold, a disinterested withdrawal from oneself and the world.

Once again, the widespread desire on the part of dentists for a relatively high degree of isolation comes into play here. Such isolationism protects dentists from the frustrating unyieldingness that characterizes hospitals and other large health care systems. But it could also be indicative of a certain degree of intolerance, that is, a less developed competence for tolerance. And yet dentists inevitably face many frustrations that require tolerance. Patients may be non-compliant, ungrateful, or outright hateful. There are ever more regulations, protocols, laws, and policies to be implemented. Continuing education demands are increasing. Private insurance companies and governmental welfare programs continue to cut rates while at the same time delaying payments. And the number of uninsured or special needs patients begging for charitable care continues to rise beyond any individual dentist's charitable capacities.

Temperance. Of the three listed competencies listed in this first category, temperance is probably the most foreign, even though it is one of the four cardinal virtues and included in many other historical catalogues. Pellegrino and Thomasma acknowledge that "traditionally, temperance is seen as a virtue that controls one's appetites for food, drink and sex." These may still be important goals but they do not appear to have much specific relevance for health care providers. However, Pellegrino and Thomasma go on "to expand this view to cover some of the more usual temptations of modern professionalism" (1993, p. 117).

Modern caregivers, far more than their predecessors, have the capacity to do much good as well as much harm. They are also confronted with the power and hence responsibility for decisions that merely half-a-century ago caregivers could not have even imagined. Paradigmatic examples in medicine include life-sustaining treatments, reproductive technologies and genetic engineering. In dentistry they include the surgical alteration of facial structure, the introduction of new teeth through implant technology, and the huge popularity of cosmetic interventions. Consequently, dentists like physicians have ever more sophisticated, invasive, elective, and expensive options available to them.

Furthermore, modern dentists work in a perfectionist culture. They are expected to provide all the latest techniques and materials without ever making mistakes. This has reinforced the already existing attitude that any treatment that is less than "the best" violates professional standards and is thus immoral. Limiting treatment for indigent patients to basic oral health care not only is an injustice to them; it is also considered an affront to the integrity of dentists.

The virtue of temperance enables dentists not to fall into this perfectionist trap. All of the warnings of old – first and foremost, do no harm; when in doubt, abstain – still hold true today. The ADA Code of Ethics insists that dentists must know their own limitations and know when to refer to a specialist or other professional. It is equally important – particularly now that the divide is growing between those who can afford the "best" on the one hand, and on the other hand the poor, the young, the old, the disabled, and the many other vulnerable patients who do not even have access to basic oral health care – that dentists resist the powerful lure of the latest technological and scientific advances when their use would be frivolous. These advances have an important place in oral health care, but they must not be normative. Not everything that can be done must be done. It requires the competence of temperance to retain one's moral selfhood in the face of such powerful external pressures.

Moral Competencies That Foster the Connectedness Between Dentist and Patient

Trustworthiness and honesty. The foundation of the therapeutic relationship between dentist and patient is trust. The patient must be able to trust the dentist. Trust is so important to the dentist-patient relationship that even the law considers this relationship to be fiduciary (from the Latin "fides" for trust). For the patient does not have the knowledge and expertise to diagnose her own condition and design a good treatment plan, let alone implement it. And yet, patients in pain are in dire need of such treatment. Thus they are vulnerable. The consumer looking for a new home theater system can shop around for the best deal, compare different options, fix his old system, or spend the money on a new TV instead. Most dental patients do not have the same freedom. They do not simply *want* treatment; they *need* it. They have no choice but to trust that the dentist will offer the right kind of treatment, and neither less nor more than is necessary to effectively treat the condition. They have no choice but to trust that the dentist will keep all of the provided personal information confidential and not sell the records to life insurance or research companies.

But such trust is not a given. It must be earned (and can also be lost). In large part, the trustworthiness of the individual dentist depends upon the trustworthiness of the profession at large. A new patient does not trust the dentist because (s)he has experienced the dentist's trustworthiness. After all, she is a new patient. All she has to go on are the recommendations of other patients and, more importantly, the trustworthy status of the profession of dentistry as a whole. But the dentist will have to live up to that new patient's expectations. If the dentist fails, he will quickly lose this patient's trust and, worse, damage the profession's overall status of trustworthiness.

Establishing and maintaining trust is not always easy. It takes time to get acquainted. But there is ever less such time, and on top of that, patients tend to change dentists frequently. Increased patient autonomy and assertiveness can foster a mutually respectful relationship between dentist and patient, but when patients become overly demanding or threaten with malpractice suits it becomes very difficult to maintain trust. The dentist will be tempted to guard his or her words, withhold information about mistakes, and insist instead on more and more forms and signatures. In addition there are the pressures of business. Sustaining one's patient pool increasingly demands the use of advertisements, particularly when other dentists in town embrace such techniques. But advertisements are not held to the same standards of honesty as are dentists in their therapeutic relationship to patients. It is a challenge to remain honest and trustworthy under such exerting circumstances.

Respect. Earlier we discussed the moral competence of tolerance, of accepting other people's otherness and not becoming perturbed by the fact that much in this world cannot be changed to meet our own ideals. Tolerance is about letting be and letting go. Respect, on the other hand, goes one step further. Respect literally means "looking at or after" the other person. It's about a genuine interest in the other person's otherness, trying to understand who the other person is, maybe even learning something from the other person. Cultural competency nowadays is a staple among all competency listings in higher education. In essence, cultural competency is a subcategory of the moral competency of respect.

In our pluralistic societies, tolerance is a necessary competency. But in the practice of dentistry, tolerance does not suffice. In order to develop an effective therapeutic relationship with patients, dentists cannot limit themselves to treating patients as mere statistics. They must make an effort to know their patients as unique individuals. Again, this is not easy to do, particularly if patients exhibit behaviors that are rather at odds with those of the dentist. Exhibiting genuine respect for each and every patient is truly a moral competency.

Compassion. Many of those who visit the dental office are "patients" in the original meaning of the term, which is to say they are suffering. Others come to prevent such suffering in the first place. And still others see the dentist not because they are (at risk of) suffering in some way, but because they want to appear more attractive. Therefore, in many dental offices the range of compassion that is required is broad.

All patients, however, require the dentist's ability to discern and acknowledge the patient's existential needs, as opposed to their optional wishes. In that sense, the potential for compassion establishes the therapeutic relationship (Welie 1998). It also sustains that relationship. Dentists who are unable to become emotionally engaged with the patients they treat and in the care they provide, will appear cold to their patients despite their level of technical competence. These patients may not be motivated to comply with instructions and ultimately may lose trust in their dentist.

Moral Competencies That Foster Connectedness between Dentist and the Profession, Community and Society

To the extent that moral competencies already figure in dental ethics, whether explicitly or implicitly, they tend to belong in the first two categories of competencies discussed above. This is consistent with dentistry's tendency towards "isolationism," to think in terms of *individual* dentists and their relationship with their *own* patients. Most assuredly, the competencies in these two categories are necessary for an ethical practice of dentistry. But our thesis is that they are not sufficient. As we have entered the 21ˢᵗ century, it is important that dentists expand their connectedness to include the profession they have joined, the community in which they practice, and society at large.

That is not to say that this third set of competencies is novel, or even new to the profession. Earlier, we referenced the new book by Rule and Bebeau entitled *Dentists Who Care: Inspiring Stories of Professional Commitment* (2005). Many of the competencies exhibited by the dentists described in this book fall in our third category (and when we next discuss those moral competencies, we draw heavily on these exemplars). It is important to note that the ten dentists in these interview-based stories are not imaginary dentists. They are all real dentists who exhibit these ideals. And more importantly, they were identified not by the authors but by their colleagues as moral exemplars for acting upon ideals that are fundamental to the profession of dentistry.

Altruism. Altruism, placing the interest of the other above one's own, has long been hailed as a hallmark of professional health care practice [³]. Why is it that dentistry, indeed all health care professions, traditionally have placed much emphasis on altruism? After all, we generally applaud people who are very generous, placing other people's interests above their own; but it's not considered immoral to first look after your own interests. Are dentists expected to be extraordinarily nice people?

The importance of altruism in dentistry is related to the unbalance in power between patients (who generally are truly in need of oral health care and thus vulnerable) and their dentists (who are the sole providers of the needed treatments and thus in a position of power). Hence, the call for altruism is not a call to be extraordinarily nice. Rather, dentists are expected not to capitalize on the vulnerability of their patients when their own interests tempt them to do so.

A classic example of an altruistic dentist is Dr. Brent Benkleman, an oral and maxillofacial surgeon who practiced in Manhattan, Kansas. Brent sees all people in pain, whether they can pay or not. And he has given specific instructions to his staff not to be told who they are. He explains: "What I would like to do is to present them the best possible treatment plan and give them the alternatives and let them make the choice. I think that's what everybody should do." Occasionally patients turn down necessary treatment because they cannot afford it. Instead of simply accepting their decision, he tells patients that 'this just needs to be done; let's do it.' He then puts the bill away, telling them that 'this is what you owe me; I'm not going to send you any bills; if you ever want to pay me, you can.' "I've had a few people pay me two or three years or four years down the road," Brent says; but then again, "we all have a certain amount of dues that we need to pay, you know. It's not like I'm going to suffer if I give a few things away" (Rule & Bebeau 2005, p. 31-43).

Dr. Jerry Lowney, an orthodontist in Norwich, Connecticut, uses every bit of power, privilege, position, and knowledge he has (and he has plenty), but not for his own self-interest. Instead he uses his talents to serve the poorest of the poor in Haiti. Rule and Bebeau describe how Dr. Lowney accompanied his friend, a Roman Catholic Bishop, on a survey trip to Haiti in 1981. He performed some extractions for the poor during that trip, but it really was a world-changing event for him. Ever since, he returns at least three times each year. What he does now is much different than in 1981. Through grant writing, connections with Mother Teresa's religious order, fundraising, the donation of much of his own money, and a huge investment of time, he now runs a multimillion dollar general health facility in one of the poorest areas in Haiti. Besides dentistry, his activities include the creation of centers for high-risk pregnancy and malnutrition, hiring physicians, training local nurse practitioners, creating and operating a piggery to replace pigs that died from an epidemic of swine fever, and the formation of an Adopt-a-Family program run by his wife, Virginia (Rule & Bebeau 2005, p. 75-92).

Another example is Dr. Donna Rumberger, a practitioner in Manhattan. She was nominated for her dedication and effectiveness in launching programs that helped others. These include the Smiles for Success Foundation with the American Association of Women Dentists and, as president of the New York County Dental Society, the Skate Safe program for inner city children in Harlem. Donna feels that her major accomplishment at that New York County Dental Society has been to use organized dentistry to encourage volunteer activity on behalf of others – rather than to promote their own self-interest (Rule & Bebeau 2005, p. 93-110).

The competency of altruism is not restricted to the area of clinical dentistry. As Dr. Mandel, nominated for his moral leadership in science, explains: "Unfortunately, there are many examples of a growing tendency to secrecy in science, especially in clinical trials, which vitiates the openness needed when patients' interests come first. Universities and dental schools have a responsibility to avoid over-commercialization and restrictions that could impinge on patients' benefits, as well as academic freedom" (1997, p. 134).

Finally, it is important to emphasize that altruism is a "shared" competency. The individual dentist will only be able to restrain his or her own power if fellow dentists do the same. When other dentists fail to be altruistic, capitalizing instead on the vulnerability of patients, it becomes virtually impossible for the individual dentist to sustain this competency. It is extremely difficult for altruistic dentists to continue caring for low-income patients when many of their peers are not so inclined, catering instead to the wealthier patients.

Gratitude. Whereas altruism is generally acknowledged to be an important moral competency for dentists, gratitude is seldom mentioned. Yet there is a risk in viewing dentists as the sole benefactors and patients and society as the sole beneficiaries. Healthy relationships are mutual relationships. As a matter of fact, dentists do not only give, they also receive a lot.

We already encountered Dr. Donna Rumberger from New York in our discussion of altruism. Interestingly, her nominator wrote: "From the minute she graduated from dental school, she believed in contributing back to society in the only way she knew how: using her skills, her dedication, and hard work to volunteer to help as many people as possible" (Rule & Bebeau 2005, p. 94-95). Thus, Donna's altruistic passion was fueled and sustained by her sense of gratitude.

Dr. Jack Echternacht practiced general dentistry in Brainerd, Minnesota. He was best known for his decades-long struggle to fluoridate his home town. However, a parallel story highlighted the role that gratitude played in his overall professional life. After only a few years in practice, Jack realized that he was thriving, and he felt acutely aware of the community's contribution to his success. He said: "I believe that if one lives in the community and makes his livelihood from it, he should return that benefit by participating in the activities of the community to better it in any way that he can" (Rule & Bebeau 2005, p. 16). Jack put his convictions into actions with megaprojects, in cooperation with the Young Men's Christian Association, the Chamber of Commerce, the Brainerd Civic Center, and others. His favorite was the Civic Center, the site of the town's hockey rink, among other things. Jack conceived the idea, organized partners, bought the property, and built the building. He and the others owned it all. At first the enterprise was working at a deficit. But, in a few years, when the Civic Center became profitable, at Jack's suggestion, the partners gave it all to the town (Rule & Bebeau, 2005, p. 7-17).

The ability to recognize and appreciate all that is good in life – one's own hard-won successes as well as the many gifts received – is not always easy. But appreciation is the fuel that keeps the altruistic engine running. If dentists – rightly or wrongly – perceive that all the giving is done by them, they will quickly – and justifiably – conclude that altruism is not a defining characteristic of professional dental practice but merely an option, a matter of charity.

Care. As the term expresses, all health care is a form of caring. However, when we talk about a "caring" dentist, this adjective does not simply reflect the dentist's ability to care *for* patients. Rather, it reflects the ability to care *about* others.

Caring about somebody else is not the same as loving that person or even liking him or her. Indeed, what makes caring about patients often difficult is that many patients are virtual strangers, and some are actually not very likable at all. The stress of daily practice, increasing patient loads, rising oral health disparities, and malpractice suits by patients all render it difficult to continue caring *about* patients. In fact, this process of erosion may start as early as dental school. A 2005 study by Sherman and Cramer shows that dental students become less caring and cynical in the course of their years in dental school.

But dentists who manage to retain or regain their capacity for genuine caring also end up liking the practice of dentistry itself much more. A good example is Dr. Jack Whittaker, a pediatric dentist from Bowling Green, Ohio. Treating poor children as a matter of course, while realizing that most of his colleagues were not doing so, in the 1990s he began a two-pronged drive to effect change. He campaigned to encourage his colleagues to accept Medicaid patients. At the same time, working together with an influential state politician, new legislation was created that increased the rate of dental Medicaid reimbursement – all for the sake of increasing access to care (Rule & Bebeau 2005, p. 45-60).

In his interview with authors Rule and Bebeau, Dr. Whittaker explained that the reason he treated Medicaid patients was simple: "They are kids, and I didn't think it made any difference" (2005, p. 46). He had grown up in a family where caring for others and fairness to all were mantras, and he had always thought of himself as a caring person. When he first entered dentistry, he felt that he certainly cared about his patients. However, he now feels that the depth of his feelings in his early years were superficial and that his capacity for caring has deepened. Jack says: "A lot of it is related to my work, and (the children with extensive disease) I take care of, and realizing that when you do care, something can get done. I cared about things, and I wanted things to get done, and wanted things to change. When I saw changes take place, that's when I realized how important it was. It's like I was given a whole new life. It's too bad I couldn't have learned that about 25 years ago. I've missed a lot. I'm serious. There's been a change" (p. 58).

Justice. In a nutshell, the competence of justice is the habit of rendering what is due to others. It is possibly the most global of all moral competencies, showing up in almost every catalogue of virtues.

We frequently use the term "justice" to refer to rights and righteousness. It is unjust if people cannot enjoy the goods that are rightfully theirs. It is unjust if insurance companies force dentists to accept increasingly lower reimbursement rates. But the virtue of justice goes beyond this kind of tit-for-tat fairness. The virtue of justice is the moral competency to acknowledge and respond to one's role in the community and in society at large. It goes beyond the respect and compassion that a morally competent dentist exhibits towards his/her patients. It goes beyond the altruism and care for patients in general that defines a good dentist. Conscious of his/her intellectual, technical, and practical abilities, of his/her expertise, power, and social status, but equally conscious of the many unmet human needs in society, the pain and sufferings of so many fellow humans who remain voiceless and unknown all too often, the just dentist accepts his/her responsibility – not as one more annoying chore, but as one more way of realizing his/her calling as a dentist.

We already encountered Dr. Jack Whittaker. He readily admits that the Medicaid system is difficult to work with, and that some of its negatives are related to the patients themselves. But he also says: "I'm frustrated because I really care about the kids. When there's an injustice done, or when people are in need of help, you've got to do it. If you're in the kids business, I think you should take care of kids. It's just too bad that I can't help them all." And later, in a slightly different context, he adds: "You get tired of seeing these little kids being pushed all over the place" (Rule & Bebeau 2005, p.47).

Dr. Whittaker found that the best way for him to contribute to a more just society was in the practice of pediatric dentistry itself. But because of their social status, dentists are often placed in other kinds of leadership roles. Dr. Hugo Owens is a black dentist who lives and practiced in the Chesapeake/Portsmouth Virginia area. Apart from running an excellent practice, he also served as Vice Mayor of Chesapeake for 10 years, as President of the National Dental Society, and as a board member of several Virginia universities. Moreover, he was a major civil rights leader in his region. The interesting aspect of his work in this area is that he never looked for it. But whenever the need knocked on his door, he answered. The course of events would often unfold as follows: (a) A patient tells him about a problem such as not being able to use the library; (b) together they visit the head of the library; (c) after being turned down there, they see the library board, perhaps with a larger group; (d) after being turned down there, they see the mayor. Always they try to negotiate. (e) Sometimes negotiation succeeds; when it fails, they sue, and Owens almost always wins. Often he funds the lawsuit himself from his dental practice. Because of his willingness to respond, Dr. Owens ended up, almost singlehandedly, desegregating all of Portsmouth and its environs (Rule & Bebeau, 2005, p.19-30).

As mentioned, Dr. Owens did not seek such social activism. Even more interestingly, his interviewers report that he never spoke about righting wrongs. Instead he spoke about helping others and in doing so help them develop self-sufficiency. As a young man he went to just about every lecture he could find that was given by a black man who had achieved success. These were all great orators, and he called them "The Giants." Collectively, they had a profound effect on him. He explained that the distillation of all their messages was, "First excel, then help others" (Rule & Bebeau 2005, p. 22).

This final wisdom from Dr. Owens underscores yet again the importance of role models, whether they be faculty in dental schools, senior dentists, or non-dental leaders. To be a just dentist is not an easy task. It requires insight, sensitivity, motivation, right judgment, and practical wisdom, much of which can only be learned from role models. Of course, by the same token, role models can also instill harmful traits. Dr. Janet Johnson was a dentist who worked in a hospital-based general practice residency program. She remembers how outraged she was, and is, for the way that patients were being harmed and for her supervisor's unconscionable treatment of the lowest income groups in our society. She says, "The major thing that runs through my life is, I can't stand a bully!" (Rule & Bebeau 2005, p.71)

Fortunately, Dr. Johnson realized that her supervisor was role-modeling injustice (and she even went a step further, as we will see in our discussion below of fortitude, by taking action against such unprofessional behavior). But that kind of insight assumes a certain degree of moral maturity that not all dental students or even junior dentists can be expected to have. It is a competency to be acquired.

Fortitude. Many of the competencies listed above concern tasks that not only are challenging and demanding but often involve going against personal routines, professional etiquette, or social patterns. To leave one's "comfort zone" generally will require a certain degree of "moral guts." The dentist will have to be "capable of acting on principle in the face of potential harmful consequences without either retreating too soon from that principle or remaining steadfast to the point of absurdity" (Pellegrino & Thomasma 1993, p. 111). The classic example is the treatment of patients with dangerous infectious diseases such as HIV/AIDS. But there are many other forms of engagement that require such fortitude.

Dr. Jack Echternacht, whom we already encountered in the section on gratitude, exemplifies the moral competence of fortitude. By the mid-1950s Dr. Echternacht's practice was doing very well. By 1954 research had been published showing that fluoridated drinking water offered huge benefits. In that year, the Junior Chamber of Commerce in Brainerd, as part of a national campaign, chose to promote the fluoridation of municipal water supplies. Jack volunteered to do it. What had seemed to be a simple task turned out to be a decades long struggle, with Jack Echternacht being the point man and the target for vilification by local antifluoridation groups. He even received threats of bodily harm and once his office, with him in it, received a nighttime gunshot. He views himself as someone who avoids conflict, "But, if there's a just cause involved," he says, "that's another matter, then we go to war" (Rule & Bebeau 2005, p.13).

Yet another example is Dr. Irwin Mandel. Fueled by daily dinner time discussions on themes of social justice, a father who lived the ideas he talked about, and a university that provided backgrounds both in science and social activism, Irwin Mandel himself became a social activist. From his days in dental school, through his years in practice, and his decades as a world-class salivary researcher, he never stopped. On issues of education, housing, employment, anti-Semitism, racial discrimination, freedom of speech, and nuclear safety, Irwin gave speeches, led rallies, spoke on the radio, held public assemblies, worked on legislation, lobbied in the state legislature, and even in Washington. Irwin says, "Selecting an activist agenda is like selecting a research project. Your feel; you read; you care; you do" (Rule & Bebeau 2005, p.151). But this simple algorithm obscures the moral courage that enables the final step: doing it, and continuing to do it.

Maybe no action by a dentist requires more moral courage than blowing the whistle on a colleague. Shortly after Dr. Janet Johnson (a fictitious name) took a job in a hospital-based general practice residency program, she saw that her supervisor was flagrantly disregarding the basic rules for safe sedation. In addition, he used untrained dental assistants – or none at all – for his deep sedation cases. Worst was his failure to request medical consultation for his medically compromised patients prior to sedation. Some patients later developed brain damage. After repeated attempts to discuss her observations with her supervisor, and later with the administrators of the hospital, Dr. Johnson took steps that resulted in the filing of a complaint with the state board of dental examiners. Ultimately more misconduct was discovered, and her supervisor lost his license for two years. Dr. Johnson received extensive and unwarranted criticism, even physical threats because of what was thought to be the frivolous reporting of a colleague. Unfortunately, this is the kind of treatment that many whistle-blowers encounter, even from colleagues who should have supported and celebrated her fortitude (Rule & Bebeau 2005, p. 61-73).

Concluding Remarks

Before the problem of disparities can be meaningfully improved, a more basic issue must be addressed: the longstanding lack of "connectedness" between individual dentists and their colleagues, the profession, their community, and society at large. The isolation continues to be one of dentistry's defining characteristics. Since the problems associated with oral health disparities are symptomatic of the overall issue of "connectedness" (or rather, the lack thereof), any attempts to "fix" the problem of oral health disparities must deal with this more encompassing problem. In order to boost dentists' ability to get "connected," we have proposed to expand the list of technical competencies with a series of moral competencies. The idea of a "moral competencies" is actually one of the oldest ethical concepts, that is, virtues.

As the forgoing descriptions have made clear, none of the virtues listed are a matter of being kind or nice. There is good reason to call them moral *competencies*. For the task at hand is always challenging, demanding and generally complex. Granted, the kind of skills that are required to perform an implant are very different from the skills required to sustain one's compassion for a complaining stranger, let alone to fight an unjust insurance company. But to perform the latter tasks successfully, it does not suffice to be a "nice guy" or a "decent person." Rather, these tasks demand certain competencies which we have labeled "moral competencies," analogous to the many technical competencies that dentists must also acquire to become good dentists.

There is, however, one added benefit of acquiring these moral competencies: The dentist who acquires and sustains them not only is a better dentist for it, but is also bound to be a more satisfied practitioner. From the perspective of virtue ethics, caring for the underserved and vulnerable is not a chore, an obligation that must be fulfilled for the greater good of all, for God and country, or simply for duty's sake. Rather, it the fulfillment, at times demanding, at times exhausting, but always rewarding, of the dentist's freely chosen identity.

Notes

1. Rubin uses the term "cultural competence to indicate "a process whereby students gradually build cultural awareness, knowledge, and skills that result in changing of their attitudes" (2004, 461). Though we appreciate his encompassing definition, we suspect that many dental educators will probably connote this term with the much more specific and hence limited ability of practitioners to relate effectively and respectfully with patient of different ethnic backgrounds. Hence, we have not adopted that term, but chosen connectedness instead.

2. "Standards for Privacy of Individually Identifiable Health Information" or "Privacy Rule" issued in 2003 by the US Department of Health and Human Services to implement the confidentiality requirements included in the 1996 Health Insurance Portability and Accountability Act or HIPAA.

3. There does not exist universal consensus that altruism is indeed an essential moral competency for dentists. Recently, Bertolami (2004) a dental school dean, argued against considering altruism a hallmark of dental professionalism. However, he appears to be an exception rather than the rule.

Bibliography

Beauchamp TL, Childress JF. *Principles of Biomedical Ethics*. 5th ed. New York: Oxford University Press, 2001

Bertolami C. Why Our Ethics Curricula Don't Work. *Journal of Dental Education* 2004, 68(4): 414-425

Bretzke JJ. The Tao of Confucian Virtue Ethics. *International Philosophical Quarterly* 1995, 35: 25-41. Cited here from the on-line version at: www.usfca.edu/fac-staff/bretzkesj/TaoVirtueEthics.pdf (access verified on 10/31/05)

DePaolo DP. Higher Education and Health Professions Education. Shared Responsibilities in Engaging Societal Issues in Developing the Learned Professional. *Journal of the American College of Dentists* 1994, Fall/Winter: 34-39

DePaolo DP & Slavkin HC. Reforming Dental Health Professions Education: A White Paper. *Journal of Dental Education* 2004, 68(11): 1139-1150

Fenton SF. If only we all cared. *Journal of Dental Education* 2004, 68(3): 304-305

Haden NK, Bailit H, Buchanan J et al. *Improving the oral health status of all Americans: Roles and responsibilities of Academic Dental Institutions. Report of the ADEA President's Commission.* Washington DC: American Dental Education Association, 2003

Hershey GH. Profession and Professionals: Higher Education's Role in Developing Ethical Dentists. *Journal of the American College of Dentists* 1994, 61(2) 29-33

Mandel ID. Oral Health Research and Social Justice: The Role and Responsibility of the University and Dental School. *Journal of Public Health Dentistry* 1997, 57(3): 133-135

Mieth D. *Die neuen Tugenden. Ein ethischer Entwurf.* Duesseldorf: Patmos Verlag, 1984

Pellegrino ED & Thomasma DC. *The Virtues in Medical Practice.* New York/ Oxford: Oxford University Press, 1993

Pellegrino ED & Thomasma DC. *The Christian Virtues in Medical Practice.* Washington: Georgetown University Press, 1996

Pieper J. *the Four Cardinal Virtues.* Notre Dame: University of Notre Dame Press, 1965

Rubin RW. Developing Cultural Competence and Social Responsibility in Preclinical Dental Students. *Journal of Dental Education* 2004, 68(4): 460-467

Rule JT & Bebeau MJ. *Dentists Who Care: Inspiring Stories of Professional Commitment.* Quintessence Publishing Company: Chicago, 2005

Sherman JJ & Cramer A. Measurement of changes in empathy during dental school. *J Dent Educ* 2005, 69(3): 338-345

Welie JVM. *In the Face of Suffering. The Philosophical-Anthropological Foundations of Clinical Ethics.* Omaha: Creighton University Press, 1998

Welie JVM. Is Dentistry a Profession. Part II: Hallmarks of Professionalism. *Journal of the Canadian Dental Association* 2004, 70(9): 599-602. Also online at www.cda-adc.ca/jcda/vol-70/issue-9/529.html

Jos V.M. Welie

The Preferential Option for the Poor.
A Social Justice Perspective on Oral Health Care

Introduction

In October of 2000, some 400 delegates from the 28 Jesuit colleges and universities in the US convened at Santa Clara University, California's oldest institution of higher education, to discuss the pursuit of social justice as a central theme for Jesuit higher education. This education-for-justice conference followed three years of self-study at each institution, identifying the extent to which the institution had successfully developed educational programs that educate students to be "men and women for others," concerned about and able to effectively participate in the struggle against social injustice. The Superior-General of the Jesuits, Peter Hans Kolvenbach, SJ, reminded the gathered delegates that, "Jesuit universities have stronger and different reasons than many other academic and research institutions for addressing the actual world as it unjustly exists and for helping to reshape in the light of the Gospel." He challenged each university and college, each school and program, to revisit all of its teaching, research and service missions as well as its processes, systems and structures in light of the Jesuit university's "responsibility for human society that is so scandalously unjust, so complex to understand and so hard to change" (2001, Part IV).

Kolvenbach's reflections, when specifically applied to the context of health sciences education, suggest that Jesuit health sciences schools are charged to deliver graduates for whom care for the poor and vulnerable is not a matter of optional kindness and charity but a defining aspect of their professional practice. This moral ideal is better known as the "preferential option for the poor."

A Counter-Cultural Notion

The concept of a "preferential option for the poor" can easily be mis-interpreted. First, the term "poor" refers not only to people of meager financial means. It also refers to individuals who for reasons other than indigence are vulnerable or live at the margins of society. Secondly and more importantly, unlike charitable care which is optional, "the prefer-ential option for the poor is not simply an 'option' for Christians. It is an obligation to choose to care for the poor to a greater extent than that found in secular society" (Pellegrino & Thomasma 1997, 121).

Pellegrino and Thomasma's statement makes clear that the prefer-ential option for the poor is a most unusual moral ideal. Society in general and indeed most dentists will grant that the existence of many poor and vulnerable patients who do not have access even to basic oral health care is most unfortunate. Thus it is righteous and admirable for dentists to provide charitable care to such patients. A 1998 survey undertaken by the American Dental Association reported that more than half of the responding private dentists provide some charitable care (US Public Health Service 2000, p. 239). The profession should celebrate such generosity and encourage all dentists to follow suit. But it is generally believed that no dentist is *obligated* to do so. The various codes of dental ethics are rather clear on this point. For example, the Canadian Dental Association (CDA) in its Code of Ethics insists that "dentists by virtue of their education and role in society, are *encouraged* to support and participate in community affairs, particularly when these activities promote the health and well-being of the public." (Section on Responsibilities to the Public, Article 6: Community Activities; emphasis added).

The American Dental Association's Code of Ethics in the section on justice specifies that "professionals have a duty to be fair in their dealings with patients, colleagues and society." The ADA Code does not specify what "fair" entails, but goes on to explain that "under this principle, the dentist's primary obligations include dealing with people justly and delivering dental care without prejudice." Thus, justice is essentially a matter of non-discrimination. This, in and of itself, would actually preclude giving priority to poor patients – i.e., positive discrimination – as the preferential option for the poor appears to require. Moreover, other articles in this Code of Ethics make clear that the ADA is pri-marily concerned about negative discrimination, that is, *not* treating certain patients because of characteristics unrelated to their medical condition. In the article on patient selection, the Code reiterates that "dentists shall not refuse to accept patients into their practice or deny dental service to patients because of the patient's race, creed, color, sex or national origin." Note that the patient's financial status is not included in the list. Apparently, dentists may refuse to accept patients into their practice when and because the patients are poor.

Free-Market Liberalism

The cited sections from the CDA and ADA ethics codes reflect a liberal philosophy of justice – provided the term "liberal" is understood in the classic sense of "freedom-enhancing" (and not as "socialist" as typically happens in the United States). This political philosophy of justice, when operationalized, generally results in free-market economics. The freedom of the trading partners is believed to be the best assurance that the interests of all involved are maximized. Some freedom-limiting rules are necessary to assure that nobody is unfairly disadvantaged. For example, trading partners may not deceive, coerce, or negatively discriminate. But otherwise, the freedom of the trading partners should not be restricted. Thus, patients should not be restricted in their choice of dentist or treatments, and dentists may not be restricted in their selection of patients or in their advertising strategies.

From such a liberal free-market perspective, health disparities are most definitely unfortunate. After all, the very purpose of the free market is the maximization of the interests of all, not just part of society. However, the disparities are not necessarily unfair. We are all responsible for the many choices we make for ourselves each day, whether to labor or linger, save or spend, invest or enjoy. Differences in affluence that result overtime from these free choices are essentially of our own making and hence fair. Conversely, a duty imposed on dentists to give preferential treatment to any group, whether rich or poor, would constitute a violation of the dentists' freedom and thus undermine the free market. In contrast, volunteerism and charity, precisely because they arise from the free will of the donors, support both the poor and the free market.

This liberal theory of social justice may easily convince entrepreneurs and politicians opposed to government imposed taxes. But in its purest form, the theory also has evident shortcomings. It is one thing to argue that poverty is the result of one's own free choices, but quite another to argue that one's gender, age, and race are. And yet, elderly black women as a group have significantly less access to health care than almost any other population in the US. The same would be true for congenital disabilities, epidemic illnesses, criminal trauma, or environmental diseases. Even if the causes of these health infractions can be blamed on some identifiable person(s), those who suffer the resulting illnesses generally are blameless. They had no choice in the matter. Consequently, their plight not only is unfortunate; it is also unfair. Justice requires that each individual at least has a fair starting chance, an equal opportunity at achieving and maintaining health and well-being.

Equal Opportunity Theories

The theoretical problem now arises which differences in people's state of being are unfair and hence merit a corrective adjustment of the free market, and which differences are merely unfortunate. Various argumentative strategies have been proposed, the best known of which probably is the one developed by the American philosopher Rawls (1971). He points out that in making these kinds of allocation decisions, it is virtually impossible not to be biased by one's own state of being. Thus, an older person will inevitably be tempted to safeguard the interests of the elderly, a rich person the interests of the affluent, a paraplegic person those of the disabled. The only way to protect against such biases is to decide from "behind the veil of ignorance." That is, one should ignore all of owns personal characteristics and only then ask oneself the question: What conditions would I want to have adjusted if I did not know where I would be born, from what parents and into what family; if I did not yet know my gender or race, genetic make-up or nationality, my IQ, physical abilities or talents? According to Rawls, participants to such a debate would come to agree – hence the term "contractarian" theory of justice – that social and economic inequalities are unjust, unless they are actually advantageous to all, and particularly those at the margins of society. But advantageous in what way? According to Daniels (1985), having ample opportunities to realize one's life goals and to participate in society, is advantageous to all.

From such an equal-opportunity perspective, diseases and traumas that significantly restrict people's opportunities to function, warrant a distributive correction, particularly if the patients cannot be blamed themselves for their conditions. Note, however, that this special care for the poor and stricken does not really arise out of a concern for them. Rather, it results from a kind of enlightened self-interest: It could have been me! This kind of enlightened self-interest underlies all insurance schemes. I buy insurance just in case some catastrophe befalls *me*. Others should also buy insurance, for else *my* premium will become too high. However, *I* only need as many other people to join me in the plan as are necessary to keep the plan solvent; those who have a high probability of consuming more benefits than they contribute in premiums should be deselected from the plan.

Evidently, such cherry-picking is only possible if we know who, because of age, genetic make-up, or other factors, poses a greater risk. Rawls' veil of ignorance is intended to prevent exactly that bias. But then again, can we ever shed such knowledge about ourselves? As long as we are healthy, it is truly difficult to imagine life as a severely disabled person. Once a certain state of affluence has been gained, it is quite difficult to make do with less. The very attractiveness of the equal opportunity approach – its appeal to rational self-interest – also reduces its real-life applicability.

Equal Rights

There are alternative theories of justice that do not build forth on individual freedom and self-interest. Or more precisely, given each person's tendency to foster his or her own freedom and interests, even at the potential detriment of others, these theories of justice use a different, non-egoistic starting point. Most such theories assume a fundamental equality of all human beings, out of which arise certain rights that each person is endowed with and that are inalienable. The best-known catalogue of such rights is the 1948 *Universal Declaration of Human Rights*, issued by the United Nations. The Declaration does not mention oral health care, but it does list a right to medical care necessary to maintain health and well-being.

As Chambers (in his contribution to this book) points out, such a declaration of rights is generally a "discussion stopper." And indeed, universal rights language is exactly intended to do this. The very idea of a fundamental human right is that it is not up for discussion. It is not conditional upon the maximization of the interests of some or even all individuals. This is the very strength of rights language.

But again, its strength is also its weakness. For there are few fundamental rights that enjoy world-wide or even wide-spread consensus. Those that do, either are phrased rather vaguely, or are negative. That is to say, they guarantee freedom from some kind of evil (such as the freedom to practice one's religion without restrictions by third persons or government). Positive rights, also called entitlements, are rare. The right (of all children) to basic education is one of the few entitlements that enjoys widespread consensus, but the right to basic health care does not. In this respect, the 1948 UN Declaration is the exception instead of the rule.

Undoubtedly, the hesitance to acknowledge positive rights is caused at least in part by the fact that such rights entail a loss for those who have to guarantee the entitlement, either in the form of labor by specified individuals or taxation income to be allocated by the government. For example, if we were to acknowledge a fundamental right to basic oral health care, dentists would automatically become obligated to provide such care, possibly supported therein with public funds (predictably at low reimbursement rates). This seems unfair to dentists, at least prima facie so. Moreover, in a world increasingly dominated by free market economics, egalitarian theories generally are not persuasive. In the United States, even those who are less well-off, tend to shun such views, driven by the dream to still "make it" and the fear that this dream will be squashed in any political system that merely reeks of socialism.

But even in countries where social-democratic ideologies have gained a stronger political foothold, any egalitarian theory that would require each and every person to be provided with the best oral health care available, would be economically unfeasible. As Winslow (in his contribution to this book) points out, it would not make much political sense to exert equality by prohibiting the more affluent from buying more expensive care. Instead of a ceiling approach, Winslow therefore advocates a floor approach beneath which nobody should sink. The challenge then is to reach agreement on the existence of a fundamental right to *basic* oral health care. And this is not a challenge easily met. The fact that in a country with a decidedly social-democratic tradition such as The Netherlands, the national commission established explicitly to study the issue of basic health care excluded dental care does not bode well for any alleged right to basic oral health care (Dunning et al. 1991)

And yet it is also clear that these egalitarian theories of justice capture a basic moral sentiment. It may be unfortunate but not unfair that large segments of society cannot afford orthodontic care. But it is decidedly unfortunate *and* unfair that so many people do not have access even to primary preventive oral health care and get to enjoy only extractions. The significant efforts on the part of individual dentists, local dental societies and, increasingly, national dental associations to improve access to basic oral health care, cannot be explained adequately by free-market theories of justice or even a Rawlsian adjustment thereof. Self-interest, even rational and enlightened self-interest, cannot account for the widespread indignation about the staggering oral health disparities and the manifold efforts to provide for the most needy. In contrast, egalitarian theories of justice that emphasize the intrinsic dignity of each human being can account for such indignation and the subsequent response.

From an egalitarian perspective, people who are severely ill, in pain, or significantly disabled must be provided with the necessary (oral) health care, not because we (who are lucky not to be so afflicted) could have ended up in their shoes, but simply because they are human like us. Their not-being-so-lucky does not reduce their humanness. Note, however, that the decisive principle, i.e., the level of basic health care, is a rather abstract and to some extent arbitrary principle of equality. The "poor" are only deserving of care because and to the extent that they have slipped under the agreed-upon level of basic oral health care.

The preferential option for the poor takes us yet a step further, that is, further away from our own interests (as in libertarian theories of justice) and even past generic human interests (as in egalitarian theories of justice). Instead of sameness to us, it is the otherness of the poor that invokes moral obligations on our part. It is precisely because they are indigent (unlike us), vulnerable (unlike us), sick or disabled (unlike us) and powerless (unlike us) that we are called to act on their behalf. But before we expand on this counter-cultural idea, let us first examine the historical origins of the preferential option for the poor.

Historical Origins

Very little has been written about the preferential option for the poor in health care. The only comprehensive overview is the recent collection of papers entitled *Jesuit Health Sciences and the Promotion of Justice*. And even here, the editors felt it necessary to add the subtitle *An Invitation to a Discussion*, so as to emphasize the explorative nature of the book (Welie & Kissell 2004). In this collection, Massaro provides an excellent summary of the historical and theological foundations of the preferential option for the poor, on which I rely heavily here.

The notion of a "preferential option for the poor" was first proposed and contextualized by the Roman Catholic bishops from Latin America at their 1968 conference in Medellin. It captured the bishops' concern about the staggering economic disparities and economic injustices in their respective countries. While the terms chosen were new, the concern was not. Throughout the history of the church, a concern for the poor and socially marginalized is evident, most tangibly in saintly figures such as St. Francis, St. Damian, and more recently, Mother Theresa.

More structural efforts arose towards the end of the 19th century as the western world was rapidly being industrialized. In the 1891 encyclical *Rerum Novarum*, Pope Leo XIII "analyzed the new challenges of the industrial age and placed the church on the side of the workers in their struggle for decent working and living conditions" (Massaro 2004, p. 77). These developments accelerated during Vatican II. Pope John XXIII, one month before the opening of the Council, declared: "In the face of the undeveloped countries, the church is, and wants to be, the church of all, and especially the church of the poor" (1988, p. xxvi). Among the documents resulting from this Council, *Gaudium et Spes* most explicitly addressed the issues of social justice, as evidenced already by its opening statement: "The joys and hopes, the griefs and anxieties of the men and women of this age, especially those who are poor or in any way afflicted, these too are the joys and hopes, the griefs and anxieties of the followers of Christ. Indeed, nothing genuinely human fails to raise an echo in their hearts" (Pope Paul VI 1992, par. 1).

Pope Paul VI offers this paraphrase: "In teaching us charity, the Gospel instructs us in the preferential respect due to the poor and the special situation they have in society: the more fortunate should renounce some of their rights so as to place their goods more generously at the service of others" (1992, par 23). Massaro's analysis of encyclicals written by Pope Paul VI such as *Populorum Progressio* (1967) and *Evangelii Nuntiandi* (1975) leads him to conclude "that the scope of his suggestions for rigorous corrective measures to benefit the poor knew no bounds, reaching to the international economic system, political procedures, land reform and even the church's own methods of evangelization" (2004, p. 78). And this concern for social justice was taken up yet again by Pope John Paul II during his lengthy pontificate.

To be sure, John Paul II also expressed concerns about the possibility that the church fail in its mission as church if it would engage itself too deeply in socio-political causes.

> Emptied of its full content, the Kingdom of God is understood in a rather secularist sense: i.e., we do not arrive at the Kingdom through faith and membership in the Church but rather merely by structural change and sociopolitical involvement. Where there is a certain kind of commitment and praxis for justice, there the Kingdom is already present. This view forgets that "the Church receives the mission to proclaim and to establish among all peoples the kingdom of Christ and of God. She becomes on earth the initial building forth of that kingdom" (Pope John Paul II, 1979, p. 62).

Specifically, the church must always foster reconciliation, so it must not in any crass way take sides, whether with the rich or the poor – hence the Pope's opposition to any liberation theology that translates the option for the poor in a Marxist-type class struggle. The "option for the poor" is not an adversarial slogan that pits one class or group against another (United States Catholic Bishops 1992, pars. 86-88). Pope John Paul II therefore preferred alternative phrasings such as "preferential yet not exclusive love for the poor" and "option or love of preference for the poor" (Pope John Paul II, 1987, par. 42).

The Great Reversal

Even if we grant that exclusive concern for the poor would constitute an injustice towards all others, Pope John Paul II's modified expression signifies the same moral core of the original adage, that is, the poor evoke a special moral obligation on the part of the well-off. And the question therefore remains why that is the case. None of the secular ethical theories of justice presented above justifies such "favoritism" of the poor. At most, an egalitarian perspective would call for equal treatment of the poor. That perspective is itself already rather radical for the most popular contemporary theory of justice, that is, free-market liberalism, tends to consider poverty an unfortunate but not unfair side-effect of an economic system that increases overall affluence so much so that probably even the poor are better off now. The preferential option for the poor thus constitutes the "great reversal" (Massaro 2004, p. 72).

Indeed, the moral foundation for this perspective is not secular but biblical. In the Judeo-Christian tradition, it is God himself who appears to have a preferential option for the poor. It captures "God's special relationship with disadvantaged people" (Massaro 2004, p. 69). There are ample references in both the Jewish Bible and the Christian Scriptures for this divine predilection (see also Table 1). "A continuous

Table 1. Biblical Selections Suggesting God's Preferential Option for the Poor

- God "executes justice for the orphan and the widow and befriends the alien, feeding and clothing him. So you too must befriend the alien, for you were once aliens yourselves in the land of Egypt" (Deuteronomy 10: 18-19).

- God has "thrown down the rulers from their thrones but lifted up the lowly. The hungry he has filled with good things; the rich he has sent away empty" (Luke 1: 52-53).

- God "chose those the foolish of the world to shame the wise, and God chose the weak of the world to shame the strong, and God chose the lowly and despised of the world, those who count for nothing, to reduce to nothing those who are something, so that no human being might boast before God" (I Corinthians 1: 27-29).

- "Whatever you did for one of these least brothers of mine, you did for me" (Matthew 25: 40).

- "Blessed are you who are poor, for the kingdom of God is yours" (Luke 6: 20)

All biblical fragments in this chapter are taken from the Catholic Study Bible, Oxford University Press, 1990

strand in the biblical witness to God's self-revelation highlights how divine favor has been heaped time and again upon the poor, the lowly and the outcast" (Massaro 2004, p. 72). Winslow (in his contribution to the book) already referenced the 8th c. BCE prophet Amos who scolded those who "trample the heads of the weak into the dust of the earth and force the lowly out of they way" (Amos 2: 7). But best known is probably Christ's lists of Beatitudes which appears in slightly different form in both the gospel of Matthew (5: 2-12) and of Luke (6: 20-26). As Massaro summarizes, "each version in its own distinctive way singles out the poor, weak, humble, meek, hungry and sorrowing as finding favor with God" (2004, p. 73). And to make matters even worse for the well-off, "Luke follows his Beatitudes ('Blessed are the . . .') with a series of condemnations ('But woe to you rich . . . ; you who are full . . . ; you who laugh now . . .')" (Massaro 2004, p. 73).

At the risk of arrogantly trying the impossible, one may wonder why God imparts such favors on the poor. The evangelist Mark reminds us that "those who are well do not need a physician, but the sick do" (2: 17). However, the subsequent verse shows that those in need of a "physician" are not the poor but the sinners, and these evidently are not synonyms – although there was in biblical times and still is in our modern capitalist societies a definite tendency to equate socio-economic success with moral quality. Burghardt explains that "[b]iblical justice is fidelity to relationships, especially those that stem from a covenant with God. God's intent in creating was not to fashion billions of monads, isolated individuals, who might at some point come together through a social contract. God had in view a family, a community, wherein no one could say to any other, 'I have no need of you'. The Jews were to father the fatherless, mother the motherless, welcome the stranger, not because the orphan and the alien deserved it, but because this was the way God had acted with Israel" (2004, p. 103).

It is one thing to stipulate a divine predilection for the poor and society's marginalized. It is quite another to clarify what that means in practical terms for us humans. Massaro readily concedes that the Scriptures do not provide an "economic blueprint" (2004, p. 75). It is quite clear which approaches are *not* consistent with the Judeo-Christian tradition. First, any economic theory that dehumanizes or otherwise lessens the intrinsic dignity and value of the poor is unacceptable. Massaro gives the example of Social Darwinism. This theory extrapolates Darwin's biological rule of the survival of the fittest to the social sphere: Supporting the poor, that is, the non-fit, risks undermining human progress. Social Darwinism in this most radical form nowadays has few advocates. However, the sentiment that the poor are somehow less worthy or less deserving appears deeply rooted in humankind and has a way of influencing many social policies. If we grant that the poor are of equal dignity and worth, if we grant that they too are created in the image of God, the second unacceptable approach is apathy. But exactly how we must be involved, is not spelled out in the Scriptures. Unfortunately, there is very little positive structural advice to be found in the Bible, particularly advice that is applicable to 21st century global economies.

Higher Educationn

Translating the moral imperative of a "preferential option for the poor" into practical strategies will yet require much visionary thinking and creative experimenting in the many different domains that make up society, from engineering to trade, from war fare to social security, and from health care to the legal system. One area in which much visionary thinking and creative experimenting has already taken place, is higher education, specifically in the colleges and universities sponsored by the Society of Jesus. Shortly after the founding of the order in 1556, the Jesuits got involved in education. By the end of the 16th century, they were already running nearly 300 schools and colleges, earning them the nickname "School Masters of Europe," even though that label fails to acknowledge that their school system was in fact global. After the papal abolishment of the order in 1773, virtually all of the existing schools and colleges had to be closed or turned over to secular authorities. Although the order was reestablished by a subsequent pope in 1814, the damage was already done. Still, with 202 institutions of higher education worldwide, 79 technical and professional schools, 444 secondary schools and 123 primary schools (2005 statistics), the present network is probably the single largest global educational system. But what matters for the purposes of this chapter is not the number but the nature of these schools.

As Welie & Kissell already have pointed out, "ever since the founding of the Society of Jesus by the Basque soldier-convert Ignatius of Loyola in the mid-16th century, the Society has been engaged in social activism, caring for the poor and marginalized, striving to improve their lot through practical care, education and political engagement" (2004, p. 9). The 1773-1814 abolishment of the order had caused its members to become much more socially restraint. But the order's overall social direction changed yet again by the mid-20th century, instigated first and foremost by the 28th Superior General of the Society. A former medical student, eye witness of the horrors of Hiroshima, Father Arrupe (1973) challenged:

> Have we Jesuits educated our alumni for justice? We will have to answer, in all sincerity, that we have not. This means that, in the future, we must make sure that the education imparted in Jesuit schools will be equal to the demands of justice in the world . . . . What kind of person is needed today by the world? My shorthand is "men and women for others". . . . Only by being a man or woman for others does a person become fully human. Only in this way can we live in the Spirit of Jesus Christ, who gave of himself for the salvation of the world, who was, above all others, a man-for-others.

Two years later, the delegates to the Society's 32nd General Congregation affirmed that the Society's mission was "the service of faith, of which the promotion of justice is an absolute requirement" (*Decrees* 1977, p. 411). Daoust (1999) lists three ways in which Jesuit universities can promote justice. (1) Accompanying the poor and making services available to them. (2) Political engagement towards a more just society. And (3) developing awareness of the demands of justice and the social responsibility to achieve it. But Daoust also warns the first two are not paradigmatic of higher education; these are the missions proper of soup kitchens and political mobilization campaigns. Essential to higher education is the third way: developing social consciousness and conscience, or "conscientization."

Indeed, the prototypical justice-oriented Jesuit university is in Latin America, the Universidad Centroamericana José Simeón Cañas (UCA for short) in San Salvador, the capital of El Salvador. Founded in 1965, its charter, bylaws and composition of the board of directors underscore that the university seeks to transform social structures. As Massaro has pointed out, the university's "research projects that focused on issues of justice, poverty and human rights were favored over merely technical ones that did nothing to challenge the oppressive status quo of the nation. Even the architecture and layout of the campus was deliberately selected to encourage a mingling of personnel and a cross-fertilization of departments intended to overcome the tendency of faculty to isolate themselves into quarreling academic fiefdoms" (Massaro 2004, p. 86) UCA's social engagement, based on high level research and promoted through its scholarly journal, *Estudios Centroamericanos*, soon gained it a reputation in the country and disrepute among the powerful elites.

Menaces and military occupations of the campus were but a forebode. On November 16, 1989, six of UCA's Jesuits and two female employees were assassinated by the Atlacatl Battalion of the El Salvadoran army.

Dental Education

Even if most of the other Jesuit sponsored universities fortunately do not face such daunting dangers, it remains a difficult task to translate the preferential option for the poor into an academic program. The task is even more challenging for health sciences degree programs. Some have evaded the problem, arguing that health care, health sciences education and biomedical research, when done well, already realize this justice mission. The greatest service one can do for the marginalized and poor is to simply educate the very best health care providers (see, for example, Hrubetz 1993). But the staggering oral health disparities in the US make clear that training truly excellent dentists and hygienists simply does not suffice.

Others have pointed out that Jesuit sponsored schools of dentistry, like other non-Jesuit Catholic institutions, have always been and still are, heavily involved in indigent care. But the question remains whether this service to the poor constitutes so-called "service-learning" as well. It is not at all clear that the health sciences students who treat indigent and other marginalized patients typically do so in the context of a structured course that specifically focuses on the problems of indigent and marginalized patients (see also the chapter on service-learning by Henshaw elsewhere in this volume). For example, are dental students trained foremost to perform high-end dental procedures that their indigent patients can only afford because the school has substantially discounted the fees in order to attract patients? Or are they trained to efficiently provide the kind of effective basic oral health care that, upon graduation, they can offer those same patients in their private practices at a price the patients can afford?

Similar questions can be raised regarding the area of biomedical research. Scientific programs heavily rely on the subsidies and grants from the medical and pharmaceutical industries. These companies are not primarily interested in the health care needs of the indigent and marginalized in society. They are not the ones who spend fourteen per cent of the national gross product on health care goods and services.

They are certainly not the patients who can afford the latest implants, veneers, and orthodontics.

A dental school desiring to help in the fight against injustices will first have to ask a similar question as did the UCA when it was founded: Who are the vulnerable and marginalized in the modern world that tend to be neglected by the oral health care system at large as well as by individual dentists? We can distinguish two main categories of vulnerable patients.

There are those who by virtue of social, economic or other non-medical factors become vulnerable. Their medical symptoms and conditions may not differ from those of patients in general, but because of these non-medical factors they are unable to reach the health care system, communicate with caregivers or afford the care they need. In order to address these needs, we must train health care providers to provide basic care, wherein the term "basic" has multiple connotations: basic as in low-tech; basic as in comprehensible; basic as in affordable; basic as in universal.

The second category of vulnerable patients are those whose very medical condition causes them to be at risk for medical neglect. This is because the medical system tends to focus on certain diseases, treatment modalities and categories of patients while paying relatively little attention to others. There are many reasons for this "favoritism" and it tends to vary by historical period and country. At present, it would seem that western medicine tends to focus on acute medical needs, curative care, interventions that are technologically advanced and elective treatments that are commercially profitable. Consequently, patients with incurable illnesses that demand a symptomatic palliative approach tend to be marginalized. So are mentally disabled patients, elderly with chronic illnesses and children in need of preventive care.

The more difficult subsequent question is how dental schools can best prepare graduates to meet the needs of these vulnerable patients. Pending a scientifically supported proposal, I submit that the a dental curriculum for justice would place heavy emphasis on preventive and community dentistry, basic dental care, dental care for patients with mental or physical disabilities, geriatric dentistry and nursing home oral health care. The courses in these disciplines, in addition to regular scientific and technical training, should be further enriched with service-learning projects.

Evidently, it would not be possible to simply expand the time allotted to the aforementioned subjects without cutting into the curriculum elsewhere. Most dental curricula are already overfilled, leaving students little time to engage in extracurricular formation activities or even with their families. This condition of permanent stress does not favor an attitude of concern for the least among us (Stempsey 2005). But as soon as we begin to list disciplinary areas that are to be sacrificed in order to make time for justice-related subjects, the suggestion is made that those disciplines fail to contribute to more justice in health care; or, even worse, they counteract justice.

The suggestion that certain health sciences courses could counteract justice is most certainly false. All of health care can contribute to the care of the poor and vulnerable in society and when properly applied, no health care causes injustice. No specialty disqualifies its practitioners of service for the poor and vulnerable. Even esthetic dentistry, though increasingly used to cater to the vanity of patients who have money to spare, can also be practiced in the service of those whose deformities, traumas or tattoos have rendered them socially vulnerable. In fact, this discussion is not about the disciplines themselves but about the patient populations on which they tend (not) to focus. It is about shifting emphases. Instead of focusing on the health care needs of people who have a voice and are already being listened to by the many other health sciences degree programs, schools subscribing to the preferential option for the poor must listen to the silent outcries of the voiceless in society.

Bibliography

Arrupe P. *Address, International Congress of Jesuit Alumni in Valencia, Spain on July 31, 1973.* Available on-line at http://www.sjweb.info/education/documents/arr_men_en.doc

Burghardt W. Biblical Justice and the "Cry of the Poor": Jesuit Medicine and the Third Millennium. In Welie JVM & Kissell JL (Eds.). *Jesuit Health Sciences and the Promotion of Justice. An Invitation to a Discussion.* Milwaukee: Marquette University Press, 2004; pp. 95-109

Daoust J. *Faith and Justice at the Core of Jesuit Education: Of Kingfishers and Dragonflies.* Keynote address to the attendees of the Western Regional Conference on Justice Education, 1999. Available on-line at: http://cms.

scu.edu/bannancenter/eventsandconferences/justiceconference/western-conference/daoust.cfm (access verified on 11/3/05)

Decrees of the 31st and 32nd General Congregations of the Society of Jesus. St. Louis: Institute of Jesuit Sources, 1977

Daniels N. *Just Health Care.* New York: Cambridge University Press, 1985

Dunning AJ et al. *Kiezen en Delen. Rapport Van De Commissie Keuzen in De Zorg* [in Dutch; Report of the National Commission on choices in health care]. The Hague: Ministerie van Welzijn, Volksgezondheid en Cultuur, 1991

Hrubetz J. Nursing education in Jesuit universities and colleges. The art of science and caring. *Conversations* 1993, Spring: 18-19

Kolvenbach PH. *The Service of Faith and the Promotion of Justice in American Jesuit Higher Education. Address at Santa Clara University, 6 October 2000.* Printed in *Studies in the Spirituality of Jesuits* 2001, 35(1): 13-29

Massaro T. A Preferential Option for the Poor: Historian and Theological Foundations. In Welie JVM & Kissell JL (Eds.). *Jesuit Health Sciences and the Promotion of Justice. An Invitation to a Discussion.* Milwaukee: Marquette University Press, 2004; pp. 70-92

Pellegrino ED & Thomasma DC. *Helping and Healing: Religious Commitment in Health Care.* Washington DC: Georgetown University Press, 1977

Pope John XXIII. Allocution of September 11, 1961. In Gutiérrez G (Ed.). Introduction to the revised edition. *A theology of liberation, fifteenth anniversary edition.* Maryknoll NY: Orbis Books, 1988

Pope John Paul II. Opening address at the Puebla conference, 28 January 1979. In Eagleson J & Scharper P (Eds.). *Puebla and beyond: Documentation and commentary.* Maryknoll NY: Orbis Books, 1979

Pope John Paul II. Sollicitudo rei socialis. In O'Brien DF & Shannon A (Eds.). *Catholic Social Thought: The Documentary Heritage.* Maryknoll NY: Orbis Books, 1992

Pope Paul VI. *Gaudium et Spes.* In O'Brien DF & Shannon A (Eds.). *Catholic Social Thought: The Documentary Heritage.* Maryknoll NY: Orbis Books, 1992

Pope Paul VI. *Populorum progressio.* In O'Brien DF & Shannon A (Eds.). *Catholic Social Thought: The Documentary Heritage.* Maryknoll NY: Orbis Books, 1992

Rawls J. *A Theory if Justice.* Cambridge: Harvard University Press, 1971

Stempsey WE. Forming Physicians for the Poor: The Role of Medical and Premedical Eductation. In Welie JVM & Kissell JL (Eds.). *Jesuit Health Sciences and the Promotion of Justice. An Invitation to a Discussion.* Milwaukee: Marquette University Press, 2004; pp. 131-151

United States Catholic Bishops. *Economic Justice for All.* In O'Brien DF & Shannon A (Eds.). *Catholic Social Thought: The Documentary Heritage.* Maryknoll, NY: Orbis Books, 1992

U.S. Public Health Service. *Oral Health in America: a Report of the Surgeon General.* Washington DC 2000. Available on-line at http://www.surgeon-general.gov/library/oralhealth/(access verified on 11/3/05)

Welie JVM & Kissell JL. A Matter of Identity: The Role of Jesuit Health Sciences Centers toward the Promotion of Justice. In Welie JVM & Kissell JL (Eds.). *Jesuit Health Sciences and the Promotion of Justice. An Invitation to a Discussion.* Milwaukee: Marquette University Press, 2004; pp. 9-15

Welie JVM & Kissell JL. (Eds.). *Jesuit Health Sciences and the Promotion of Justice. An Invitation to a Discussion.* Milwaukee: Marquette University Press, 2004

David W. Chambers

Distributive Justice

Distributive justice is concerned with the way common benefits should be distributed within the group to which they are common – bluntly put, who gets what from the common stock (Audi 1999; Edwards 1967)? The question has two parts: Which benefits are common (as opposed to private) and how is the allocation to be made? This paper will not address issues of retributive justice (fair punishment), substantive justice (what is fair to ask for), or formal or procedural justice (fair procedures) – although there is some evidence that such questions are regarded as more telling for the public's sense of satisfaction (Alexander & Ruderman 1987; Folger 1977).

Issues of distributive justice can be raised with regard to oral health. For example, are dental treatment (or certain kinds of dental treatment), a specific level of oral health, or information about or diagnostic and other public health measures community goods and should action be taken to distribute them differently from what results from forces currently in place? In addition to voluntary contributions from industry and donated services by dentists (which the ADA estimates to be approximately $10,000 per dentist, or 0.5 percent of dental services), the U. S. government purchases about 4 or 4.5 percent of all dental care for redistribution through Medicaid, the uniform services, the Indian Health Services, prisons, etc. In addition, the government funds, to a small extent, public health measures such as public water fluoridation, oral health promotion, and research. Some of the questions that arise include: Is this the right amount? Are the resources optimally distributed? Are the allocation mechanisms meaningful, clear, and efficient?

The plan for this paper is to mention briefly the shortcomings of individual and universal solutions to problems in social justice and to focus on game theory, including Pareto optimality and six alternative rational approaches for discovering the justice criterion – the fair way to distribute resources. In the end, it will appear that this task is complex, and more importantly, necessarily possible only in limited ways. Such a conclusion points to the value of discursive ethics – the creation of ethical communities through mutual promises – as the best way forward.

The Sense of Justice

"Just" is different from other adjectives such as "big" or "benign." It is morally suasive. One could not say, "I prefer to be unjust" – but it is acceptable to strive to be small or even have a "deadly" jump shot. If one is accused of injustice there is a social obligation to defend one's actions or change them. There is a corresponding obligation for anyone who makes such an accusation to place his or her differing views in the lists. Because the term "should" is admitted to discussions of justice they become moral questions.

Discussions of justice take the form of comparisons among alternative future world views that are believed to be feasible and possibly attainable. When the dentist says Medicaid insurance should reimburse for crowns on lesions covering multiple cusps, he or she is taking the position that the world would be better (for some group of individuals) if this were the case. Because the insurance carrier takes a contrary position, we can assume that some others would prefer a different world. Both the dentist and the insurance company are willing to take action to increase the chances of their world becoming the future reality. Often the action is low-grade complaining; sometimes more resources are attached (as in lobbying or marketing); or there may be escalation to research or litigation. The point is that ethical conflict over issues of distributive justice are collisions between future world views that are at least partially incompatible and which call forth some level of response on the part of those who hold these different alternatives.

There are four general approaches for addressing such conflicts over competing world views of distributive justice.

1. *A Personal Approach.* A strictly individual view is really only workable when there is no cost in taking a position. The dentist who eschews Medicaid patients could proceed along these lines. One writing an editorial or even a journal article or making a speech to an audience holding friendly views could work this angle. There may be some personal reward to be harvested, but no views of justice are likely to be changed.

A variation is to argue from a superior position. Theoretical justifications, such as philosophers and academic writers might take, and "rights" language are examples (Brandt 1979). Claims that one party is coming into the discussion with a universally appropriate position typify a century's-old quest that has so far produced only contenders and no champions (Kane 1996).

2. *Oral Health As Right.* With the exception of a recent presidential commission of the American Dental Education Association (Haden et al. 2003), arguably the United Nations, and possibly a few others, no one has held that oral health or oral health care are rights. Rights are a special class of ethical assertion that apply to individuals by virtue of who they are and not what they have done (Edwards 1967). Human rights (such as life and liberty) apply to all people without qualification, civil rights (such as *habeas corpus* and adult suffrage) apply to citizens of the country in question – different countries, different rights. The rights and privileges of membership in a group (such as using the initials FACD in certain contexts if one is a fellow of the American College of Dentists) are specific community rights. Rights imply an obligation on the part of the community as a whole (the human race, the country, or the organization) to ensure that its members' rights are redeemable. Almost all rights are negative, such as freedom from unlawful search and seizure, or opportunities (the pursuit of happiness), rather than positive, as perhaps a right to a specific income.

Evoking rights tends to be a discussion stopper. "We hold these truths to be self-evident . . . ," boldly stated in the US Declaration of Independence was not intended to invite analysis or debate. As Norman Daniels remarks, "One problem with this somewhat pragmatic appeal to rights is that is does not carry us past our disagreements and uncertainties about the scope and limits of such rights claims" (Daniels 1985, p. 5). Both Daniels and John Rawls (1971; 1993) are explicit that healthcare is not a right. (Daniels suggests that "prudent deliberators" would seek health care as a social benefit to the extent that it "protected individuals' normal opportunity range at each stage in life" (1985, p. 103). The 1948 United Nations Universal Declaration of Human Rights mentions that everyone has "the right to a standard of living adequate for health and well being of himself and his family, including food, clothing, housing, medical care, necessary social services, and the right to security in the event of unemployment, sickness, disability, widowhood, old age, or lack of livelihood in circumstances beyond his control." It also states in

Article 23-3 that "everyone who works has the right to just and favorable remuneration ensuring for himself and his family an existence worthy of human dignity."

Comprehensive philosophical positions on justice, such as those advanced by Plato in the *Republic* (1983), René Descartes (1979), Jean Jacques Rousseau (1978), John Locke (1988), David Hume (1966), or Immanuel Kant (1958) are no longer fashionable. Current thought leans to clarifying specific issues such as property rights, conflicting interests of nudists and communities, and various welfare policies (Aday, Andersen & Fleming 1980; Bayer, Caplan & Daniels 1983; Sandel 1983; Sterba 1980; Veatch & Brayson 1976). Some rights are held to be prima facie – they are in effect to the extent that other rights don't trump them. Because rights are unqualified and beyond discussion, this view results in a standoff between arbitrary positions.

3. *Discursive Approaches.* The discursive view of ethics lies between the individual and the universal approaches. Ethics is a reflection of communities (MacIntyre 1984). In fact, the discursive or rhetorical process of searching for generally meaningful world views and making promises to other members of the community to behave in predictable fashion is intrinsic to creating community. This method will be taken up at the end of this paper.

4. *Game Theory.* A fourth approach has gained popularity among academics and offers an advantage of being content neutral. About the only assumptions necessary in game theory are that the question can be reasonably well structured and that people will act in ways that maximize their self interests (Luce & Raiffa 1957). Game theory can be used to reveal the structure of a very large number of situations because it can be shown that, generally speaking, issues involving many individuals can be converted into two-person games (one party vs. all others as a group) and that complex courses of action involving many steps can be converted into decisions involving one strategy vs. all others. (There are differences among games that do and do not have equilibrium points such that one strategy always dominates, whether a zero-sum game is being played – a person can only win what others lose, and whether communication among players takes place, but such nuances are beyond this paper.)

Writing in the ethics of distributive justice generally proceeds along one of two lines: (1) a characteristic of the current distribution that annoys a writer is documented and a principle is presented that justifies the teleological position of the writer or (2) a principle is selected and its implications are worked out. This paper differs in addressing what it means to evaluate alternative distributions of social goods. In the sections on game theory and the justice criterion that follow, it is demonstrated that no universally appropriate standards exist and thus there will always be valid reasons for and against individually favored positions. These are difficult arguments to follow and difficult for some to accept. The reader who is willing to concede this point may want to skip to the section on on Making Resources Common.

Game Theory

1. *Outcomes Envelope.* Consider a very improbable world view that distributes oral health resources in lavish ways to all individuals. Anyone who wants it is entitled, at no fee, to any dental procedure deemed beneficial by a panel of dentists, including all elective procedures such as orthodontics, veneers, and whiting. Further, users are compensated for lost income while receiving care, and transportation and childcare are reimbursed. This unrealistic distribution gives all the benefits to the patient and places heavy burdens on others, such as dentists and the public. The opposite extreme would involve some form of guaranteed benefits to dentists, with prohibitions against some people receiving care (even if it could be paid for personally as would happen if treatment were denied to undocumented aliens) and patients could be required to spend time waiting and be embarrassed with bureaucratic work. This costs the government or the public nothing. Some might argue that a worse alternative would be this scenario with patients receiving iatrogenic care, and that in fact such examples currently exist. This system offers nothing for the patient and everything for others. These extremes are indicated in Figure 1 as Points P and O.

Between the extremes of Points P and O there is a vast array of alternatives, each involving some better balance between the patient and others. Not every one of these combinations of outcome makes sense, however. For example, it is not possible to support everything the patient wants and everything everyone else wants at the same time, the utopian Point U. The dashed line on the left indicates a boundary of economic infeasibility for the public or the profession. Anything to the left of the line could not be sustained. The dotted line represents

Figure 1. Outcomes Envelope relating Joint Potential Benefits to Patients and Others; Pareto Optimal Set is Depicted by the Havy Line.

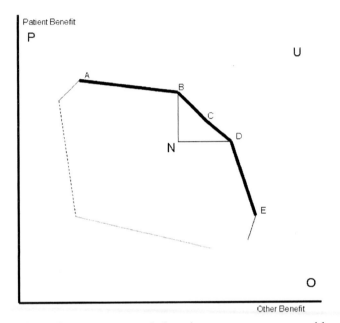

the standard of care. Outcomes below this point are unacceptable, and a pattern of practice that makes such outcomes probable requires the intervention of society.

Generally, any outcome within the envelop would not cause concerns of a policy nature. Naturally, an outcome at point N would be seen as an opportunity for the patient that something more toward the top would be preferred; while the dentist or public might like to see something nearer the right. These are non-zero-sum opportunities because improvements can be made that do not require a sacrifice from others. The possibility of such outcome signals an inefficient system. The dentist could use better materials or be educated in more up-to-date approaches; the patient could find a dentist closer to home or use better personal hygiene.

2. *Pareto Optimality.* The upper-right border is of special significance. These are the expected outcomes that leave nothing on the table for either party. These are zero-sum combinations – any advantage for

patient or dentist and the public comes at the expense of the other. This upper-right boundary is called the Pareto optimal set, named for an Italian economist who first discussed it extensively (he also invented the 80:20 rule). Two things are important about Pareto optimality. First it is an operational definition of a maximally mutually beneficial strategy in a game situation. Second, it is not a single point; it is a set of strategies – depicted in Figure 1 by the heavy line from points A through E – which meet the mutually optimal strategic criterion.

3. *Interpretation of the Outcome Envelop.* The figure represents a theoretical abstraction rather than the actual American oral health-care system or any part of it. It is important to realize that there has been virtually no research designed to draw this picture in reality. The question of scale has been begged. We do not know whether these are dollar or personal satisfaction units; but it is theoretically sufficient to hold that something like relative value units are assumed to be involved. Changes in scale (to reflect personal preferences) will have the effect of twisting the envelope to some extent. There will still be an economic and a standard of care boundary and a Pareto optimal boundary, and they will be in the same general positions. It is appropriate to note that the diagram achieves a two-person game structure by combining the interests of dentists and the public in opposition to patients' interests. It would be equally appropriate to combine the public and patient interests in opposition to dentists. This would most likely twist the envelop, but the landmarks would probably retain their relative positions.

It should be noted that there is lack of closure in the lower right-hand side of the diagram. This is intentional. The benefits and burdens of providing care to the historically underserved are not well understood; nor do we well understand the value these individuals place on the services they do not use. Despite rhetoric regarding a single standard of care, a multiple standard exists now and may make excellent sense. If this were not the case, differences along the Pareto optimal line in the vertical dimension would be nonsense. Isn't orthodontic care for those who can afford it and no care for those who cannot afford it a differentiated standard of care? Equally, the possibility must be considered that typical dental care represents a net negative value for some individuals. Even when care is provided at affordable costs (free), many individuals avoid it. Equating pain control (emergency room visits for extractions) with oral care is a distortion. Such individuals are not using the oral health care system; they are using the medical system. At the very least, it is risky beyond responsibility to extrapolate from one part of the diagram to others. To assume that individuals in the lower right-hand segment of the diagram have the same values as patients in the upper left or the same values that dentists have is irresponsible.

The Justice Criterion

We have not yet identified a just distribution of benefits and burdens among parties even though we have described the set of possible outcomes and explored in a general way which are impossible, which are undesirable, which are too poorly understood to work with, and which are most efficient (the Pareto optimal set). Although the Pareto optimal set offers the most promise for finding a point of just distribution, it normally includes many alternatives, and nothing has been said that favored one point over another. For example, no one has proposed 100 percent fee coverage for all dental needs. The welfare economist Amartya Sen makes the case against the other extreme: "An economy can be optimal in [the Pareto sense] even when some people are rolling in luxury and others are near starvation as long as the starvers cannot be made better off without cutting into the pleasure of the rich" (Sen 1970, p. 121). We must investigate various alternatives on and near the Pareto optimal set to see what is entailed in various criteria for setting the justice point. However, there is no generally accepted solution to this problem.

   1. *The Utilitarian Principle.* English social philosophers such as John Stuart Mill and Jeremy Bentham proposed, beginning in the late eighteenth century, a general approach that society thrives when, or even exists for the purpose of, maximizing the utility of its members (Bentham 1970; Mill 1956, 1972; Sidgwick 1907). The utilitarian principle states that social justice is the greatest good for the greatest number. The power of this formulation rests in its appeal to individuals determining their own values and the possibility of using factual data to inform policy. It should be remembered that Utilitarianism was born in the formation of the great principles of liberalism, such as the French 1789 Declaration of the Rights of Man and of the Citizen ("Liberty consists in the freedom to do everything which injures no one else; hence the exercise of the natural rights of each man has no limits except those which assure to the other members of society the

enjoyment of the same rights"). Adam Smith's contemporary theory of markets required only "an invisible hand."

Its strengths are also the vulnerabilities of the Utilitarian approach. Philosophers have long enjoyed giving examples of anti-social individual utilities. Should we, for example, count in establishing policy for the distribution of common benefits, the law-breaking personal preferences of counterfeiters or those who engage in civil disobedience? The utilitarian advice given by the dental establishment to its new recruits, "All you need to know about ethics is that you should treat every patient as though he or she were your mother" fails on the grounds that some people's mothers are sociopaths, or at least have uncomplimentary views about poor people. The troublesome side of the Utilitarian base in fact is the possibility it raises that justice is an empirical rather than a philosophical question. Are we to decide what is "just" by counting actual utility preferences rather than thinking about what they should be? In philosophy this is known as the Naturalistic Fallacy – the mistaken belief that "what ought to be" can be determined from an examination of "what is."

The result of several hundred years of work with the Utilitarian criterion for determining just distribution of resources has been its acceptance as a general guideline only. No one proposes to resolve disputes over justice with opinion polls, but references to "the benefit of the many over the privileges of a few" carry weight in debates. The pure form of Utilitarianism is indefensible – people are not to be trusted as individuals or collectively (other than in political speeches) – so legislators, bureaucrats, academics, and pundits have arisen and organized for the purpose of making a few necessary adjustments in the system. Modern politics can be largely understood in terms of the amount of improvement in human nature necessary through law and regulation – with "the right" referring to those that favor small corrections and "the left" referring to those who see greater opportunities to improve human nature through greater intervention.

There is also an argument against Utilitarianism on the ground that it is impractical. It would be extremely cumbersome to measure the preferences of a large number of people, definitions of the units of preference (known to decision scientists as "utiles") are still being debated, and people change their minds. The mathematics of utility decisions can become too complex for the typical person to perform or even understand. In fairness, these criticisms can be leveled against all attempts to find the justice criterion (with the possible exception of the voting method).

2. *Majority Vote.* Under certain conditions, simple vote is an excellent method for determining the just will of a group. It is assumed that the preference of each person should be given the same weight. Election of the American President and senators approximates this model. This approach is simple.

Some chafe at the constraint that all are assumed equal when there are clear differences in political qualifications. For example, idiots and bigots get the same consideration as those who are civically engaged and have studied the issues. Machine politics is an obvious abuse. So is the concern that senior citizens can vote benefits for themselves while children cannot.

Majority vote works well when there are two choices; but problems arise when there are three or more alternatives (Bodily 1985). For example, A might be preferable to B and B preferable to C, but it sometimes happens that C would be preferred over A. After all, comparisons are made among alternatives that have many features. Or A might be more desirable than B, except when C is present. This is known among decision scientists as the transitivity problem (Kenney & Raiffa 1993). The outcome of a vote or other system for establishing group preference depends on which options are presented, with the possibility that options not chosen determine the outcome selected. Recently, this was seen in the Oregon presidential primaries where Republicans petitioned (unsuccessfully) to place Ralph Nader on the ballot in hopes that enough liberal Democrats would vote for him to give the Republican Bush the plurality over Democrat Kerry. An analogous argument is currently circulating in the debate over patient access to care. Advocates are attempting to shift the balance of opinion in the profession toward more open access by raising the prospect that a "third party," the political process is prepared to weight in.

A principal shortcoming of majority vote as a method for determining the justice criterion is that appropriate groups simply do not vote on such matters. Perhaps the board of an insurance company could vote, or a large group practice might vote concerning policy within its purview, but almost all decisions that might collectively be taken as the expression of social justice are at best representative democracy, where a group elected for general purposes is asked to decide a test case rather than a comprehensive principle. There are no plebiscites on dentistry; decisions about oral health are not referred to all the people with teeth.

3. *Maximin (John Rawls).* The recently deceased American social justice philosopher John Rawls (1971, 1993; see also Moskop 1983) was concerned that efficiency in a social system (Pareto optimality) does not define justice. In fact, he argues that justice is a higher principle than efficiency, so the justice point might not even be in the Pareto optimal set (even though that is where the search begins).

Rawls' Difference Principle – his key to defining social equality – states: "The social order is not to establish and secure the more attractive prospects of those better off unless doing so is to the advantage of those less fortunate." Among decision theorists, this position is known as the maximin principle – changes should be made in the distribution of multi-party strategies until no further improvement can be expected in the prospects of the group that begins in the least favored position. The argument is more complicated than it may appear at first. For example, it is not proposed that those with many benefits should give them away so everyone has the same level (communism). Successful dentists are necessary to maintain a successful oral healthcare system. Boris Pasternak's novel *Dr. Zhivago* is a study in what happens when a profession is stripped of its prerogatives.

Rawls' analysis focuses on the question, "What is the proper level of superior benefit for the more privileged?" His answer is that justice can be achieved by establishing systems that benefit privileged classes if those increases benefits also result in greater benefits for the least advantaged in society, and systems should be established that reduce benefits for privileged groups when their benefits are not translated into advantages for those groups worst off. Rawls proposes a "trickle down" theory of social justice, one where social advantages are valued to the extent that they benefit others. States use something like Rawlsian logic when deciding whether to establish dental schools (Lightner & Zwemer 1999). Oral health is a social benefit and the tax base provided by professionals is attractive. Rawls would imagine (there is no evidence in his writings that he actually proposes this specific test) that legislatures debate whether it is more advantageous for the long-term oral health of the state for those with the worst oral health to fund programs for the underserved or to invest in more dentists (through schools or through transfer systems such as WICHE) – or to improve the lot of the poor through food stamps, education, job training, etc.

It is possible to argue that Rawls would have had little concern with the American fee-for-service dental system based on the fact that dentists as a group pay approximately twice the annual amount of federal income taxes as the government spends on all oral healthcare programs. The current concern over access to dental care is not straightforward. The oral health status of the poorer segments of America is roughly the same (in absolute and relative terms) as it was twenty years ago, as is utilization of services. If we have an "access issue" now, we had one two decades ago, and probably a worse one still fifty years ago. What has changed during this time is the proportion of dentists' income derived from services that are not health-related – bleaching, orthodontics, veneers, and other cosmetic services. These do not benefit the least advantaged in society. For the past twenty years, the income of dentists has increased at 150 percent of the American economy generally (Guay 2005), and the amount of oral health care provided to the poor has remained a constant proportion of the healthcare budget. Rawls would probably favor policies to curb the recent shift of a privileged group benefiting from serving another privileged group.

A peculiarity in Rawls' maximin approach is his insistence on treating levels in society as classes, represented by single individuals, "the representative man." Lawyers equal members of the working class equal the unemployed; each class having the same weight in his analysis. On this framing of the issues, Rawls suggests that his maximin principle is more liberal (kindly to the least advantaged) than the position of his archrivals, the Utilitarians (Rawls 1993). Weighting classes by their numbers or their economic impact seems defensible and certainly changes the order of the rules for finding the justice criterion. In fact, among all the rules to be considered in this paper, Rawls' maximin rule or Difference Principle is the most conservative – his view of justice allows the greatest range across benefits and burdens.

4. *Harsanyi's Additive Utility.* A much more liberal definition of the justice criterion is offered by John Harsanyi (1955), who proposes an elaboration of Utilitarianism to allow for the possibility that all individuals are not of the same value or importance to society. His formula is simple: the preferences (utilities) of each involved individual are to be weighted by some factor that reflects each individual's significance in the decision. The weighted preferences are then tallied. For example, a consortium of organizations that funds healthcare clinics for the underserved would vote on several alternatives for the distribution of

their common benefit, but each organization's vote would be weighted by the dollar contribution it has made to the common fund. Alternatively, the directors of the programs that might receive such funds would vote based on the number of patients they could deliver. The American Association of Retired Persons is exactly an example of Haranyi principle. It is a self-defined lobbying group that actively recruits members for the purpose of gaining weight in the political arena (Putnam 2000). A similar process is involved in organizations such as the American Dental Education Association, the American Dental Association, and so forth when policy positions on social issues are taken, along with representations about their numbers or the influence of their members, to "decision makers" in other settings, such as legislatures.

The liberal bias of the Haranyi (weighted utility) rule for finding the justice criterion is made more apparent by considering another rule developed by Vilfredo Pareto. It is no joke that he developed the 80:20 rule (80% of the problems are caused by 20% of the people, etc.). As an economist, he studied the distribution of wealth in Europe at the end of the nineteenth century and discovered that it was a severely positively skewed distribution (Pareto 1909). Small numbers of people have large amounts of resources. Such distributions are known as Matthew curves (a misinterpretation of the verse in Matthew 13:12 about those who have been given more). Later work in the field has shown that such distributions develop spontaneously in systems where the benefits accrued at Time 1 can be carried over in same way to Time 2. Such multiplicative relationships as compound interest, education, or health always result in positively skewed distributions over time. Any weighting of positions that does not exactly match the criteria that created the skewed distribution in the first place will tend (by the rule of regression toward the mean) toward a more uniform distribution – reallocation of resources toward those who do not have them now. (This is a characteristic of numbers, not of social benefits and burdens.)

The second great principle of social justice proposed by Rawls (besides the Difference Principle) was that "social and economic inequities are to be arranged so that they are attached to offices and positions open to all under conditions of fair equality of opportunity" (Rawls 1993). In a word, Rawls urges that no systems or structures should be created that codify or prevent the reversal of gains in benefits through exercise of the multplicative principle of the Matthew curve.

The problem with the Harsanyi approach is determining how weights should be assigned in a fair manner. Naturally occurring mechanisms – such as larger population groups among those on the left and more money to buy media and closer personal connections with influential individuals on the right – are at play in American politics. Haranyi developed his ideas originally in the limited context of small groups (such as committees), and he proposed the generally unworkable solution of having a third party determine the allocation of weights. The court system does on occasion play this role, but it is not regarded as a satisfactory sufficient approach.

5. *Nash Bargaining Solution.* A useful and intuitive approach for fixing the justice criterion was suggested in the 1950s for the two-person case by John Nash (1950) and subsequently generalized by a number of decision theorists (see Luce and Raiffa 1957). Nash's insight was that those who have the most must give up the most to maintain a relationship. Consider the metaphor of a Caribbean hurricane. The same unfortunate event costs many times as much in Florida as it does in Haiti. What is the likelihood that a dentist will sue a patient compared to the likelihood of a patient suing the dentist?

To implement a Nash solution (or to capture the power of this view without formally solving specific problems) we need to know what each party stands to gain (or to lose if the transaction does not take place). A dentist with empty chair time looks at a capitation plan differently from a dentist who has a full schedule. The economic analysis of marginal utility for the plan is not the same – there is no intrinsic value in outcomes independent of what they add to the utilities of others. (This point will become critical in discussions below). Writers in the theory of negotiation refer to the baseline position as the BATNA – the best alternative to a negotiated solution (Fisher & Ury 1991). Those with large relative BATNAs have a strong negotiating position. As the situation with international terrorism demonstrates, those with nothing to lose are in the strongest position. Formally, the Nash solution is to maximize the product of the potential gains for each strategy under consideration.

The Nash solution to defining the justice criterion introduces three new ideas. First, the marginal utility perspective (gain rather than outcome) is important. It matters where each party is at the beginning of any considered change in strategy. The Nash approach is the best known of this class of decision rules called von Neumann-Morgenstern bargaining solutions (von Neumann & Morgenstern 1944). These two mathematicians demonstrated that there is no need to consider the entire range of potential outcomes or even the entire Pareto optimality set when searching for fair solutions. Each party can be presumed to rule out all alternatives that are worse then their current position. The negotiation set, shown in Figure 1 as the area N, B, D describes the outcomes that are mutually no worse than the current joint situation, N, presumably the only outcomes that should be considered. The Nash solution will always be in the von Neumann-Morgenstern negation set.

Second, Nash's view is described as a "bargaining" solution because it lends itself to iterative approximations of a mutually optimal resolution. This is in contrast to theoretical positions such as Rawls' or Harsanyi's views where a one-time insight into the optimal solution (usually by a third party) is desired. The view of social policy formation as a give and take, extending over time and even into the future, is intuitive. Theorists have correctly noted that the iterative nature of a bargaining approach contains the inherent potential for reaching only local maxima (Luce & Raiffa 1957). That is a valid criticism and one that explains why revolutions occur from time to time.

The third unique characteristic of the Nash approach is that it depends on an understanding of what others stand to gain or lose. Technically, the Nash maximization of utility gains is calculated over all other parties, holding one's own position constant. This is a shift in perspective from choosing what is good for oneself in the abstract to finding what is best for oneself by considering the impact of one's position in terms of its effect on all others. The Nash approach might be avoided precisely because of this characteristic. A faux Nash solution is typically advanced instead, where individuals decide what they think is best for other parties. In thirty years of attending meetings on the allocation of oral health resources, the author has never met anyone who was present only in the capacity of a patient, let alone an individual who had not regularly received dental care. There has been no shortage of individuals, however, who have been willing to explain what they thought these absent Americans needed.

The Nash solution applies only in those cases where the parties value continued participation in the group. Bodily (1997) has demonstrated that, for any common set circumstances about a decision, the Nash solution will always lie between the conservative Rawls solution and the liberal Harsanyi solution.

6. *Third-Party Solutions*. The final alternative approach for finding the justice criterion on the distribution of benefits and burdens partially abandons the two-party game structure assumed until now. Especially in situations were outcomes are uncertain or where there is substantial ambiguity, parties may agree to submit the determination of a fair decision to a third party. The courts are often thus engaged. In other circumstances, third-parties insert themselves into differences regarding just distribution without being invited, as in the case of regulators.

Except, perhaps, in the case of "last best offer" arbitration (where the arbitrator is constrained to choose only between the two final offers made by the parties and is not free to introduce any alternatives), a third-party solution will never be found in the Pareto optimal set (French 1990). A fair resolution is some point on a straight line between two positions on the Pareto curve offered by the two parties. In "splitting the difference" as some sense of justice, the arbitrator sacrifices efficiency for justice (Chambers 1995).

Third-party solutions to the issue of justice have the important characteristic of sacrificing efficiency. Mutually, the parties to an arbitrated solution enjoy less than they would have mutually in a two-party solution. Although either party might get more or less in the two-party solution to justice, cumulatively they receive less. Third parties take benefits out of the social system – always. There are two costs: one is the direct costs of keeping the third-party in business, the other is the lost opportunity of unrealized benefits. It is always better in the long run to settle; the short run is what costs. It is not always the case that a third-party solution to the distribution of social benefits falls in the von Neumann-Morgenstern negation set. Imagine a tangent between points A and E on Figure 1. All arbitrated solutions represent losses for one or both parties. The collapse of communism and the United States government's sometimes attempts to drive down healthcare costs by increasing supply are examples. Charles Dickens's novel *Bleak House* describes the tragedy of a court fight between two parts of a family that entirely consumed the disputed inheritance and destroyed lives.

Making Resources Common

Most of the attention devoted to questions of social justice is focused on the fair division of the pie; there is less concern with how big the pie should be (Daniels 1985; Sen 1973, 1982). The public purchase of oral health is almost entirely from undifferentiated sources – taxes. There is no requirement that specific groups within society contribute directly to oral health – as there is in medicine where the residency system provides subsidized care. Also unlike medicine, there are no direct obligations for patients to participate in pro-health behaviors. The public is required, for example, to show proof of certain inoculations to enter school or to wear motorcycle helmets or automobile seat belts in order to reduce the general health burden.

Most "rights" begin in the common domain (Audi 1999; Edwards 1967). Liberty, the pursuit of this or that, and freedom of something else need not be taken from one person to be given to another. Freedom to follow healthy lifestyles – involving such behaviors as dietary choices, exercise, and flossing – are possibly of this category. But oral health treatment is not in the common domain, it must be brought in from various private sectors. Robert Nozick (1974) develops a theory of social justice that has as its first principle the ownership of personal property.

Society has three primary means for converting personal resources to common ones. These include (1) agreement, (2) eminent domain, and (3) incentive (Kane 1996). Income tax and compulsory military service are examples of agreement. In almost all such cases, the group making the decision is a representative for the community. Members of the community agree in advance to be bound by all decisions of the group, even if made by representatives or if they object to some decision, in exchange for a voice in the process. Alternatively communities may also decide that specific personal resources are needed for the public good and they can take them (under conditions of due process and compensation). This category includes specific behaviors such as required health practices, attending school, and having fluoridated drinking water. The public decides where the common good trumps private interests. The final category includes tax breaks for environmental practices, Medicaid, and public support of education (including the education of dentists). This approach to increasing the size of the common pool of resources functions by the public "investing" with a view to attracting "matching" private resources by making it advantageous to transfer them for common use. Harden's 1986 essay, "The tragedy of the commons" describes how depending on private self-interest will invariably lead to draining of common resources.

Although little work has been done on this issue, it is possible that game theory, discursive ethics, and other approaches to distributive justice described in this paper for use in solving allocation problems for community assets of a fixed size could also be used to determine some useful characteristics of the boundary between private and public resources. At first glance, intimidation, embarrassment, and confiscation would appear to be unjust practices for this purpose. It is unclear how voluntary contributions of private resources should be regarded. Biological economics theorists, such as Hirshleifer (1997), who attribute benefits to altruism would not regard this as a problem; but game theory requires an assumption that each party seeks to maximize its long-run benefits.

The Impossibility Argument

Readers who have worked their way to this point in the paper have likely begun to form a feeling that distributive justice is a difficult topic. If this is already a profound feeling, you are encouraged to skip this section. It will be demonstrated here that decisions regarding social justice are at best arbitrary across some specific group for some period of time. Strictly speaking, distributive justice can never be a coherent system that is consistent and complete. Evidence will be reviewed showing that decisions regarding social welfare are necessarily indeterminate and that the human nature of would-be decision makers is inherently inconsistent, arbitrary, and distorted.

1. *Indeterminacy.* In 1951 the economist Kenneth Arrow published the first of his explorations of an ideal system of social welfare (Arrow 1963). His general topic was how should individual choices be made to ensure a fair distribution of social benefits. He began by laying out reasonable conditions for such a welfare system: (1) there are at least two decision makers and three or more alternative plans for allocating resources; (2) patterns of preferences among existing alternatives will not be altered by the discovery of new, options not chosen or the removal of others; (3) if individuals do not change their order of preferences,

the order will not be changed in society; (4) no citizen can impose his or her will on others; and (5) no one person is empowered to choose on behalf of society.

Although the five conditions of Arrow's theorem make sense individually, taken as a whole they are inconsistent. No method for making welfare allocations simultaneously satisfies all requirements. Amartya Sen (1970, 1973, 1982) offers other variations on the impossibility of fair and consistent welfare allocations. Luce and Raiffa (1955) provide a summary and proof of Arrow's theorem and suggest that the easiest way out of the paradox is to relax one of the conditions. The preferred approach is normally to sacrifice the second, intransitivity, condition. In other words to permit inconsistencies in the just distribution of benefits and burdens. Examples include federal support for end-stage renal failure, but not for other terminal conditions or the prohibition of charging higher fees for the same services to members of protected groups but not unprotected groups, while simultaneously holding that all groups are equal.

Arrow's indeterminacy theorem is only one of many such demonstrations that our understanding of the world cannot be simultaneously consistent and complete. Einstein's relativity theories and Heisenberg's indeterminacy principle in physics are seminal demonstrations. Gödel's Proof that elementary number theory cannot be both complete and consistent is yet another example (Nagel & Newman 1958). This general class of proofs does not claim that collective human activity is irrational, just that all solutions are local (not universal) or temporary (open to change on next consideration). This is only discouraging to anyone who thinks he or she has discovered a grand slam solution to issues such as social justice or who feels that what is clear to them must be equally inescapable to others.

The warning in Arrow's theorem is not against the futility of general solutions to problems such as the distribution of oral healthcare resources; it is against thinking that these have been achieved. As Luce and Raiffa remind us, "If a welfare function satisfies conditions 1, 2, and 3 [rationality], then it is either imposed or dictatorial" (1957, p. 339). Both dangers are real. Organized dentistry, as have all professions, has labored diligently to achieve a position where they can impose a solution (contra condition 4) (Chambers 2004b). Alternatively, critics have sought to carve out territories (sometimes existing only as theoretical kingdoms) where their solution is sufficient (contra condition 3) (Chambers 2004a).

2. *Imprecision*. It has already been shown that decisions about distributive justice are necessarily local or temporary. Now it will be argued that they are necessarily inexact. Anyone who has tried to work out coherent oral health systems or has argued with those who have tied to do so understands how the discussion tends to fade in and out of focus. It's like eating Jell-O with four-foot-long chop sticks. There is sufficient evidence that communities cannot solve the problems of justice adequately because we, as individuals, lack the cognitive equipment to do so. Three examples of this fundamental shortcoming will be mentioned: bounded rationality, heuristic insufficiency, and non-linearity of personal utility functions.

Nobel-prize-winning economist and cognitive psychologist Herbert Simon (1957, 1973) was not the first, but certainly he has been among the most persistent in pointing out that rational decision-making is an atypical human activity. Most of the time we use well-worn and unthinking couplings of stimulus and response. When confronted with important and novel challenges we attempt a variety of approaches until we find one that seems to work. We accept approximations rather than insisting on optimization. This "satisficing" is necessary because we lack the capacity to remember, discover, and simultaneously consider all that is needed to solve even simple problems and because the difference between optimal and satisficing solutions is typically not worth the additional effort. Shapira (1995) has studied successful executives and discovered that they are more likely to divide or redefine problems into ones that can be easily solved than to attempt complex or risky solutions. March (1995) has proposed a "garbage can" theory of organizational decision making in which actors, problems, and solutions float, almost at random, and are only recognized as problem-solving solutions when an actor associates himself or herself with a serendipitous confluence of a problem and a solution.

The psychologists Amos Tversky and Daniel Kahneman and their colleagues (Gilovich, Griffin & Kahneman 2002; Kahneman, Slovic & Tversky 1982) have made a life-long study of how individuals actually solve problems instead of how they are supposed to do so. We consistently overestimate the occurrence of important things, attempt to explain complex events in terms of single causes, underestimate the baseline in diagnosing conditions based on evidence, and exaggerate archetypes.

Two favorite examples are their early research showing that individuals are much more likely to say that pink resembles red than vice versa and that a daughter looks more like her mother than the other way around. The author has summarized some of these "holes in our heads" as they pertain to dentistry (Chambers 1997).

Finally, there is the problem of non-linear utility functions (Kahneman & Tversky 1979). It would be unusual to find a person whose net worth is in the millions of dollars who is as excited about the prospect of earning $50 on a small errand as it would be to find a person on welfare to be excited about that prospect. Value changes depending on where the baseline is. Typically, larger amounts are needed to achieve the same utility as the base amount increases (a negatively increasing curve). A similar pattern exists for potential losses, except that most people are more concerned to protect against losses than they are to earn benefits. Loss has a negatively decreasing curve, but it is deeper than the curve for gain. For example, most people would not take a bet for a 50:50 chance of winning $100 or losing $100. The chances of finding anyone who would go for $100,000 on these odds are even smaller.

The problem of non-linear utility functions is that they differ in shape from one person to another and they depend significantly on where baseline is. One of the advantages of the Nash solution to the justice criterion problem is that it alone makes adequate adjustment of baseline. A danger exists in projecting values at one point in the solution set of alternative oral healthcare outcomes any distance across the set. Even the values that create equilibrium at one point in the Pareto optimal set may not travel well to other points on the set. It is risky in the extreme to assume that the utilities that one party holds as justifying its position apply to other parties at other points. Lacking clear knowledge of the values of individuals who are not regular users of the oral healthcare system is not sufficient justification for imputing to them the values of either patients generally or, worse, of politicians or healthcare professionals.

A Discursive Way Forward

As wonderful as it might be to discover the pot of gold at the end of the rainbow of distributive justice, this is unlikely to happen. It should be recalled that no one has found it yet despite numerous cases of philosophers and politicians who say they have seen it clearly and demonstrably pointed out where it is. The thesis of this paper is that there is no general solution to the problem of distributive justice – at large or in oral health care – and that all approaches to it are, at best, complex approximations. Under such conditions the only reasonable course open to us is to proceed forwards with vigor.

But the game has changed. We should no longer be looking for the general solution to the problem of distributive justice that we will than share with other who weren't as clever as we have been. The new program is to create ethical communities in which members see mutual advantage in allocation of resources toward general goals. The communities may not be comprehensive and may overlap; they will all be provisional – lasting only as long as they are useful; and they will be loosely coupled, probably even sloppy as they seek to balance the effectiveness of the group with its cohesion.

This is the program known as discursive ethics (Chambers 1996, 2000). Rhetoric or rational discourse, the proposing of alternative world views in hope of fashioning ones that are large enough to host the world views of members, is the means for creating such community. Local communities engage in discourse with other communities, again with hope of finding common ground and mutual advantage.

This approach has been most prominently associated with the German liberal political philosopher Jürgen Habermas (1984, 1996). He draws heavily on the German intellectual tradition of unfolding layers of social institutions and the English linguistic philosophers who believe that language has the capacity to perform acts as well as describe them – in particular, promises are acts that show the way toward mutually fulfilling cooperative action.

It is not the purpose of this paper to develop discursive ethics, but it will be useful to mention several features that relate directly to the discussion of distributive justice.

1. *People can say only what they believe to be true.* This rule binds the speaker to his or her word. It is a promise to behave in ways that are predictable based on what has been said. It is a way of minimizing the damage Arrow warns us of in his condition (2) on transitivity of options. Test positions communicate mistrust. The devil's advocate was an ecclesiastical appointment to challenge candidates for sainthood. The role as such does not exist otherwise.

2. *Anyone affected by the outcomes of a decision, who is competent, should be allowed to speak on their own behalf.* Again the purpose of this rule is to bind individuals and their word. It is also a protection from having others speak on someone's behalf, an especially dangerous problem in distributive justice. We must never presume that individuals cannot speak for themselves with regard to what is in their best interests. When they do speak, we must believe them until that proves impossible.

3. *What is held to be true is only true in the community.* We cannot extend our concepts of expected behavior to those outside the community. We will surely want to negotiate with other communities to see whether we can reach common understanding, but the concepts of right and wrong do not cross community boundaries.

4. *What is true in one situation is true in all similar situations.* This is a protection against capriciousness and hypocrisy. Without such protections groups cease to function or function inefficiently.

5. *Those who assert a position must be prepared to redeem their claims.* Reasons need not be given in advance for everything, but if questioned, we have to explain why we hold our views and to give acceptable explanations for behavior that appears to deviate from what we have said. Because rights language closes conversation, it is incompatible with discursive ethics.

6. *Those who do not abide by the mutual understandings of the group are not entitled to the benefits of the group.*

A final note that is more practical than philosophical – the most conspicuous obstacle to creating a system of distributive justice in oral health is the lack of participation in policy discussions by those who currently stand outside the system. It is not an acceptable substitute for others to speak for them. There is a tremendous need to engage them in the discourse. There is a separate need to conduct research that clarifies their values, rather than assuming that these values are the same as the values others in the system hold. As Rawls notes: "Arrow and Sen are surely right that the same index for everyone would be unfair" (1993, p. 183).

Bibliography

Aday LA, Andersen R & Fleming, GV. *Healthcare in the US: Equitable for Whom?* Beverly Hills: Sage, 1980

Alexander S & Ruderman M. The Role of Procedural Justice and Distributive Justice in Organizational Behavior. *Social Justice Research* 1987, 1: 177-197

Arrow KJ. *Social Choice and Individual Values.* New Haven, CT: Yale University Press, 1963

Audi R (Ed.). *The Cambridge Dictionary of Philosophy.* Cambridge: Cambridge University Press, 1999

Bayer R, Caplan Λ & Daniels N (Eds.). *In Search of Equity: Health Needs and the Health Care System.* New York: Plenum, 1983

Bentham J. *An Introduction to the Theory of Morals and Legislation.* London: Athlone Press, 1970

Bodily SE. *Modern Decision Making: A Guide to Modeling with Decision Support Systems.* New York: McGraw-Hill, 1985

Bodily SE. A Delegation Process for Combining Individual Utility Functions. *Management Science* 1997, 25(10), 235-239

Brandt RB. *The Good and the Right.* Oxford: Clarendon Press, 1979

Chambers D.W. Beware the Fourth Party. *Journal of the American College of Dentists* 1995, 62(2): 2-4

Chambers, DW. Looking for Virtue in a Virtuous Society – Discursive Ethics and Dental Managed Care. *Journal of the American College of Dentists* 1996, 63(4): 39-42

Chambers DW. Holes in Our Heads – WNL. *Journal of the American College of Dentists* 1997, 64(1): 40-44

Chambers DW. Promises. *Journal of the American College of Dentists* 2000, 67(3): 51-55

Chambers DW. Rhetoric. *Journal of the American College of Dentists* 2004a, 71(3): 36-44

Chambers DW. The Professions. *Journal of the American College of Dentists* 2004b, 71(4): 57-65

Daniels N. *Just Health Care.* Cambridge: Cambridge University Press, 1985

Descartes R. *Meditations on First Philosophy.* Indianapolis, IN: Hackett, 1979

Edwards P (Ed.). *The Encyclopedia of Philosophy.* New York: MacMillan, 1967

Fisher R & Ury W. *Getting to Yes: Negotiating Agreement with Giving.* In New York: Penguin, 1991

Folger R. Distributive and Procedural Justice: Combined Impact of "Voice" and Improvement on Experienced Equity. *Journal of Personality and Social Psychology* 1977, 35: 108-119

French W. *Human Resources Management.* Boston: Houghton Mifflin, 1990

Gilovich T, Griffin D & Kahneman D (Eds.). *Heuristics and Biases: The Psychology of Intuitive Judgment.* Cambridge: Cambridge University Press, 2002

Guay AH. Dental Practice: Prices, Production, and Profits. *Journal of the American Dental Association* 2005, 136 (March): 357-361

Habermas J. *The Theory of Communicative Action. Vol I: Reason and the Rationalization of Society.* Boston, MA: Beacon Press, 1984

Habermas J. *Moral Consciousness and Communicative Action.* Cambridge, MA: MIT Press, 1993

Haden NK et al. Improving the Oral Health Status of All Americans: Roles and Responsibilities of Academic Dental Institutions – The Report of the ADEA President's Commission. *Journal of Dental Education* 2003, 67(5): 563-581

Hardin G. The Tragedy of the Commons. *Science* 1996, 162: 1243-1248

Harsanyi JC. Cardinal Welfare, Individualistic Ethics, and Interpersonal Comparisons of Utility. *Journal of Political Economy* 1955, 63: 309-431

Hirshleifer J. Economics from a Biological Viewpoint. *Journal of Law and Economics* 1997, 20(2): 1-52

Hume D. *An Enquiry Concerning the Principles of Morals.* LaSalle, IL: Open Court, 1966

Kahneman D, Slovic P & Tversky A (Eds.). *Judgment under Uncertainty: Heuristics and Biases.* Cambridge: Cambridge University Press, 1982

Kahneman D & Tversky A. Prospect Theory: An Analysis of Decisions under Risk. *Econometrica* 1979, 47: 263-291

Kane R. *Through the Moral Maze.* Armonk, NY: Sharp, 1996

Kant I. *The Critique of Pure Reason.* London: MacMillan, 1958

Keeney RL & Raiffa H. *Decisions with Multiple Objectives: Preferences and Value Tradeoffs.* Cambridge: Cambridge University Press, 1993

Leightner JE & Zwemer JD. Dental Education: An Excellent Investment for the Government. *Journal of Dental Education* 1993, 63(9): 704-708

Locke J. *Two Treatises on Government.* Cambridge: Cambridge University Press, 1988

Luce RD & Raiffa H. *Games and Decisions: Introduction and Critical Survey.* New York: Dover, 1957

MacIntyre A. *After Virtue: A Study in Moral Theory.* London: Duckworth, 1984

March JG. *A Primer on Decision Making: How Decisions Happen.* New York: The Free Press, 1994

Mill JS. *On Liberty.* Indianapolis, IN: Bobbs-Merrill, 1956

Mill JS. *Utilitarianism.* London: Dent, 1972

Moskop J. Rawlsian Justice and a Human Right to Health Care. *Journal of Medicine and Philosophy* 1983, 8(4): 329-338

Nagel E & Newman JR. *Godel's Proof.* New York: New York University Press, 1958

Nash JF, Jr. The Bargaining Problem. *Econometrica* 1950, 18: 155-162

Nozick R. *Anarchy, State, and Utopia*. New York: Basic Books, 1974

Pareto V. *Manuel D'Economic Politique*. Paris: Giard, 1909

Plato. *The Republic*. Hammonsworth, England: Penguin Books, 1983

Putnam RD. *Bowling Alone: The Collapse and Revival of American Community*. New York: Simon & Schuster, 2000

Rawls J. *A Theory of Justice*. Cambridge: Harvard University Press, 1971

Rawls J. *Political Liberalism*. New York: Columbia University Press, 1993

Rousseau J-J. *The Social Contract*. Hammonsworth, England: Penguin Books, 1978

Sandel M. *Liberalism and the Limits of Justice*. Cambridge: Cambridge University Press, 1983

Sen A. *Collective Choice and Social Welfare*. San Francisco: Holden-Day, 1970

Sen A. *On Economic Inequality*. New York: W. W. Norton, 1973

Sen A. *Choice, Welfare, and Measurement*. Cambridge, MA: MIT Press, 1982

Shapira Z. *Risk Taking: A Managerial Perspective*. New York: Russell Sage Foundation, 1995

Sidgwick H. *Methods of Ethics*. London: MacMillan, 1907

Simon HA. *Models of Man: Social and Rational – Essays on Rational Human Behavior*. New York: John Wiley, 1957

Simon HA. Organization Man: Rational or Self-actualizing? *Public Administration Review*. 1973, 33: 346-353

Sterba J (Ed.). *Justice: Alternative Perspectives*. Belmont, CA: Wadsworth, 1980

Veatch R & Branson R (Eds.). *Ethics and Health Policy*. Cambridge, MA: Ballinger, 1976

von Neumann J & Morgenstern, O. *Theory of Games and Economic Behavior*. Princeton: Princeton University Press, 1944

Part II

International Perspectives

Kimberly McFarland

Care for Native American Patients

As a female dentist working on an Indian Reservation shortly after having graduated from dental school in the 1980s, I felt like I was making a difference. I was the only dentist in a rural county where there were approximately 5,000 tribally enrolled Native Americans who very much needed my services. Each day the appointment book was full to capacity and the four dental chairs in the clinic were utilized. The staff of three dental assistants, an office manager and myself worked hard to meet the dental health needs of the community in a respectful and caring manner. Each day we went home feeling very self-actualized, convinced we were truly making a difference.

Imagine my shock and horror one day, when a tribal elder asked me if I was having my period. If so I couldn't treat him because he considered me unclean. At first, I wanted to tell him it was none of his business. He had no right to ask such a question and he should not discriminate against a female dentist. It's difficult enough being a woman in a male dominated profession, let alone being singled out by patients who feel I am somehow inferior because of my gender. As a Native American, who probably knew firsthand how it felt to be singled out and discriminated against, I thought this man should posses the sensitivity and understanding of how inappropriate his question was. I also admit I thought about telling him he needed to look in the mirror and check his own hygiene status.

After a somewhat extended silence on my part, he volunteered that he was a medicine man. His belief system was that women who were having their periods somehow diminished his power as a medicine man. He also had an upcoming cleansing ritual he needed to lead so he wanted to make sure his powers were strong.

Fortunately I was not having my period. I informed him his powers were safe and we could proceed with his dental treatment. He needed a tooth removed and afterwards was grateful to be rid of the pain he had endured for so long. To gain the respect and appreciation of a medicine man was an accomplishment that I would not fully comprehend until many years later.

The ethical dentist strives to do that which is right and good, no matter who the patient may be. But when that patient is from a culture we know little about and brings a rich history of customs, treaties and practices foreign to us, we must assume the role of student. We must learn as much as possible about those we are called to serve. The Native American culture and history is no exception. Likewise, a knowledge of the health status of Native Americans is critical in providing ethical care. Only then will the ethical implications of treating this underserved population be apparent.

Historical Perspective

Prior to Europeans arriving in North America, more than 10 million original inhabitants, now known as American Indians and Alaska Natives, lived and flourished throughout what is now referred to as the United States of America (Nies 1996). By the mid to late1800s, their population had diminished to less than 500,000 (Kneeland 1864). This was due largely to the contagious and infectious diseases Europeans brought to the Native peoples as well as the war they waged against these original inhabitants for control of the land.

In fact, it was the United States War Department who administered Indian Affairs until 1849 when those duties were transferred to the newly formed Department of the Interior (National Library of Medicine 2005). At that time most Native Americans were being forced to reside on reservations or plots of land the federal government had designated for the various tribes. Reservation land was usually extremely remote and often times deemed undesirable by the general public. Reservation life was challenging beyond belief. In 1907, Susan La Flesche Picotte, the first Native American woman physician, wrote a letter to the Commissioner of Indian Affairs, Francis E. Leupp, describing the poor living conditions, lack of food and the people's inability to practice their cultural way of life, on her own reservation in Macy, Nebraska (Leupp 1907). Many Native Americans perished on the reservation because of the conditions.

The administration and provision of health care to Native Americans has been the responsibility of the federal government through the various Treaties and agreements it signed with the tribes in exchange for land or the use of the land. Some Native Americans can quote actual wording contained in the Treaties and tell of how their family members and elders have shared this information with each generation over many years. Words like, "As long as the rivers run and the grass grows, we will provide for your people," are a part of the Native American culture and expectation of what is owed as a result of these Treaties. The legal basis for federal services to American Indians and Alaska Natives is summarized in Table 1 (U.S. Department of Health and Human Services 2004).

Table 1. Legal Basis for Federal Services to American Indians & Alaska Natives by year (please note this list is not all inclusive)

YEAR	LEGISLATION
1787	United States Constitution
1921	The Snyder Act
1954	The Transfer Act
1959	Indian Sanitation Facilities & Services Act
1975*	Indian Self-determination & Education Assistance Act
1976	Indian Health Care Improvement Act
1986	Indian Alcohol & Substance Abuse Prevention & Treatment Act
1990	Indian Child Protection Act 1990

* enacted

Consequently, present-day Native Americans have a long legal history of subsistence provided by the United States of America. Even in the early 1900s when the Office of Indian Affairs was given the charge to oversee the needs of Native Americans, the Office was poorly equipped to handle the assignment (Neave 1894). The reservations were plagued by cases of small pox, tuberculosis, and other infectious diseases. The federal government's plan of assimilation of Native Americans into the white culture impacted all aspects of reservation life, including child rearing, education and health care. The original plan was to provide health care including the transportation of Native Americans off the reservation to receive care. When this proved problematic, Indian hospitals were ultimately constructed.

While physicians at the time may have harbored some curiosity about Native American medicine, they did not recommend its practice even among the most culturally devout Native Americans. European physicians considered themselves and their techniques superior to Native American "medicine men" or " Indian cures." The general public, however, did not share this sense of cultural imperialism. The public was intrigued by "Indian cures." The possibility of perhaps a natural compound providing healing relief for their ailments was appealing and oils and medicaments marketed as such, readily sold. This original "alternative medicine" experience among the American public and Native Americans actually began to shape our national health policy. Native American medicine was judged as uncivilized by the medical establishment and the Office of Indian Affairs shared this viewpoint. To this day, alternative medicine is viewed as somewhat suspect by the medical establishment. Nevertheless, the general public continues to have an intense interest in healing herbs, elixirs and vitamins.

In 1954, Congress transferred all Native American health care programs to the Department of Health, Education and Welfare's Public Health Service and by 1964 congressional hearings were held to examine the poor quality of care provided to Native Americans (Reader's Digest Association 1995). In 1955 the Indian Health Service was established to better meet the needs of Native Americans. Many hospitals were built during the early years of the Indian Health Service and remain in use today (U.S. Department of Health and Human Services 2004).

The following narrative, "Adapting White Medicine to Indian Culture," from a 1959 Orientation Guide to Health on the Navajo Indian Reservation, illustrates how Western medicine providers were starting to comprehend the importance of culture as it relates to the practice of healing:

> If Western medicine is to help and not harm the Navajos, it must get them to accept our pertinent and practical knowledge without undermining their faith. Their faith must not be ruthlessly attacked simply because it offers some obstacles to medicine. Instead, Western medicine should be expressed to the Navajos in terms of their own culture, in ways that accord with their understanding of the world and their values. If a public health worker wins the friendship of a few Navajos and takes time to listen to them, he will learn much that will be of practical use in adapting treatments, procedures, and teachings to the Navajos.

However, many Native Americans to this day harbor concerns about the care they receive on Indian Reservations and question the motives of those who provide that care.

Health Status

According to the 2000 U.S. census, 2.7 million (1.3%) of the adults in the United States are American Indian or Alaskan Native or a combination thereof. There is a substantial network in place for serving some of the health care needs of Native Americans and Alaska Natives.

The Indian Health Service has approximately 230 hospitals and clinics with more than 1800 dentists, hygienists and dental assistants. Approximately 55 percent of tribally enrolled Native Americans rely on the Indian Health Service as their only source of health care (US Dept. of Health and Human Services 2004).

Understanding the health needs and status of Native Americans is necessary if high quality, ethical health care is to be provided both within and outside the traditional network of Indian Health Service facilities. Most notably, Native Americans experience an array of health challenges including higher mortality rates from tuberculosis, chronic liver disease, cirrhosis, accidents, diabetes, suicide and homicide compared to other Americans (Barnes et al. 2005).

In regard to oral health, the data are equally compelling. American Indian/Alaska Native (AI/AN) children, aged 2-4 years, have 5 times the rate of dental decay compared to all US children and 6-8 year old AI/AN children have about twice the rate of dental caries experience. Periodontal disease is 2.5 time greater in Native American adults than in the general population (U.S. Department of Health and Human Services 2000). It is important to remember that the available oral health data for AI/AN applies only to those residing on reservations where services, including dental services are provided. Thus, Native Americans have striking disparities in health and oral health status when compared to the dominant culture. Only after understanding these disparities can a health care provider begin to make decisions that have an ethical context.

Personal Experience 1

As a dentist who spent several years providing dental services on a Indian Reservation, I believe the importance of this historical and health status information relative to the Native American population, is invaluable, especially if one is to provide care with justice and dignity. Just this information alone, however, would not have prepared me for my various experiences of providing ethical dental care for Native Americans. It is only after thoughtful reflection and diligent application of the principles of dental ethics that I have been able to begin to discern and work towards ethical dental care of Native American populations.

One of my first experiences in treating Native American dental patients, was a conversation I had with a mother of three children. The children were ages 2, 5 and 7. The mother had brought the 5 and 7 year old children to the dental clinic for check-ups. We encouraged the mother to also let us see her 2 year old child and the mother agreed. We provided a dental examination with radiographs and cleaned the teeth of each child. The older children had rampant dental decay. Her 2 year old son was still utilizing the bottle and had the beginning signs of early childhood caries or what used to be called baby bottle mouth.

I proceeded to provide tooth brushing instructions to the children and talked about good and bad foods with the children. The children seemed to enjoy their new toothbrushes and they knew candy was bad for their teeth. I then proceeded to visit with mom about the importance of substituting a cup for the bottle. We talked about how water can be put into a bottle at bedtime for children under the age of one. However, once the child turns one year old, he or she needs to discontinue using the bottle. Children age one and older should drink from a cup or glass. Mom smiled and nodded her head in affirmation of what I had said. She clearly seemed to understand the message and I was confident this information would prove invaluable for her 2 year old son.

Approximately 9 months later this same mother brought her now three year old son to the clinic for a toothache. The child was crying incessantly and we tried to take an x-ray of the teeth in question, but were not successful. As the child screamed I was able to view the teeth and they appeared to be decayed. The swelling present indicated that the teeth were most likely abscessed. I wrote a prescription for both an antibiotic and pain reliever, and arranged for the family to see a pediatric dental specialist. Clearly the child's numerous dental needs were more than we could handle in our general clinic.

After visiting with the mother about the next steps she needed to take, I inquired about our previous discussion nine months earlier, and specifically regarding the discontinuation of the bottle. The mother replied, "How many children do you have?" I had to say none, but I did have eight years of dental school training and several years of private practice experience. I stated that many learned people have studied these things and the scientific literature is very clear about these practices. I advised that it's best for children to discontinue the use of the bottle by age one. The mother simply smiled at me and turned to gather her children as she departed from the clinic.

I shared this experience with the dental staff and they laughed because they understood exactly what the patient was trying to tell me, namely that since I have no children I have no expertise in this area. The Native American culture values mothers and respects their expertise. Although a doctor is respected, it's the real world experience of parenting that is respected and revered as gospel. It doesn't matter how many years of training or how many learned people have written scholarly tomes on the subject of early childhood caries. The bottom line is that moms know best what children need. I needed to both understand and respect that cultural fact.

Luckily, one of the dental assistants in the clinic was the mother of five and very well known on the reservation for raising her children according to Native American ways. Her children danced in the tribe's POW-WOW which is an annual celebration of the culture and harvest. Her family also participated in the annual mushroom hunt which was revered as the highlight of spring.

After educating the dental assistant/mother of five children about the finer points of early childhood caries, dental hygiene and nutrition counseling, I was able to educate families about these topics through her. This education could occur in a respectful way and was valued by the tribal members.

Enhancing the welfare of others through acts that do good is perhaps a challenge for which even the most well-trained dentist may not be prepared. Only through thoughtful discernment and careful reflection can one balance beneficence and paternalism. Added in the mix is the element of autonomy or self-determination. The ethical dentist can facilitate this autonomy by assuring key information is provided to the patient in a respectful and culturally appropriate manner.

Personal Experience 2

Nursing homes or Long Term Care Facilities (LTCF) are not places frequented heavily by dentists. On the Indian Reservation where I worked, however, the LTCF was part of the Health Center and Dental Clinic building. The dental clinic staff were routinely called to the LTCF to assist the residents with their dental needs. Only Native American residents were served by the LTCF on the reservation and that care was provided in a manner reflective of the Native American culture. Hand games and other Native American past times were a part of the LTCF scheduled events. Native American decorations adorned the walls of the LTCF and some very respected elders of the tribe permanently resided in the facility.

Once a year the dental clinic staff were invited to come to the LTCF and provide dental examinations for all the residents. These examinations were required by the federal government's Medicare program. The findings of the dental examination had to be entered into the resident's medical chart in order for the clinic to bill Medicare and receive payments from the federal government.

When I reported to the LTCF to provide the dental examinations, I went to each resident's room and provided a thorough dental exam including an oral cancer examination. I was surprised to learn how many of the residents were edentulous and had dentures. This finding did make sense, however, when one considers the fact that approximately 50 percent of the tribal members are estimated to be diabetic. Diabetes is a risk factor for periodontal disease which often times contributes greatly to tooth loss. Of those who had teeth, many had advanced periodontal disease. I made the necessary entries in the medical chart and arranged dental appointments for those needing care.

But I was not prepared for the resident who refused to have a dental examination. As I entered his room he started to speak his native language and I could tell from the tone of his voice that he did not like my being there. I explained we just needed to look inside his mouth. The nursing staff apologized and explained he was a tribal elder from the "old school." He was very traditional in his Indian ways and would not let a women dentist look in his mouth. Although women and the role women fulfill are valued by the tribe, Indian tradition does place men ahead of women in regard to status. I also learned from the women of the tribe that only recently had a woman been allowed to serve as the tribal chairmen or leader of the tribe. Historically this was a position reserved only for men.

As a woman dentist and the only dentist in the entire county, I was shocked that this gentleman did not want me to look in his mouth. As the dental director for the tribe, I felt I had an obligation to secure the dental examination both for the patient's sake and also so the tribe could bill the Medicare program and keep its certification.

After visiting with the staff of the long-term care facility, I was able to determine that the gentleman in question was competent, healthy and well nourished. He participated in social activities regularly and spoke mainly to other male residents of the facility. He had no real family and no one came to visit him. When he did require medical attention, the resident would request a male physician. The health center easily accommodated this request because there were several male physicians available to provide care.

After reflecting on the various options available, I did offer the resident the opportunity to travel to a neighboring reservation to receive his dental care from a male dentist. He declined. Therefore we simply noted in the chart the resident refused a dental examination or treatment. A notation was also made that alternative care was offered to the resident and he declined. The Medicare program accepted this good faith attempt to provide care and continued to reimburse the tribe for the resident's long-term care expenses.

Patient consent is often taken for granted. Dentists sometimes feel as though we know what is best for patients and assume all recommended care will meet with the patient's approval. When competent patients refuse treatment or even the dental examination itself, a provider must be willing to respect the patient's autonomy. The provider may attempt to contact the patient's family members to assist in securing consent or provide alternative treatment in a manner acceptable to the patient. In this example the patient was not in distress or harmed by not having an annual dental examination on a particular day. Although no family members were available to assist in securing consent, by offering the patient the opportunity to receive care in a neighboring community, the patient had full autonomy in self-determining his care.

Personal Experience 3

As the only dentist on an Indian Reservation, with a population of approximately 5,000 Native Americans, the dental clinic was always busy. One day a Native American man presented to the clinic with a toothache and demanded immediate dental care. We had the patient complete the health history form and seated him in a dental chair for an emergency dental examination. A molar tooth appeared to have a large carious lesion and a radiograph was ordered.

The patient was a large man, every bit of 6'5" (183 cm) tall and most likely weighed at least 300 lbs (135 kg). He had multiple health history problems involving his heart, lungs, liver and kidneys. He was not a happy individual and seemed at times argumentative in his comments and interaction with the staff.

After reading the radiograph and confirming his tooth was abscessed, I informed him of the need for a root canal or extraction. Upon learning of the diagnosis, he became very agitated and started yelling. He did not want a root canal or removal of the tooth. He wanted a filling placed in his tooth and he wanted the filling placed immediately.

I explained a filling was not an option in this case. The disease process had progressed too far into his tooth. The only appropriate treatment was a root canal or extraction. At this point he became extremely upset and jumped out of the dental chair. He began pounding his fist on the counter and demanded I place a filling in his tooth.

As I watched his display of anger, a part of me wanted to run out of the clinic and another part of me wanted to stand up and yell back at him. I determined a third approach was needed. When he finished, I quietly sat there and acknowledged how painful and frustrating it was to have an abscessed tooth. I also explained that while I would like to place a filling in his tooth, it would not make his pain go away. He could yell and pound his fist on the counter top, but it wouldn't change the fact that he had an abscessed tooth. He could even put his fist through the wall and all it would do is give him a sore hand to go with his painful tooth. I explained that I went to school for eight years to be a dentist and worked very hard to learn how I could help patients. The care I provide must match the diagnosis. If someone had a broken arm, a physician would not place a band-aid on it. Similarly, when a tooth is abscessed or dying, I can't place a filling. It's not needed. What's needed is a root canal or extraction. I explained I would be happy to write a prescription for medication so he could think about which treatment he would prefer. When he was ready he could return to the clinic for treatment.

To my surprise, he quietly sat down in the dental chair and said he didn't want a prescription, he wanted his tooth taken out. He was a cooperative patient and we provided the care he needed. I often think how many people would have simply provided a filling in face of the threat for their personal safety. Clearly a dentist could have felt justified in lying to the patient about his need for a filling. The ethics of honesty can be a test, especially when serving underserved patient populations.

Conclusion

In treating underserved patient populations the concept of fidelity or faithfulness to the doctor-patient relationship is key. The duty to provide patients with information they need to know and to provide that information in a culturally appropriate manner is essential if ethical dental care is to be provided. Likewise, patients cannot exercise their obligations of fidelity without complete knowledge and understanding.

The ethical dentist must appreciate the culture and community he or she is serving. The ethical dentist needs to have an awareness of the history, customs, practices and beliefs of the community being served. When this awareness is transformed into an appreciation, then the doctor-patient relationship can become more than a casual acquaintance and provide for an environment in which a dentist can truly do that which is right and good.

Similarly understanding the health status and needs of those being served is important to building the doctor-patient relationship. The American Dental Association in its Code of Ethics calls upon all dentists to provide competent and timely delivery of quality care within the bounds of the circumstances presented by the patient. Only by building a strong doctor-patient relationship through a complete understanding of the health needs and an appreciation of the culture of underserved populations can one truly meet the ethical challenges of serving the underserved.

Bibliography

Barnes PM, Adams PF & Powell-Griner E. *Health Characteristics of the American Indian and Alaska Native Adult Population: United States, 1999-2003.* Advance data from vital and health statistics; no 356. Hyattsville, Maryland: National Center for Health Statistics. 2005:1

Kneeland J. On Some of the Causes Tending to Promote the Extinction of the Aborigines of America, *Transactions of the American Medical Association*, Vol. 15, 1864

Leupp FE. Response to Picotte's letter. November 20, 1907. Available at the National Archives and Records Administration

National Library of Medicine. *The History of Medicine: Health Care to Native Americans.* Bethesda, MD: U.S. Department of Health and Human Services, National Institutes of Health; 2005

Neave JL, An Agency Doctor's Experiences Among Frontier Indians. *Cincinnati Medical Journal*, Vol. 9, 1894; 875-6

Nies J, *Native American History*. New York, NY: Random House; 1996

Reader's Digest Association, *Through Indian Eyes: the untold story of Native American peoples*. Pleasantville, NY: Reader's Digest; 1995

US Department of Health and Human Services, Indian Health Service Fact Sheet, Rockville, MD: US Department of Health and Human Services, Indian Health Service, 2004

US Department of Health and Human Services, *Oral Health in America: A Report of the Surgeon General*. Rockville, MD: U.S. Department of Health and Human Services, National Institute of Dental and Craniofacial Research, National Institutes of Health, 2000. Available on-line at: http://www.surgeongeneral.gov/library/oralhealth/ (access verified on 11/3/05)

Sefik Görkey

The Changing Face of
Turkey's Dental Profession

A Short History of Dentistry in Turkey

Turkey has had a long and illustrious history in dentistry. Most books about the early history of dentistry have emphasized the success of the Etruscans in making dental prostheses (Hoffmann-Axthelm 1981, Lyons & Petrucelli 1987, Atabek & Görkey 1998), but few articles have been written about the "lower anterior bridge," dating back to the 7th century BC that was found in Western Anatolia, Turkey (Terzioglu & Uzel 1987). In this exceptional piece, artificial teeth were affixed to the mandibular second incisors with a gold bar. Considering the time period, it is truly impressive that both the function and the esthetic quality of the patient's teeth were restored. We cannot be sure that this artefact represents the beginning of the dental profession in Anatolia, but it shows that early Anatolians were already very skilled in making artificial dental prostheses.

We do not have clear chronological or systematic information about the history of dentistry in Anatolia. Bronze spatulas from the ancient Greek period and dental forceps from the Byzantian age give us some information about the profession's long history in the country (Uzel 2000). According to Uzel, the first known dentist in Anatolia is thought to be Antipas from Pergamum who lived during Roman times. During the Islamic period, physicians in Anatolia paid attention to medical as well as dental problems problems. The first known Turkish medical monograph of Hekim Bereket from the 11th century has a section on dentistry.

Further advances were made during the Ottoman period. Serefed-din Sabuncuoglu was one of the most important figures in Ottoman medicine. He was born in 1385 in Amasya, where the Ottoman princes used to live. He became a physician at the hospital there and wrote three medical books, *Aqrabadin, Mucerrebname* and *Cerrahiyet ul Haniye*.

Three copies of the last book exist today; two of them were actually handwritten by Sabuncuoglu himself. The importance of this book for dentistry is that it includes chapters on tooth diseases. The author gives information about their treatment and illuminates the text with miniatures about his treatment methods (Dizdar 1981; Uzel 1987, 1999).

Musa bin Hamun is another important figure in dental history. A descendent from a Jewish family, he served Süleyman the Magnificent (who ruled from 1520 to 1566) as a court physician. According to Terzioglu and Krebs (1980), Musa bin Hamun's father emigrated from Spain to the Ottoman Empire after Granada was conquered by a Spanish king. Musa bin Hamun wrote a Turkish manuscript about dentistry for Suleyman the Magnificent. This unique manuscript is considered one of the oldest books on dentistry. Chapters in the book cover gingival diseases, dental surgery, treatment methods for tooth and gum diseases, the importance of using a toothbrush (*misvak*), anatomy of teeth, how to stop a toothache, etc. (Terzioglu & Krebs 1980; Terzioglu 1974; Terzioglu 1977). Musa bin Hamun's contribution was very important for dental history in general. The dental forceps, produced by the Ottoman Empire during the 17th century (Uzel 2000), and some other equipment from this period show that the practice of dentistry reached an important level compared to other parts of the world during that period (Gurkan 1974; Uzel 1999).

The first known dental association was established among dental students in 1912. Since that date other associations have been established in the country such as Darülfunun Osmani Tip Fakültesi Discilik Subesi Mezunin ve Talebe Cemiyeti, and Turk Dis Tabipleri Cemiyeti. Many also publish periodicals on a regular basis. Dis Tabipleri Cemiyeti Mecmuasi is one such example (Efeoglu 1992, Mugan 1994). The Turkish Dental Association (TDA) was established by law in 1985. The Turkish Dental Association Law regulated the establishment of a National Dental Association, dental chambers in the country and even subchambers, as well as their activities, elections, administration, and responsibilities of the chambers and the members. Today 32 chambers exist in the country that work under the TDA.

The first international Dental Congress was held in 1992 in Izmir. Ever since, the TDA has organized an international dental congress annually. The 2004 congress drew an audience of some 2,500. In addition, there have been various national meetings about the problems of dentists, some of which have resulted in white papers on such topics as dental education, patients' rights, and dentists' rights.

Regulations

The year 1923 represented a new beginning for Turkish society when Turkey became a secular state. Since that date many laws have come into force, some of which are specific to health care. The first was enacted in 1928 as a general health law and remains in force. The Medical Deontology Regulation was enacted in 1960. It regulates relationships among physicians as well as between physicians and patients, but applies equally to dentists. A variety of issues are covered, such as private clinics, employment by state hospitals, advertisements, patient confidentiality, and informed consent. This Regulation has not been updated since. Yet Turkey in 2005 is very different from Turkey in the 1960s. For example, advertising by dentists has always been an important topic in medical deontology texts. But the 1960 Regulation evidently does not cover the internet, which has become an important venue for dentists to advertise. In 1999, the presidents of the various regional chambers of dentistry met in Abant to discuss a new *"Draft of Dental Deontology (Ethics) Regulation."* This document covers an expanded and updated series of issues, including ethical principles (Article 5), objectivity of the dentist (Article 7, 8), confidentiality (Article 10 and 26), respect for patients' rights (Article 29), the patient's right to choose a dentist (Article 30), human experimentation and clinical trials (article 37), and ethical issues for publication (article 38). Unfortunately the draft still awaits parliamentary action to take effect.

Since the late 1970s, more specific legal regulations governing medical procedures have come in force, such as laws on organ transplantation (1979), abortion (1983), and in vitro fertilization (1987, 1996). Whereas these laws have not had much direct relevance for dentists, the recent law on the establishment of Research Ethics Committees (1993) has. Research Ethics Committees (REC) have been evaluating clinical trials since the mid 1980s, but following the 1993 law, REC approval has become a legal necessity for clinical trials. Today RECs work and evaluate the project proposals in a more professional way. Unfortunately, this 1993 regulation is tailored to medical research in general, and many dentists who are involved in research struggle with the guidelines. Obtaining approval from a medical school REC, which tends not to be familiar with dental research, is often rather difficult.

In 1959 Turkey applied to the European Economic Community to become a member. After a long waiting period and much political discussion, candidateship of Turkey was officially approved in 1999 in Helsinki. Turkey has begun negotiations in 2005. Many new legal regulations are coming into force, causing many changes in the field of dentistry as well. For example, the 78/686/EEC directive addresses the diplomas and circulation of dentists in the European community. A TDA Commission has been working since 1997 on this issue (Oktay 1997).

Another new law of importance to dentists is the 1998 law on Patient Rights which closely follows the Amsterdam and Lisbon Declarations on Patients Rights (Aydin 1999, 2001, 2004, Sert 2004). Turkey has also signed the Convention of Bioethics (Oviedo) from the Council of Europe.

In 1999, the law on Private Oral Health Centers (1999) took effect that regulates multi-dentist private clinics and private medical clinics with dental departments. This regulation also created a standard for advertisements in dental practices, replacing the old regulation from 1960 that applied to both physicians and dentists.

In addition to the various legal regulations listed above, the TDA has developed white papers on such topics as disciplinary activities, honorary positions, educational programs and specialization in dentistry. Today a dentist can specialize in any dental field. The dentist has to complete doctoral level education. In medical fields, the system is different. If a young physician would like to specialize in a field or specific area, he/she must pass a central exam given countrywide. Recently, the Turkish government has drafted a policy to adopt this system for dentistry as well, but the TDA has resisted.

Interest in Dental Ethics

Turkey's medical education system has a strong tradition in "medical deontology," that is, the code of conduct for physicians. The lectures on medical deontology have been compulsory since the Ottoman period. When dental schools first opened as part of medical facilities, this tradition influenced the dental curriculum. Indeed, *dental deontology* is a compulsory topic as well. In the mid 1980s the medical deontology lectures began to include topics on medical ethics. Atabek's 1983 textbook on *"Topics in Medical Deontology,"* includes chapters about medical ethical issues such as abortion, human experimentation, and euthanasia. Soon thereafter, doctoral dissertations on medical ethics began to be published, and ever since interest and expertise in medical ethics has been growing steadily.

The dental community has likewise exhibited a strong interest in ethical issues and dilemmas. The Turkish Dental Association congresses generally include sessions on dental ethics. A special TDA Ethics Committee was established in 1992. Subsequently, two nationwide meetings were organized by the TDA to discuss dental ethics, and representatives of all regional chambers attended. Most recently, the Committee has developed guidelines concerning the websites of dentists (Yildirim 2005).

Additionally, some dental schools have begun to establish their own Dental (Hospital) Ethics Committees. Although few cases are discussed, lectures and informational sessions about those committees tend to draw attention in dental schools. Many deans have shown to be supportive, consulting the committee and promoting it to others in the school. Moreover, sometimes patients directly apply to an ethics committee themselves. The Patient's Rights movement that followed the 1998 legal regulation, and discussions in the mass media seem to have had a positive effect on attitudes towards ethics.

Dental Education in Turkey

Archival documents that survive from the Ottoman period suggest that prior to the 19th century, there existed no special education for dentists. Dentists worked with experienced colleagues in order to learn the practice and learned from their own experiences. In the 19th century, young dentists were expected to obtain a testimonial from a senior dentist with whom they had practiced before they could begin to practice on their own. (Uzel 1999).

According to recent research, during the December 9, 1894 session of the council of Ministers, there were discussions on the reform of dental and pharmacy education (Yildirim 2003). Discussions continued with the goal of establishing a modern dental education system. Finally, in

1909 the first school of dentistry was established in Istanbul as a part of a medical school. Professor Halit Sazi (Kosemihal) opened the School of Dentistry, and he taught dentistry until his death (Uzel 2000). The first dentists graduated in 1911, and graduates from this school practiced not only in Turkey but in Bulgaria, Greece, Yugoslavia and Romania as well (Uzel 1999).

Although there were women healers who pulled teeth during the Ottoman era (Uzel 2000), Sadiye Guvendiren, a 1927 graduate from Istanbul University School of Dentistry, was the first licensed woman dentist in Turkey (Dolen, 1998; Uzel 2000). She was born in Istanbul and graduated among 175 students as 35th in her class. After her graduation she practiced dentistry with her husband. In 1935 she went to Afghanistan and helped to establish modern dental education in that country (Uzel 1999). In the early 1930s Turkey had close relationships with Afghanistan, and there existed a policy to contribute to the modernization of that country by the young Turkish republic. As a part of this policy, physicians, dentists and pharmacists went to Afghanistan. Dentist Celal Faik was the first dentist to go to Afghanistan as part of this program and Sadiye Guvendiren was the first woman dentist who went to Kabul (Denli-Atac-Aray 2005).

The year 1933 was an important turning point in higher education. The founder of the Turkish Republic, Kemal Ataturk, invited successful professors of Jewish origin, who had problems with the Nazi government in Germany, to come to Turkey. One hundred and fifty professors and their assistants came to Istanbul in 1933. They represented not only the field of medicine, but also the fields of zoology, botany, etc. They brought about academic reform in Turkey. Today we call this period the 1933 University Reform (Yildirim 1993).

Alfred Kantorowitz (1880 – 1961) was among those professors. Kantorowitz was a successful academician in Germany, but had problems with the Nazis because of his Jewish identity. According to Yildirim (1993), he was already jobless and in a concentration camp in Germany when he was invited to come to Istanbul University. Today, dental historians and senior dentists agree that Alfred Kantorowitz made important contributions to the academic life of modern dentistry during that period. He lectured on many topics, wrote books and educated young dentists and assistants who went on to become academicians themselves. He stayed 17 years in Turkey and returned to Germany in 1950 (Yildirim 1993).

Today 18 dental schools exist in the country. According to data from 2003, there were 5,306 students in dental schools and 747 academicians in teaching positions. The government has issued a draft in order to establish two new dental schools. However, it is not clear whether these plans are motivated by the shortages in dental personnel (which do in fact exist; see below) or by electoral motives of politicians (e.g., the promise of more higher education opportunities for youngsters and of new economic progress in the towns that will host the schools). Consequently, this plan has met with some resistance from TDA and academicians who insist on maintaining academic rigor and fear that the new dental schools will only produce more jobless dentists in big cities rather than increase dental services in rural areas.

Access to Oral Health Care

Of the 19,991 dentists who live in the country, 12,231 of them have private practices, 3,510 work both for state and in private practices, 2,690 work for the state, 637 are in the army, and 887 dentists do not practice dentistry (TDA data). Dentists, it seems, mostly practice in the western parts of the country and there exists a geographic disbalance in the spread of dentists throughout the country.

Data from the TDA from 2003 show that 40 percent of the population visit dentists, 47 percent do not, 12 percent did not respond to the questionnaire, and 17 percent of children experience decay before the age of 6 (Taskin 2003). Those data unfortunately show that there are a lot of unmet oral health needs in Turkey.

As in all countries facing the problem of oral health disparities, the question arises whether and to what extent the dental profession carries responsibilities for these unmet oral health care needs. Turkish dentists who work in state hospitals are employees of the state and are required by law to take care of every patient applying to that hospital or state clinic. But dentists who own private clinics have the right to choose which patients (not) to accept into their clinics (except for emergency care which must be provided by law). Moreover, dentists can open a private clinic anywhere in the country. Spurred, amongst others, by the high cost of purchasing dental equipment and the need therefore to earn a sizeable income, they mostly choose big cities, causing a significant maldistribution of dentists throughout the country. So far, the government has not issued any policies encouraging young dentists to open private practices in rural areas.

There continue to be significant distribution problems in Turkey, but there is also evidence that the dental profession is taking a more active role towards the resolution of these problems. The new code of ethics drafted by the TDA (which still awaits parliamentary approval) for the first time mentions the principle of justice – a hopeful sign.

Bibliography

Aydin E. *Tip Etigine Giris*. Pegem A yay. Ankara 2001

Aydin E. Bioethics Regulations in Turkey. *Journal of Medical Ethics* 1999, 25:404-407

Aydin E. Rights of Patients in Developing Countries: The Case of Turkey. *Journal of Medical Ethics* 2004, 30:555

Atabek EM. *Tibbi Deontoloji Konulari (Topics in Medical Deontology)*, Yenilik Basimevi. Istanbul 1983

Atabek EM & Görkey S. *Baslangicindan Ronesansa kadar Tip Tarihi*. İstanbul University Cerrahpasa faculty of Medicine Publ. 1998

Denli M, Atac A, and Aray N. Afganistanda Turk Hekimleri. IV. Lokman Hekim Tip Tarihi ve Folklorik Tip Gunleri. Manisa., Bildiri Ozetleri Adana 2005, s.25

Dizdar A. 15. yuzyilda Turk Distababeti ve Serafeddin Sabuncuoglu. I. Uluslararasi Turk Islam Bilim ve Teknoloji Tarihi Kongresi. ITU 14- 18 Eylul 1981. Bildiriler Cilt II. ITU Mimarlik Fak. Baski Atolyesi. Agustos 1981:38-45

Dolen E. Cumhuriyet'in Ilk Onbes Yilinda Istanbul Universitesinde Kiz Ogrenciler. Saglik Alaninda Turk Kadini Cumhuriyet'in ve Tip Fakultesine Kiz Ogrenci Kabulunun 75. Yili (ed) Prof. Dr. Nuran Yilidirim. Istanbul 1998. s. 8-47.

Efeoglu A. *Dishekimligi Tarihi*. Istanbul: Yuce Dagitim A.S., 1992

Mugan N. *Turk Dis Hekimligi Tarihi* I.U. Yay. Istanbul: Edebiyat Fakultesi Basimevi, 1994.

Görkey S. Etik Komiteler ve Dishekimligi (Ethics Committees and Dentistry) *I.U.Dishek Fak Derg* 1995, 29:74-77

Gurkan SI. *Kanuni Sultan Suleyman Devrinde Yazilmis Discilige ait El Yazmasi Kitap*. Yazan Musa bin Hamun. İstinsah eden S.I. Gurkan, I.U. Dishekimligi Fakultesi Yayinlari, 1974

Hoffmann-Axthelm W. *History of Dentistry*. Tokyo: Quintessence, 1981

Lyons AS and Petrucelli RJ. *Medicine. An Illustrated History.* Hong Kong: Abradale Books, 1987

Oktay I. Avrupa Birligi Sürecinde Diploma Denkligi Calisma Grubu. *TDBD* Temmuz 1997. sayi 38, s.10-11

Sert G. *Hasta Haklari (Patient Rights).* Uluslararasi Bildirgeler ve Tip Etigi Cercevesinde. Babil Yay: 2004

Taskin T. Yeni Dishekimligi Fakulteleri Hangi Ihtiyaca Yanit Verecek? *TDBD* Aralik 2003 sayi 78, s. 74-76

Terzioglu A. Eine bisher unbekannte türkishe Abhandlung über die Zahnheilkunde aus dem Anfang des 15. Jahrhunderts. *Südhoffs Archiv,* Bd. 58

Terzioglu A. *Moses Hamons Kompendium der Zahnheilkunde aus dem Anfang des 16. Jahrhunderts.* Muenchen, Dissertations und fotodruck frank., 1977

Terzioglu A & Krebs LM. *The History of Old Turkish Dentistry.* Munich: Demeter Verlag, 1980

Terzioglu A and Uzel I. Die Goldbandprothese in Etruskischer Technik. Ein Neuer Fund aus Westanatolien. *Phillip Journal für restaurative Zahnmedizin.* 1987 (April), 2:109-112

Turk Dishekimleri Birligi Kanunu (Turkish Dental Association Law) 1985

Uzel I. Sherefeddin Sabuncuoglu. A Dental Surgeon of the Fifteenth Century and his Interpretation of Abulcasis Notes on Oral Surgery. *Hamdard* 1987, XXX (4):3-20

Uzel I. Osmanli – Turk Dishekimligi. XIII: Turk Tarih Kongresi. Ankara 4-8 Ekim 1999, 633-660

Uzel I. *Anadolu Uygarliklarinda Dishekimligi (Dentistry in the Anatolian Civilizations. An Illustrated History)* Adana Ofset Baski (T.C. Kültür Bakanligi katkilari ile basilmistir) Printed with the contribution of Republic of Turkey, Ministry of Culture, 2000

Yildirim N. Istanbul'da Disciler Mektebi Kurma Girisimi (1894 – 1904). I. Turk Dishekimligi Tarihi ve Etigi Kongresi Istanbul 20-22 Kasim 2003. Poster Bildiri Ozetleri. S. 8-10

Yildirim M. Ulkemizde 19. yuzyilda ve 20. yy basinda Dishekimligi Egitiminin Gelismesi. I.U. Saglik Bilimleri Enstitusu. Deontoloji ve Tip Tarihi ABD. (Doktora Tezi) Danisman: Prof. Dr. A. Terzioglu. Istanbul 1993

Yildirim CK. President of Turkish Dental Association (TDA) Personal interview May 19, 2005

Sinikka Salo and Matti Pöyry

Access to Oral Health Services in Finland. A Review of Recent Legal and Policy Changes

Introduction

Finland is a Nordic country with a population of about 5.2 million people (year 2005). Regional government is organized through 6 provinces and 452 municipalities. The national parliament has 200 members, elected under a system of proportional representation. The President of the Republic is elected by direct popular vote. In the regular course of events, a presidential election takes place every six years. In Finland healthcare is funded largely through general taxation, with an additional special tax for health which is paid by everyone including those who are retired. The Primary Health Care Act (PHC Act) of 1972 reformed the planning of primary health services by establishing a network of health centers funded by the municipalities. These provide a range of local public services, including medical services, radiology, laboratory and dental services – although the latter vary between health centers. In 2002 the proportion of GNP spent on general healthcare was 7 percent, including dentistry.

In Finland the responsibility for planning oral healthcare lies with the Ministry of Social Affairs and Health, but the actual service is usually provided by municipalities. The government social insurance agency (KELA) also provides some assistance in paying for healthcare, again under the strategic direction of the Ministry. The agency is self-regulating, under the supervision of the Finnish parliament, has its own budget, and 328 branch offices in municipalities. However if the KELA has a budget deficit, the government is obliged by law to make up the total spent from taxation.

The dental services are delivered either through the system of public health centers, or by private dentists, dental technicians and dental laboratories.

Access to Oral Health Services before 2002

Before December 2002 it was possible to limit public dental services to special age groups only. Municipalities in Finland are very independent, and some limitations for services were in use in many of them. The situation in oral health care was highly unequal and would vary according to age, general health status, and geographical region.

Of the total population of 5.2 million, approximately 2 million people (40%) used private dental services and paid all the costs for their oral healthcare themselves, with no assistance from state bodies such as the KELA. Of the remaining 3 million, about 1 million were children under the age of 19 who mainly received municipality based care in health centers free of charge (Table 1). A further 1 million adults were also

Table 1. Oral health services in Finland before December 2002

Population	Establishments and cost
Adults (2 million)	Private practice: 100% cost
Under 19s (1 million)	Health centers: Free of charge
Adults (1 million)	Health centers: 33% costs
Adults (1 million)	Private practice: 100% fee reimbursement from Kela

treated at municipality health centers which provided care on average at one third of the cost compared to fees of the private services. These were mostly health centers in rural areas or in small towns. Health centers of big cities were able only to treat under 19 year olds and some special patient groups, e.g. diabetic, disabled or older persons. The remainder paid full fees to private practitioners, but got reimbursed by the KELA at 60 percent of the KELA's rate. By law, those reimbursed were citizens born after 1956, or patients with systemic disorders. War-veterans had some better benefits as well, and their reimbursement varied from 60 to 100 percent depending on the type of treatment (e.g., clinical examinations and preventive measures were reimbursed 100%). Reimbursement from dental fees was possible only for private services, because the fees of health centers were already subsidized by local municipalities.

Access to Oral Health Services after 2002

From December 2002 the age limits applied thus far in Finnish dental care were abolished. At that time public health centers treated about one third of the adult population, and local authorities had been free to decide, for example, that only those under 40 years of age would have access to this care. After 2002 it was no longer possible for the centers to select patients on the basis of age, and it is anticipated that public health centers may come to treat one half of all adults. Despite the banning of age limits, municipalities retained some autonomy in organizing their services. The main principle that municipalities must adhere to when structuring their program for service delivery is that they are responsible for the health services for people in need. The Ministry of Social Affairs and Health ensures that municipalities act within the new law. While there will be charges for treating patients over 18 years of age, such treatment will nevertheless be cheaper than private dental care. However, access to treatment and the scope of treatment provided will vary according to geographical region.

There has been a major change in Finland affecting all healthcare from the beginning of March 2005. A new Act, called *Guaranteed access to treatment*, imposes new requirements on municipalities which must organize their public health care so that patients will receive an assessment of their need for non-emergency treatment from a health care professional – not necessarily a doctor – within three days. Necessary treatment must be provided within three to six months. The new legislation also applies to public dental care. Treatment must at least be initiated within six months of the treatment assessment. Emergency treatment must be provided immediately.

As a part of the National Health Care Project, the compilation of uniform grounds for access to non-emergency care was initiated in February 2004. A management group was established with representatives from the Ministry of Social Affairs and Health, the National Authority for Medicolegal Affairs, the National Research and Development Centre for Welfare and Health (Stakes), the Finnish Dental Association, the Association of Finnish Local and Regional Authorities, the hospital districts, health centers and organizations among others. The task of the management group was to steer, guide and coordinate the compilation of the uniform criteria. Treatment criteria have been compiled for the treatment and examination of 193 diseases. The goal is to compile criteria for about 80 percent of non-emergency treatment. The work will not be completed at one go; instead the criteria are revised and developed continuously. The latest criteria are available at the website of the Ministry of Social Affairs and Health (http://www.stm.fi). The public internet access to the criteria means that citizens can study the criteria too. Physicians will be using these criteria as a guide when deciding on the treatment of patients. In addition to the criteria, the physician should always take into consideration the patient's individual living situation and need for treatment. The physician will make a decision concerning the patient's treatment in mutual understanding with the patient. The patient does not have the right to get any treatment he or she wants. Individual physicians or dentists may, if well founded, diverge from the uniform criteria.

Discussion

Public oral health care services are provided mainly in health centers organized by municipalities singly or collectively. Dental services are part of other local health services. A local chief dental officer is responsible for arrangements, together with other local authorities. Municipalities get funding for these services from the central government, but most of the financing must come from their own internal funds through taxes. Patients also pay a relatively large co-payment. Despite these fees the charges are about half of what patients pay in private sector. In Finland, in 2003 less than 1 percent of the public used private insurance schemes to cover their dental care costs.

Despite the new laws, it has not been possible to arrange all dental services in health centers because of the limited municipal resources. In 2002 there were 4,720 active dentists in Finland (Fig. 1). The public health centers employ about 2,100 dentists, and very little new dental workforce has been hired to municipal services. A slightly larger number is working in the private sector. There seem to be some unused resources in the private sector (Fig. 2). In addition, the dental workforce has been diminishing considerably. The number of dentists graduating each year is 60. That results in a decrease in the workforce as more dentists retire than are being trained. It was calculated that by the year 2020 there would be approximately 4,000 dentists in active practice, which is not an

Figure 1. Patients visiting either the public or private oral health services, year 2000.

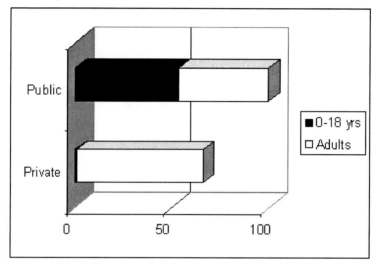

encouraging number given the already high workload of those working in public service.

It was not the intent of the new laws to move all dental services into the public sector, but rather to give patients choice. However, remaining differences in cost *de facto* limit patients' choices. According to public health insurance law, the reimbursement for fees paid by the patient to the private dentist should be 60 percent, but at the moment this

Figure 2. Dentists in health centers and private practices 2000 and 2003 (estimated)

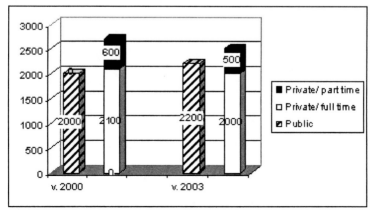

compensation amounts to only 35 to 40 percent of the fees charged by private dentists. This is due to the fact that a private practitioner is free to decide the price of treatment (fee-for-service), but the compensation is calculated from the government social insurance agency KELA's rate list. And that rate list has remained unchanged since 1989. Consequently, the fees in the public health centers that are subsidized by municipalities are about half of what patients pay in the private sector.

These significant differences in cost have raised concerns about large shifts from the private to the public sector. Private dentists had feared that their patients would start to opt for the public sector and enter the health care center waiting lists, because there they would be paying less than half of what they pay on the private market. According to a study by Nihtilä & Widström (2005) one out of every four adults in the Helsinki metropolitan area had switched or tried to switch from private to public dental services during 2003-2005. However, in the same period, the proportion of adults using public dental services had increased only by 4-5 percent.

Nevertheless, the new regulation from 2005 will cause some patient shifts with more adult and older patients being seen in health centers. Access to treatment and the scope of treatment provided will vary according to geographical region. Health centers in rural areas and small towns have always been able to offer services to all citizens. However, in big cities only children, adolescents and some special patient groups have had access to public services. In August 2005, only 17 percent of adults in the Helsinki metropolitan area were able to use public dental services (Nihtilä & Widström, 2005).

Conclusion

The aim of new Finnish laws for oral health services is to allow the citizens more equal access to publicly paid dental services and to improve the dental health of all Finnish citizens. In this early stage of implementation, it appears that access to treatment, costs and the scope of treatment provided will vary according to geographical region and the resources of municipal health centers. More importantly, the Finnish government's efforts to increase access are counteracted by decreasing workforce trends. This will render it more difficult to ensure that all Finnish citizens receive the oral health care they need.

Bibliography

http://www.stm.fi: Yhtenäiset kiireettömän hoidon perusteet: Sosiaali-ja terveysministeriön oppaita 2005:5

Nihtilä A. & Widström E. Haasteena oikeudenmukaisuus – keski-ikäisten kokemuksia hammashoitouudistuksesta pääkaupunkiseudulla, Yhteiskuntapolitiikka 3/2005, STAKES, ISSN 1458-6118

Gunilla Nordenram

Sweden's Dental Insurance System for the Elderly, Unwell and Disabled People in Sweden. Ethical Implications

Within any welfare state, there are complicated systems to protect the needy. The health of the population is an important measure, because health is a highly relevant outcome for most individuals. Both nationally and internationally, inequality in health services often constitutes an important dimension of inequality in society as a whole.

Different welfare programs are dependent on the political structure of the welfare system. In Sweden, the welfare system relies on high taxation levels. Historically, the emergence of the working class as a political power through the Social Democratic Party has been identified as central to the development of the Swedish model of the welfare state.

Around 1970, one-fifth of the adult population was receiving dental care at public dental health clinics and four-fifths from private practitioners. There was no subsidy for private dental care and private practitioners set their own fees for service. In the public dental clinics, a national table of treatment fees, determined at government level, had applied since 1938. These fees were intended to finance the clinics and any shortfalls were to be made up by the local county councils. Dental care for children up to 16 years of age was free of charge.

System Changes between 1974 and 1999

Because of substantial social class differences in both dental health and dental care utilization – in 1968, poor dental health was three times more likely among blue-collar workers than white-collar workers – a national dental health insurance scheme was introduced in 1974, with the aim of making dental care accessible to all citizens, regardless of their financial status. The insurance provided free dental care up to 19 years of age and paid 50 percent of treatment costs for all adults. The insurance covered all types of treatment and all items of service were subsidized. It covered both private and public dental care, and above a certain limit, the insurance covered the full cost of treatment. At the same time public dental services were undergoing major expansion.

The system was overhauled yet again in 1985. The overall objectives of The Dental Service Act of 1985 are good oral health and dental care for the whole population. The dental services are to be of high quality, provided on equal terms and be easily accessible to all. The services shall be based on respect for patients' integrity and their right to make their own decisions. To the extent possible, the treatment decisions should also be made in consultation with the patient. A patient is not entitled to treatment that contravenes evidence-based or proven knowledge. Patients have the right to informed consent and informed refusal. This part of the Dental Service Act concerns the mutual respect between the dentist and the patient – the integrity of both.

Although differences in dental health by socio-economic status continued to exist, by 1991 blue-collar workers were only one-and-a-half times more likely than white-collar workers to have poor oral health. Surveys from 1974 to 1991 also showed a decrease in edentulousness and an increase in the proportion of people with multiple restorations, including fillings, crowns and bridges. Increased dental care utilization contributed to the decrease in edentulousness. Age-specific comparisons have shown that the change was most pronounced among the elderly. This has meant that dental care needs have risen among older people in particular (Ahacic 2002).

In 2003, Thorstensson and Johansson published the results of a study on the oral status of Sweden's oldest population segment, that is, octogenarians (and older). A population-based randomized sample of 357 subjects was studied. The median age was 86 years, 80 percent lived in ordinary housing, 13 percent in some form of assisted living and 7 percent in institutions. The dentate group comprised 51 percent. These 181 individuals on average had 14 teeth each; 52 percent had fixed prostheses with an average of 5 units, 23 percent had removable partial dentures and three had cross-arch implant bridges.

However, deterioration in the national economy made it necessary to reduce government subsidies for adult dental care, with initial reductions in 1978 and gradual progression until subsidies were finally abandoned in the second half of the 1990s.

The Dental Health Care System since 1999

These cuts did not coincide with public opinion. According to a 1996 study by Arnberg and colleagues of the attitudes of 3,000 randomly selected persons, 46 percent believe that heart transplants should have priority over dental care when resources are allocated. However, 45 percent agreed that all dental care should be free of charge; 32 percent agreed that all dental care should be provided by the municipal authorities.

A reformed system of dental care subsidies was introduced in 1999 with the aim of subsidizing treatment costs for certain risk groups. Dental care for all children has remained free of charge. In accordance with the "Necessary Dental Care for Patients with Special Needs" program, patients with considerably greater need for dental care due to illness or disability are protected from excessive dental expenses and their dental care is now subsidized to the same level as outpatient health and medical services, that is to say there is a cap of SEK 900 (about 100 US$) per twelve-month period.

The county councils have the financial responsibility for this insurance and decide what treatment may be charged at health and medical service rates. The reform has given rise to great variations between the rules and regulations by the different councils and the National Board of Health and Welfare now considers that there is legal uncertainty.

In 2002 a high-cost protection for fixed prosthetics was introduced for all people who are 65 years of age and older. Treatment costs above SEK 7,700 (about 850 US$) are fully covered by the insurance. The treatment plan must be approved by the social insurance office. All elderly (65+) are covered by this safety net. This system of 100 percent coverage for fees exceeding SEK 7,700 also means that the care providers' fees are fully met by publicly-funded insurance. This may have affected the behavior of the care providers and the patients, as it is not in the interest of either to limit costs. From 1999 to 2002, there has been an average rise in expenditures for dental care of about 40 percent in both the public and private sectors.

Although both the government and parliament have previously rejected proposals for regulation of fees for dental services, a committee appointed by the government recently concluded that it is unreasonable to leave fees completely unregulated when the cost is covered in full with public funds through the state or the county councils. The government declared that the care providers have a major responsibility for rationing and making their operations effective so that future expenditures are contained, and warned that if insurance claims continued to rise at the current rate, the safety net for 65+ would be in jeopardy and make it necessary to modify government subsidies (Swedish Government 2003).

Since 2002 there has been a shortage of dentists, due to retirement and a reduction in the number of undergraduate places for dental students. In some parts of Sweden it has become hard to get a dental appointment. The current shortage of dental manpower does not favor price regulations and the minister for social services has become more cautious in her comments.

Even so, too many Swedish dentists failed to heed the government's warning about the system's delicate solvency. The high-cost protection for 65+ patients drained too much money from the total insurance system and since 2004 the government has introduced a price regulation for implant treatment. The fee schedule for implants used by the county public dental clinics is now also the norm for the private dentists in the region.

System-Induced Overtreatment

The 2002 high-cost protection for fixed prosthetics was intended to make sure that elderly in need of such expensive intervention would not be precluded from receiving it because of cost. However, several features of the system appear to be fostering overtreatment.

Firstly, the high-cost protection that allows for the full coverage of fixed prosthesis does not cover periodontal treatment, endodontic treatment, preventive treatment, or the material for crowns and bridges. So in cases of partial edentulousness, conventional therapy becomes much more expensive for the patient. This price difference appears to foster overuse of fixed prostheses. Clinics for postgraduate specialist training now report an increase in referrals for fixed implant supported bridges, but a marked decrease in referrals for periodontal consultations and endodontic treatment.

Secondly, dentists generally consider fixed implant-supported bridges to be superior to conventional bridges, overdentures, removable dentures and the shortened dental arch-concept. Kronström and colleagues (2003) investigated the provision of mandibular implant overdentures at 28 Swedish specialist prosthetic clinics during 2001. Seven clinics had not provided any mandibular implant overdentures. The number varied markedly from clinic to clinic (0-22, median value 2). The number of fixed implant-supported bridges was much higher (4-100, median value 17). These results reveal the great predominance of fixed implant-supported bridges in Sweden, which is in contrast with other industrialized countries. Although there is rapidly increasing use of mandibular implant overdentures internationally, fixed implant-supported bridges continue to predominate in Sweden, and mandibular implant overdentures are relatively uncommon. Feine and Carlsson (2003) in their textbook *Implant overdentures. The standard of care for edentulous patients* emphasize two-implant overdenture as first choice of treatment for the edentulous jaw.

More worrisome is the fact that this widespread use on fixed implant-supported bridges is not fully support by scientific research. The dentist must consider what treatment is optimal for each individual; for older people it is not always the maximal treatment. Furthermore, it is not uncommon for new implant systems to be introduced after brief or inadequate follow-up studies and the dentist must be aware of the evidence base for the proposed treatment.

Thirdly, dental practioners not only tend to believe that a fixed prosthesis is preferable to a removable denture. In a study by Kronström and colleagues (2003), two thirds of the prosthodontists also thought that patients would be equally satisfied with a removable or a fixed prosthesis. Again, scientific reports contradict that view. In a controlled study on implant treatment from Canada (Feine et al. 1994), 15 patients were given the opportunity to test and choose between a removable and a fixed prosthesis. As many as 7 chose the removable prosthesis and 8 the fixed alternative for the final therapy. There was a tendency for the removable prosthesis to be chosen by older subjects (50+). In the Swedish study by Kronström and colleagues already mentioned, almost 5 percent of 667 respondents aged 55-79 years already had dental implants (Kronström et al. 2002). Again, it was shown that many subjects with removable dentures did not want to have implants instead. In fact, most did not. Of 40 patients with partial maxillary dentures, 43 percent wanted implants; and of 27 with partial mandibular dentures, 50 percent wanted implants. And of 69 patients with full maxillary dentures, 26 percent percent wanted implants, and of 54 with full mandibular dentures, 24 percent wanted implants.

Now that the Swedish public has become familiar with dental implants and such treatment is accessible to most elderly people, removable dentures appear to have become less socially acceptable. Patients of all ages expect a high level of oral comfort and this leads to a high demand for fixed implant-supported bridges.

Patients are entitled to information but information can easily be manipulated. The dentist may advise the patient that old teeth are not worth preserving and that the treatment of choice would be implants, preferably implant-supported fixed bridges.

Lately confidence in professionals has been questioned in the media, with newspaper headings such as "Dentists extract healthy teeth!" A number of complaints have been investigated by the Disciplinary Committee of the National Board of Health and Welfare, a government body that determines registration of health professionals to practice in Sweden. In some cases dentists have received a warning for malpractice.

System-Induced Undertreatment

From an ethical perspective, the cost of the proposed treatment must be economically justifiable for the patient *and* the publicly-funded insurance scheme subsidizing the treatment. At the moment the more expensive fixed implant-supported bridges are cheap for the 65 + patient, profitable for the dentist yet very expensive for the dental insurance system.

With increasing unemployment, a growing number of people cannot afford regular dental care (National Board of Health and Welfare 2002). Treatment fees are rising and dental insurance subsidies for adults in general are decreasing, so dental care has become very expensive.

Newly retired people are generally quite well-off, with reasonable retirement incomes funded by their superannuation schemes. Thus they can more easily afford dental care than younger people and the unemployed. Consequently, the fairness of the dental insurance subsidy for 65+ people is being questioned increasingly in both public and political debate.

However, even among the elderly there are subpopulations at greater risk of undertreatment. Since the introduction of the "Necessary Dental Care for Patients with Special Needs" program and the high-cost-protection for 65+ patients, it has been possible to help many chronically ill and handicapped elderly people who previously had major unmet dental treatment needs. The financial responsibility for the system rests with the county councils, not the state and national insurance office. The county officials must define what treatment is necessary and hence may be charged at health and medical service rates. Pressured by costs, there are great differences between the rules and regulations of the different councils. A good example is the provision of implants. Most patients with special dental care needs due to illness or disability do not require complicated treatment: the basic goal of treatment is usually to achieve cleanliness and comfort (freedom from pain) and as good a masticatory function as possible. Some county officials therefore have determined that fixed prostheses are not necessary for this population. However, there are cases when a fixed prosthesis is indicated, for example for a patient impaired by stroke. Due to a persistent facial paralysis, it may be impossible for the patient to manage a removable denture. With an implant-supported denture, the patient can chew, talk and smile. Such treatment is of importance for the patient's rehabilitation as well as for his/her well being. Unfortunately, the decision by county officials is final and cannot be appealed. If the patient wants more extensive treatment and is willing to pay for it, he loses all subsidies. It is not possible to receive a subsidy for a partial denture treatment and pay private fees for a bridge or an implant. This "take it or leave it" approach fosters undertreatment.

The risk of undertreatment is furthermore increased by the decreases in dental personnel resources in Sweden. Under such conditions, elderly with illness and disabilities frequently are not given precedence and their right to dental care becomes threatened.

Resource Allocation:
A New Challenge for Swedish Dentists

The Swedish political system traditionally has assumed responsibility for social issues such as health and welfare. Given the high levels of income taxation, medical and dental care are considered a state liability. The Dental Service Act defines good dental care and requires dentists to treat patients according to accepted standards of practice, following regulations by The National Board of Health and Welfare. Private and public dental care services are subsidized equally by the national dental insurance. The Dental Service Act defines the responsibility of the county councils as follows: "The County Council shall plan delivery of dental care on the basis of treatment need in the population." This also includes private dental care: "Planning shall include dental services provided by dentists other than those employed within the public dental services."

Because of the traditional role of the government in matters of resource allocation, Swedish dentists in general have never considered distribution issues to be part of their professional role. Unfairness in the distribution system is not seen as a violation of the dentists' own code of ethics. Instead, prioritization issues are seen as political issues to be discussed and decided in the parliament. However, the mounting financial pressures on the system and the evident role dentists play in generating (and limiting) costs, will force Swedish dentists to get involved in these allocation discussions and begin considering justice issues a matter of professional ethics.

Bibliography

Ahacic K. Improvements in the aging population 1968-1991. Thesis. Stockholm University, Department of Social Work 2002

Arnberg D, Söderfeldt B & Palmqvist S. Attitudes towards financing of dental care in a Swedish population. *Acta Odontolologica Scandinavica* 1996;54:81-86

Feine JS, de Grandmont P, Boudrias P, Brien N, LaMarche C, Taché R & Lund JP. Within-subject comparisons of implant-supported mandibular prostheses: Choice of Prosthesis. *Journal of Dental Research* 1994;73(5)1105-1111

Feine JS & Carlsson GE. *Implant Overdentures. The Standard of Care for Edentulous Patients.* Quintessence Publishing Co., Chicago 2003

Kronström M & Karlsson GE. Use of Mandibular Implant Overdentures: Treatment Policy in Prosthodontic Specialist Clinics in Sweden. *Swedish Dental Journal* 2003, 27(2): 59-66

Kronström M, Palmqvist S, Söderfeldt B & Vigild M. Subjective need for implant treatment among middle-aged people in Sweden and in Denmark. *Clinical Implant Dentistry and Related Research* 2002;4(1):11-15

National Board of Health and Welfare. *Yearbook of Health and Medical Care 2002.* Stockholm 2002 (In Swedish)

Swedish Government. *Dental care until 2010.* Official Reports SOU 2003:53 (In Swedish)

Thorstensson H & Johansson B. Oral health in a population-based sample of the oldest-old: Findings in twins 80 years and older in Sweden. *Swedish Dental Journal* 2003, 27(2): 49-57

Part III

Educational and Policy Perspectives

Linda C. Niessen

Oral Health and Social Justice:
Oral Health Status, Financing &
Opportunities for Leadership

> "Bleeding gums, impacted teeth and
> rotting teeth are routine matters
> for the children I have interviewed…"
> Jonathan Kozal,
> *Savage Inequalities*, 1991

In the book, *A Theory of Justice,* John Rawls wrote "Justice is the first virtue of social institutions, as truth is of systems of thought" (Rawls 1971, p.3). Dentistry is a social institution and a learned profession. As a learned profession, dentistry has adopted a code of ethics which provides guidance for the professional conduct of its members.

As a profession, dentistry has a responsibility to serve all the community. In fact, the mission of many professional dental organizations is to improve oral health for all. Unfortunately data suggest that disparities exist in oral health status and use of dental services. I argue that if dentistry is to remain a profession, it must work to insure that the most vulnerable members of society have access to basic oral health care and preventive services. This package would constitute a floor, so to speak, or a set of minimum oral health services that society believes each person requires in order to reach his or her individual potential.

This chapter explores issues in oral health and social justice and identifies where opportunities for future leadership in solving these inequities in oral health status and care delivery exist. The purpose of this chapter is threefold. First, it reviews the epidemiology of oral diseases and examines patterns and distribution of oral diseases in US. What do we know about oral health status in our US population? Do disparities exist and if so, where? Second, it examines US data on financing of dental care and access to dental services. What do we know about who accesses oral health care? Is access distributed fairly? Finally, the chapter discusses leadership opportunities for improving the distribution of oral health and oral health services. This chapter is written from the perspective of a clinician and public health dentist, one who has provided oral health care in both the non-profit (US Public Health Service, Division of Indian Health and the Department of Veterans Affairs) and private practice delivery systems.

Oral Health and Wellness

A survey done by Research!America found that 85 percent of Americans think oral health is important (Figure 1). Esthetic dentistry and recent

Figure 1. Oral Health is Important to the Public

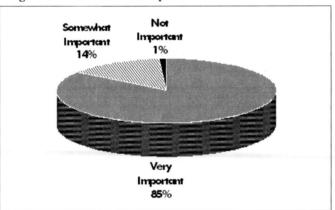

Source: Harris Interactive for Research! America- May 2000 Omnibus Survey.

television programs such as Extreme Makeover have raised the awareness among the public about oral health. In fact, consumers have begun to include oral health when they consider health and wellness.

Indeed, oral health can affect overall health. Untreated dental disease can complicate: organ and bone marrow transplants; prosthetic joint replacements; head and neck radiation; cancer chemotherapy (Public Health Reports 1993). New data are suggesting an increasingly important relationships between periodontal disease and premature low birth weight babies, between periodontal disease and diabetes, and between periodontal disease and cardiovascular disease and stroke (Jeffcoat et al. 2003; Grossi et al. 1997; Desvarieux et al. 2005). If these relationships continue to strengthen, prevention of oral disease and maintenance of oral health may contribute to preventing chronic systemic diseases and improved overall health.

In 2000, the Surgeon General published a report on oral health (US DHHS 2000). Of the 34 Surgeon General's Reports which have been published, only 5 have *not* been tobacco related. Oral health has the distinction of being one of these 5 reports. A major theme of this Surgeon General's Report is that oral health is more than just healthy teeth. The Surgeon General's report on oral health noted, "Oral health is essential to the general health and well-being of all Americans and can be achieved. However, not all Americans are able to take that message to heart" (DHHS 2000). The report noted a "silent epidemic" of oral diseases is affecting our most vulnerable citizens – poor children, the elderly, and many members of racial and ethnic minority groups." The report also defined health disparities as "…the diminished health status of population subgroups defined by demographic factors such as age and socioeconomic status, geography, disability status, and behavioral lifestyles. These disparities "reflect the diversity of the U.S. population by gender and age, racial or ethnic identity, educational attainment, income."

Overall, the Surgeon General's Report noted that oral health matters as part of an individual's well being, that general health is related to oral health and vice versa, that effective dental preventive methods exist, and unfortunately oral health disparities also exist. The Surgeon General's Report on Oral Health spotlighted oral health within the US. It is now up to society and, in particular, the dental profession to provide optimal oral health for all.

Epidemiology of Oral Diseases

"Although dental problems don't command the instant fears
associated with low birth weight, fetal death or cholera,
they do have the consequences of wearing down the stamina of
children and defeating their ambitions."
Jonathan Kozol,
Savage Inequalities, 1991

If what characterizes us as a society, and as a profession is how we care for our must vulnerable citizens, then how should we be evaluated in the US? Is oral health distributed equitably in the US population? Do all citizens suffer equally from the ravages of oral diseases? To answer these questions, we must review the epidemiology of various oral diseases in both children and adults.

Figure 2 shows that dental caries is the most common disease of childhood, five times more common than asthma (DHHS 2000).

Figure 2. Prevalence of common conditions of childhood

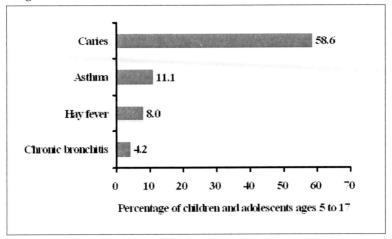

Source: US DHHS, Oral Health in America, 2000

Data on dental caries show that 25 percent of children now account for 75 percent of dental caries, with higher disease levels in poor and low income children, minority and recent immigrant children and children whose parents have less than a high school education.

Data show that poor children 2 to 9 in each racial/ethnic group have a higher percentage of untreated primary teeth than non-poor children (Figure 3).

Figure 3. Poor children 2 to 9 in each racial/ethnic group have a higher percentage of untreated primary teeth than non poor children.

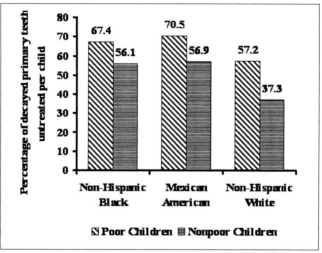

Source: US DHHS, Oral Health in America, 2000

One study reported that only 49.9 percent of children aged 5-17 had dental caries in their permanent dentition (DHHS 2000). However, when the data were disaggregated, only 24 percent of children aged 13-17 were caries free. Even more alarming, of the children aged 17 years, only 16 percent were caries free in their permanent dentition. In other words, over 84 percent of 17 year olds still suffered from dental caries.

Dental sealants provide a measure of both oral health status and access to care. Caucasian children are 4 times as likely to have sealants than African American children and twice as likely as Hispanic American children (US DHHS 2000). Figure 4 shows sealant use by income. As family income increases, the percentage of children with sealants increases. In economic terms, when the consumption of goods and services increase with increasing income, this good or service is said to perform as a "luxury" good. Is there any dental professional that wants a valuable preventive service like sealants to become a luxury good?

Figure 4. Use of sealants in US children, aged 5-17 by family income

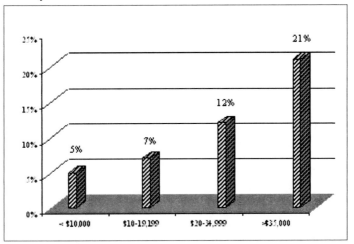

Source: USDHHS, Oral Health in America, 2000.

Would society be comfortable with immunizations becoming a "luxury" good?

If we examined outcomes of poor oral health, such as restricted days of activity, data show that as family income increases, the number of restricted days of activity decreases. Figure 5 (page 221) shows this pattern graphically.

Oral health status of adults also shows evidence of disparities based on income and education. A study by Joshi, et al. (1996) showed that as education increased, the number of natural teeth increased. National data in the US population over age 65 show that as income increases, the percentage of edentulous persons decrease (Table 1). This trend exists both in the 65-74 year olds as well as the 75+ population (see Table 1, page 221).

Oral cancer, by far the most deadly of all oral diseases, affects approximately 28,000 Americans each year, killing one person every hour every day or about 9,000 people annually. (Neville 2002) One half will die within five years, ranking it among the worst 5-year mortality of all cancers, a number that hasn't changed for the past 50 years!

Since 1950, oral cancer has seen its sex ratio shift from 6:1 male to female to a 2:1 male to female ratio in 2000 (Silverman 2001). Women's oral cancer rates have increased in the past fifty years, as a result of

Figure 5. Restricted Activity days per 100
children because of dental problems by
family income

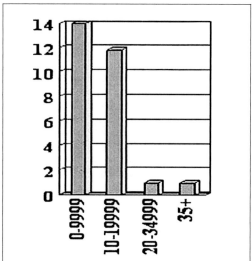

Source: National Health Interview Survey,
Centers for Disease Control, 1994.

increased tobacco use. Disparities also exist in 5-year survival rates
between Caucasian American and African Americans. White Americans
have a 53 percent five year survival rate, compared to 31 percent for
Black Americans. The question remains: is oral cancer a more aggressive disease among African Americans or do African Americans enter

Table 1. Edentulism rates in the US
population over age 65 by income levels

Income	Percent Endentulous	
	Age 65-74	Age 75+
< $10,000	46.1	56.3
$10-34,999	28.2	40.4
>$35,000	12.0	30.3

Source: Bloom B, Gift HC, Jack SS. National Center
for Health Statistics, 1992.

the care delivery system at a later stage, after the cancer has progressed? Research is necessary to answer these questions.

Oral health in 21st century America is an economic development issue and a human potential issue. Children can't learn when they suffer from dental pain or they miss days from school. Research has shown that poor oral health is related to decreased school performance, poor social relationships and less success in later life (GAO 2000). Adults don't have same employment potential when they are missing front teeth. In the 19th Century manufacturing economy, missing anterior teeth didn't affect one's ability to be employed on an assembly line. However, missing anterior teeth does affect one's ability to be hired in the 21st Century service economy on a reception line.

As the US population ages, oral health in nursing homes will become an increasingly important health issue, one that has been characterized as a "looming crisis" (Lamster 2004). Currently many health professionals when examining the oral cavity, go from the lips to the oral pharynx and overlook the 4 cubic inches in between. Why does a decubitus ulcer in a nursing home patient trigger a quality assurance audit, but a patient with a mouth full of periodontal disease or root caries is ignored? As the baby boom population ages and retains their natural dentition, oral health in nursing homes will become increasing salient as a measure of quality care in nursing homes. The contributions the oral health profession can make to educating our medical and nursing colleagues about the relationships between oral health and chronic systemic diseases remain to be seen.

Access to Oral Health Care

The epidemiologic data show that profound oral health disparities exist within our population. Access to oral health care provides another measure of oral health status in the US.

The US economy operates as a free market capitalist system. This system distributes goods and services fairly efficiently. However, it tends to creates inequities. As a society, how do we deal with these inequities? Perhaps more importantly, as a profession, what is our ethical responsibility to address these inequities?

In 2002, dentistry in the US accounted for only 5.3 percent of personal health care expenditures, but this still amounted to a $70 billion industry (CMS 2002). Approximate 50 percent of these expenditures were paid through private dental insurance, while 44 percent were out of pocket costs to the patient. Government expenditures for dental services accounted for less than 5 percent. This contrasts sharply to medical expenditures where public funds account for 46 percent of national health expenditures. This $70 billion bill for dental services averages to $247 per person, or $480 per person who used dental care (Brown & Manski 2004).

An economic analysis of the dental care market would examine the supply and the demand for oral health services. In reviewing the supply variables, several issues are noteworthy. Currently, the US dentist supply shows an aging and retiring dentist workforce. Additionally, this workforce is not nearly as diverse as the US population. Since the 1980s, the number of women entering dentistry has increased dramatically. The outcome on productivity of this demographic change is unknown at the present time. While current data show that women dentists early in their career work part time at higher rates than their male counterparts, it is not known if they will continue to work longer in the later stages of their career than their male counterparts. If the women dentists' careers prove to be longer than those of the men, this would equalize the lower productivity they demonstrate in the early stages of their careers. Only longitudinal analysis of women dentists will demonstrate if the full-time equivalents (FTE's) of "years in practice" for both male and female dentists are similar.

With more dentists retiring than entering the profession, a dentist supply problem is generated. This supply problem is not evenly distributed throughout the US and appears to affect some geographic areas more than others. Three new dental schools have opened in the past ten years (Nova Southeastern University, University of Nevada at Las Vegas, and Arizona School of Dentistry and Oral Health). Of note is that two of these three new schools are housed in osteopathic medical schools, which have a long tradition of health and wellness. It remains to be seen how these osteopathic medical schools will contribute to the culture of dental education, but the homeopathic traditions appear to be consistent with dentistry's longstanding preventive orientation.

The dental hygiene workforce has increased because several new dental hygiene programs have started in the past ten years. However, the retention issue in the hygiene workforce remains a concern. On the other hand, several state boards of dental examiners are examining the roles of dental hygienists. In some states, the boards are expanding the roles and the scope of duties of dental hygienists to assist in meeting the needs of underserved populations.

In the area of dental laboratory technology, education programs are disappearing. As dental laboratory technology becomes increasingly sophisticated, the number of trained technicians is decreasing. Furthermore, dental assistants remain difficult to recruit and hire and many are on-the-job trained. State dental boards, however, are often requiring them to become certified in radiology, infection control or other important functions within the dental office.

From the above discussion, it appears that there is a labor shortage in every category of dental professional-dentists, hygienists, assistants and dental laboratory technicians. With any labor shortage, strategies to increase supply include: opening immigration to the needed job skills, expanding the roles of professionals within the dental profession to meet the needs, and expanding the roles of non-dental health professionals to meet the oral health needs of those underserved.

In examining the demand side of the equation, approximately 70 percent of population see a dentist annually (routine and emergent care) according to the American Dental Association (ADA 2001). Use of dental services demonstrates an inverted U pattern, with the under 5-year olds and 65+ individuals having the lowest utilization. Use of dental services increases with income and education. For every child who does not have medical insurance, there are 2.6 children who do not have dental insurance.

Research on use of dental services and family income shows startling results. The data are examined using the federal poverty level ($18, 400 for a family of four). Children from families who are at or below 199 percent of the federal poverty level (FPL) are three times as likely to have an unmet dental care need as children from families who are at or above 200 percent FPL (Newacheck et al. 2000). Only 36 percent of children aged 6-18 years whose families live at or below the federal poverty level visit a dentist compared to 71 percent from families who are at or above 400 percent FPL (GAO 2000). These data suggest that use of dental care by children performs like a luxury good. As family income increases, children get more dental care.

Use of dental services by adults show similar trends. As education increases, use of dental services increases (CDC 1995). Similarly, as family income increases, use of dental services increases. Individuals with dental insurance use dental services more frequently than those without dental insurance. Table 2 shows that in adults, the use of dental services is correlated with the presence of natural teeth, with adults having teeth using dental services far more frequently than those with no natural teeth (Jones 2005).

Table 2. Percent of adults with dental visit in last year by selected characteristics, United States, 1995.

	% with visit in last year
Annual Household Income	
<$15,000	51.2
$15,000-24,999	59.2
$25,000-34,999	67.6
Insurance status	
Insured	78.3
Uninsured	57.6
Dentition status	
Edentulous	24.3
Dentate	72.5

Adapted from: Jones JA, Journal of Dental Education, in press. Original data from CDC, 1995.

In summary, demand for dental care appears to be greater than the supply. In economic terms, the dental care market provides as a luxury good. As a person's income increases, his or her consumption of dental services, or use of dental services increases. Should dentistry be a luxury good, or is it a social good required by society to achieve one's human and economic potential?

Leadership Opportunities

The Surgeon General's Report on Oral Health brought attention to this neglected area of health. As a result of this report, various organizations have examined their roles in improving oral health for the US Population. In 2003, four significant reports were released. Each contains recommendations that represent the thinking of a given constituency, from dental school faculty and federal government officials to state legislators and health policy organizations.

In March 2003, the American Dental Education Association published a report examining the roles and responsibilities of academic dental institutions in improving the oral health status of all Americans (Haden et al. 2003) This report acknowledged the important role that academic dental schools play in improving access to oral health care. The report provided guiding principles for academic dental institutions and listed a set of recommendations. These recommendations included monitoring the future oral health care workforce needs, improving the effectiveness of the oral health care delivery system, preparing students to provide oral health services to diverse populations, increasing the diversity of the oral health workforce and improving the effectiveness of allied dental professionals in reaching the underserved.

In May 2003, the Surgeon General released a "Call to Action" (US-DHHS, 2003). The vision underlying this call to action is "to advance the general health and well-being of all Americans by creating critical partnerships at all levels of society to engage in programs to promote oral health and prevent disease." The goal of this call to action was to create a National Oral Health Plan that will "promote health, improve quality of life and eliminate oral health disparities." The Call to Action envisioned partnerships at all levels of society- local, state and federal-and saw the opportunities for a variety of players to serve as partners. The Call to Action identified five actions that were necessary to improve oral health. These included:

• Change Perceptions of Oral Health
• Accelerate Building and Application of Science
• Build Effective Health Infrastructure
• Remove Barriers to Oral Health Services
• Use Public-Private Partnerships

Each of these topics provided additional ideas for actions among partners. The extent to which the dental professional acts upon the Surgeon

General's Report on Oral Health and follows up with recommended activities from the call to action will demonstrate the seriousness to which oral health disparities are viewed by the profession.

In June 2003, the National Conference of State Legislatures issued a report, entitled "Oral Health." This report reviewed strategies that states had taken to address access to oral health. They identified that increased reimbursement for Medicaid and State Children's Health Improvement Program (S-CHIP) did improve access to needed oral health services among America's most vulnerable children. The report listed examples of some novel programs to meet these needs, such as a program implemented by the state of Maine to provide loan repayment to dentists working with underserved populations. The report also identified programs that were expanding scope of practice for dental hygienists and primary care providers. North Carolina's program to increase the use of fluoride varnish among pediatric health professionals was noteworthy.

This report was significant in that it represented the thinking of policy makers rather than health professionals. It noted that dentists are the most active/visible advocates in state legislatures but they are not perceived as good advocates for children. As a learned profession, we have much to do to change this perception. I can report that during the 2005 Texas Legislative Session, the dentists of the Texas Dental Association were among those most actively advocating for the re-instatement of oral health services into the Texas CHIP program. (The 2003 Texas Legislature eliminated dental services as part of the S-CHIP program in an effort to balance the state budget.)

In June 2003, the National Health Policy Forum at George Washington University published "Improving Oral Health: Promise and Prospects." The report featured a background paper that examined issues affecting access to oral health care in the US. It reviewed public financing and privately funded efforts. It examined the changing roles of providers and primary health care providers, particularly physicians and nurses. It also reviewed the role of prevention in improving oral health among the most vulnerable citizens.

The significance of these reports is that each organization recognized that access to needed oral health services has become such a critical issue that it cannot be ignored by policy makers. The fact that two of these reports were conducted by policy makers suggests that the problem is of such a magnitude that oral diseases are problems no longer confined to the dental profession. As a result, policy makers are asking questions about how to distribute oral health more equitably. States are taking action, and are not waiting for solutions from the federal government or for federal assistance.

So what's on the table? How do policy makers see solving these problems? In times of labor shortages, policies are implemented that mitigate this shortage. Immigration laws are eased to allow individuals with the needed skill set to enter and work in the US more easily. Dental licensure laws that had been used to limit the number of dentists in a state are now being re-evaluated. Dentists from various countries are obtaining dental licenses more easily in states that previously made obtaining a dental license for a foreign dental graduate virtually impossible. State dental licensing boards are reviewing their scope of practice and asking who can do what and why. In addition, issues such as "who can bill" and "why" are being asked by insurance providers. States are experimenting with state-based loan repayment programs, in addition to the federal loan repayment programs.

At the federal level, loan repayment programs for dentists working in underserved areas are woefully underfunded. The federal-state Children's Health Improvement Program has expanded dental services to low income children but not all states participate in this program equally, creating disparities among states in terms of their publicly funded dental programs.

Professional associations play a major role in both advocating on behalf of vulnerable citizens and providing care directly. Recently, the American Dental Association has developed a program to promote voluntarism among its members. The first ADA nationwide effort, "Give Kids a Smile," was held on Feb. 21, 2003 and provided care to over one million children in 5,000 locations. This national "Give Kids a Smile" day has been increasing in scope each year as the number of dental teams participating increases and the number of patients treated increases. But as Dr. Jim Bramson, executive director of the American Dental Association has noted, "Voluntarism is not a delivery system." These efforts are admirable but not equitable. Children and families lucky enough to be seen on the respective days receive dental care, but many other children remain in need.

National foundations have also identified oral health disparities and developed creative solutions to eliminate them. The WK Kellogg

Foundation has initiated a Community Voices Program that supports 13 communities targeting activities to increase access to oral health care. The strategies are designed to meet the needs of the respective community, such as dentist recruitment programs in New Mexico and teaching families about oral health in El Paso.

Similarly, the Robert Wood Johnson Foundation developed an innovative program called "Pipeline, Profession and Practice." This program provides $15 million to dental schools to increase community externships for dental students. Each dental school participating provides a six week externship for their students to provide dental care in underserved community settings. By providing dental students the opportunity to care for patients in various community settings, they will be more likely to do so when they graduate.

Oral Health America has developed several programs to decrease oral health disparities and promote access to dental care and preventive services. From the Seal America project for increased access to dental sealants, to the National Spit Tobacco Education program, to the publication of Oral Health Report Cards for each state, these efforts shine a spotlight on oral health disparities and offer solutions.

Research has shown that community dental preventive programs are the most cost-effective, in terms of time, dollars invested, and disease avoided. Community water fluoridation could be considered a preventive program that is distributed equitably throughout the community since it benefits all the residents of a community, regardless of economic status (provided, that is, that an individual drinks the tap water, not bottled water.) Some states are promoting oral examinations prior to starting school, so dental problems can be identified early. This is similar to school districts that require immunizations prior to starting school. Can we use immunization as a model for improving oral health?

Future initiatives will require a team approach to improving oral health. It may take a village to raise a child, and it may take a team to improve oral health. Future members of the team may not be the "usual suspects" of dental professionals but may consist of professionals outside of dentistry, such as social service professionals, geriatric health care professionals, primary health care professionals, mental health professionals and elementary and high school educators, not to mention policy makers and legislators.

Improving the distribution of oral health care will require creative solutions. Workforce shortages will require thinking about how to increase the supply of oral health professionals. New workforce models will be needed. Can different personnel provide various oral health services with the appropriate dental training? Such models already exist. New Zealand and Saskatchewan dental nurses have long provided care to their respective populations. Denturists have met the denture needs of Canadians and various US citizens in states where they are legal. Expanding the scope of dental practice for individual team members is doable, provided the appropriate dental education is provided.

New delivery models may also be needed. The legal system has a "pro-bono" model for legal services for those who cannot pay. Give Kids a Smile is a first step. Can the dental profession adopt a similar program, where each dentist agrees to provide care to 10 low income patients each year and/or 10 dental Medicaid patients?

Can the reimbursement system reconnect the mouth to the rest of the body? Will some health insurance company take a risk and develop a health insurance product that reimburses the diabetic patient to have her diabetic foot treated, her diabetic eye problem treated, her diabetic heart disease treated and her diabetic periodontal disease treated? What a novel concept, one reimbursement system for one person's health care!

Oral health for all Americans shouldn't be a game of chance. We have models that work. We have frameworks for action. We have a learned profession in dentistry that requires reaching out to various members of society to meet our vision of optimal oral health for all.

In the words of Margaret Mead, "Never doubt that a small group of thoughtful citizens can change the world. Indeed, it is the only thing that ever does."

Bibliography

American Dental Association. *Future of Dentistry*. Chicago: American Dental Association, Health Policy Resource Center, 2001

Brown E & Manski R. Dental Services: use, expenses, and sources of payment. 1996-2000. MEPS Research Findings No. 20. Rockville(MD): Agency for Healthcare Research and Quality.; 2004 Report No.: AHRQ Pub. No. 04-0018

CDC. Dental Service Use and Dental Insurance Coverage – United States, Behavioral Risk Factor Surveillance System, 1995. *MMWR* weekly 1997:1199-1203

Centers for Medicare and Medicaid Services (CMS) Office of the Actuary, National Health Statistics Group. National Health, Personal and other Personal Expenditures Aggregate and per Capita Amounts, Percent Distribution, and Average Annual Percent Growth, by Source of Funds, and Type of Expenditure, Selected Years 1980-2002. In: Center for Medicaid and Medicare Services, Office of the Actuary, National Health Statistics Group; 2002

Desvarieux M, Demmer RT, Rundek T et al, Periodontal microbiota and carotid intime-media thickness. *Circulation* 111:576-82, 2005

Grossi SG, Skrepcinski FB, DeCaro T, et al, Treatment of periodontal disease in diabetics reduces glycated hemoglobin. *Journal of Periodontology* 68:713-719, 1997

Haden NK, Bailit H, Buchanan J et al. *Improving the oral health status of all Americans:Roles and responsibilities of Academic Dental Institutions. Report of the ADEA President's Commission.* Washington DC: American Dental Education Association, 2003

Jeffcoat MK, Hauth JC, Geurs NC, Reddy MS, Oliver SP, Hodkings PM et al. Periodontal disease and preterm birth: Results of a pilot intervention study. *Journal of Periodontology* 2003, 74: 1214-1218

Jones JA. Financing elders' Oral Health Care: Lessons from the Present and Innovations for the Future. Presented at the Elder's Oral Health Summit, Boston University School of Dentistry, Boston, Sept.13-14, 2004. Financing and reimbursement of elders' oral health care: lessons from the present, opportunities for the future. *Journal of Dental Education* 2005, 69(9): 1022-1031

Joshi A, Douglass CW, Feldman H et al. Consequences of Success: Do More Teeth Translate into More Disease and Utilization? *Journal of Public Health Dentistry* 1996, 56(4):190-197

Kozol J. *Savage Inequalities*. New York. Crown Publishing, 1991

Lamster IB, Oral Health Care Services for Older Adults: A Looming Crisis. *American Journal of Public Health* 2004, 94: 699-702

Neville BW & Day TA. Oral cancer and precancerous lesion. *CA Cancer Journal Clinics* 2002, 52:195-215

Newacheck PW, Hughes DC, Hung YY et al. The Unmet Health Needs of America's Children. *Pediatrics* 2000, 105:989-997

Oral Health Coordinating Committee. *Toward Improving the Oral Health of Americans: An Overview of Oral Health Status, Resources and Care Delivery.* Public Health Reports, 1993

Rawls J. *A Theory of Justice*. Cambridge. Harvard University Press, 1971; p. 3

Silverman Jr. S, Demographics and Occurrence of Oral and Pharyngeal Cancers: the Outcomes, the Trends, the Challenge. *Journal of the American Dental Association* 2001, 132 (Suppl): 7S-11S

U.S. Department of Health and Human Services. *Oral Health in America: A Report of the Surgeon General*. Rockville, MD: US Department of Health and Human Services, National Institute of Dental and Craniofacial Research, National Institutes of Health, 2000. Available on-line at http://www.surgeongeneral.gov/library/oralhealth/ (access verified on 11/3/05)

U.S. Department of Health and Human Services. *A National Call to Action to Promote Oral Health*. Rockville, MD: US Department of Health and Human Services, Public Health Service, Centers for Disease Control and Prevention and the National Institutes of Health, National Institute of Dental and Craniofacial Research. NIH Publication No. 03-5303, May, 2003

U.S. General Accounting Office. *Oral Health: Dental Disease is a Chronic Problem among Low Income and Vulnerable Populations*. Washington, DC: US General Accounting Office, 2000

James T. Rule and Jos VM Welie

Justice, Moral Competencies, and the Role of Dental Schools

The Profession's Mandate on Issues of Justice

The 2000 Surgeon General's Report *Oral Health Care in America* (US Public Health Service 2000), the first report on oral health by the nation's highest health administrator, clearly demonstrated the existence of oral health disparities in the United States. In fact, oral health disparities are about twice as large as those of general health. The report points out the "striking disparities in dental disease by income level. Poor children suffer twice as much dental caries as their more affluent peers, and their disease is more likely to be untreated" (Executive Summary, p. 11). It elaborates on the barriers to oral health care, which "include lack of access to care, whether because of limited income or lack of insurance, transportation, or the flexibility to take time off from work to attend to personal or family needs for care." Furthermore, it recognizes that additional barriers may be faced by "individuals with disabilities and those with complex health problem" (p. 11) To make matters worse, "the public, policymakers, and providers may consider oral health and the need for care to be less important than other health needs, pointing to the need to raise awareness and improve health literacy" (p. 11). As a result, the Report calls for an increased acceptance of oral health as a component of general health.

The Surgeon General's Report rightly states that meeting this goal requires changes in perceptions of the public, policymakers, and non-dental health providers. But despite its otherwise comprehensive outlook, the Report is remarkably silent with respect to dental health providers themselves. Although they receive mention, it is only in the context of patients' failing to secure care from them – as if it is the patients' fault.

The National Institute of Dental and Craniofacial Research (NIDCR) further acknowledges the importance of oral health disparities by recognizing them as a target area for funding. The NIDCR's focus on oral health disparities includes both those with medical problems and those who are poor. Neither group gets adequate levels of care, and in some instances suffers from higher levels of oral disease. Like the Surgeon General's report, the NIDCR report, *A Plan to Reduce Health Disparities*, contains subtleties of language that reveal a certain reluctance to fully confront the problem. Although it lists the many *medical conditions* demanding improved oral care, identifies the *patients* who are not adequately cared for, and describes the *financial context* for the provision of care, it is silent with respect to the *care providers*.

The above critique is not intended to suggest that dentists and hygienists are solely responsible for existing oral health disparities. However, it does suggest that many dentists and the profession as a whole may have difficulty acknowledging that the existing disparities are not solely the problem of others. The relevant codes of dental ethics are an indicator that there may be some truth to this charge. With respect to issues of justice, a look at some of the codes of ethics from both the United States and other countries that have been published throughout dentistry's history, suggests that these documents tend to be rather quiet on issues of justice (see the Digest of Codes appended to this volume).

But there is also evidence of dentistry's long time, genuine concern about social justice. William J. Gies, an influential leader in dentistry who was well-known for his 1926 report on dental education to the Carnegie Foundation, in 1937 stated his vision for the future of dentistry: "It will plan and endeavor to bring to all the people the benefits of ample oral care. As a humanitarian profession, it will help to perfect economic procedures for the benefit of all persons who cannot, or without aid could not, pay for needed oral health service. It will, by action and guidance, achieve these constructive results as a welcome professional opportunity to serve the public, rather than as a test in political servitude" (as quoted by Mandel 1997).

These optimistic predictions by one man from generations past have been echoed more recently in a 2004 white paper by the American Dental Association, in which the profession adds its unequivocal support for improving access to the underserved. "The nation's dentists have long sought to stem and turn the tide of untreated disease, as individuals, through their local, state and national dental societies, and through other community organizations. Dentists alone cannot bring about the profound change needed to correct the gross disparities in access to oral health care. But dentistry must provide the leadership that initiates change, or it will not occur" (p. 1). This forthright assumption of a leadership role by the American Dental Association is clear evidence that dentistry is beginning to take on responsibility itself for the existing oral health disparities.

Despite dentistry's clear commitment for leadership to make the "profound change needed to correct the gross disparities in access to oral health care," it is less clear how this translates into action by individual practitioners in their offices. More importantly, clarification is needed on what energizes the motivation to effect such a "profound change" in all levels of the profession. In this chapter, we argue that an essential role is to be played by the dental schools. It would be unfair to expect an untrained swimmer to jump after a person drowning in a deep and muddy lake. Likewise, it would be unfair to expect oral health care professionals to live up to this calling unless they are adequately prepared to take up this challenge. As DePaolo has pointed out, "oral health professionals often fail to achieve improvements in the oral health of the community because *they are not provided or lack the skills necessary* to share their knowledge and expertise with those beyond the dental office, the dental school, or the university setting. As a result, their oral health knowledge and skills remain within the narrow confines of the 'dental operatory' or dental school, rather than dispersed widely to members of the community at large for the purpose of improving the common good" (1998, p. 2; emphasis added). Thus the specific role and responsibility of dental schools becomes evident.

A Primary Role for Dental Schools in Fostering Concepts of Justice

The historical process by which professions develop – dentistry included – reveals how the public gradually comes to trust a particular occupation with the stewardship of a commonly held "estate" of expertise. The transition from an aspiring occupation to a profession includes the emergence of an increasingly more secure and profitable position in society. It begins with the practitioners of a given occupation coming together to form associations, the purpose of which is first to survive and then to flourish. Over long generations, they work to establish their credibility. Essential components of this credibility are requirements for the adequate training and licensure of would-be professionals. Once the public feels secure with the existing safeguards – some of which are well established, others in process – the associations may then be powerful enough to lobby for formal statutory recognition by government. If they are successful, they receive competitive advantages in the marketplace (i.e., monopoly status). Persons not having the sanctioned education and licensure would not be allowed to practice a particular expertise. The members of aspiring professions "also understood that they would not be taken seriously unless they demonstrated that they could provide dedicated service, administered with a sense of integrity" (Rule & Veatch 2004, p. 21) Thus, in this lengthy process, the establishment of a system of formal education has been a key component in the gaining of public confidence. The modern, university-affiliated and accredited dental school would simply not exist if it were not for the sanction of society.

Society not only expects the new professionals who emerge from these dental schools to have a certain level of expertise, but also an inclination to use it with integrity and for the public interest. After all, the public gives significant financial support to dental education – even at private schools. This is not an argument likely to inspire graduates who are burdened by educational debts in excess of $100,000. But neither does this unfortunate and problematic fact justify overlooking the ethical implications of receiving public support. Indeed, the public's backing of dental education extends beyond finances. If it weren't for patients willing to submit themselves to dental students, the latter would not be able to gain the level of clinical competency they now achieve in a mere two or three years. Furthermore, advancement in the biomedical sciences has been achieved in no small part by the public's willingness to submit to experiments, often non-therapeutic experiments. And historically, many research subjects have come from the ranks of the poor and vulnerable. In short, as stewards of the clinical, scientific, and technological knowledge base that belongs to all people jointly, dental schools must make sure that all people derive benefits from that knowledge.

It is obvious that dental schools believe they ought to instill at least some degree of social awareness and concern about justice in oral health care. In its seminal 2003 report entitled *Improving the Oral Health Status of All Americans: Roles and Responsibilities of Academic Dental Institutions*, the American Dental Education Association affirms the role of dental schools in promoting social justice. It states that "knowledge about oral health is not the property of any individual or organization; rather, society grants individuals the opportunity to learn at academic dental institutions with an assumed contract that this knowledge will benefit the society that granted the opportunity to obtain it" (Haden et al. 2003, p. 3).

The American Dental Association's Commission on Dental Accreditation (2004) has developed competency standards. Standard 2.25 for clinical competency states that "graduates *must* be competent in providing oral health care within the scope of general dentistry, as defined by the school, for the child, adolescent, geriatric and medically compromised patient" (p 15; emphasis in original). Furthermore, Standard 2.26 states that competency is also required for "assessing the treatment needs of patients with special needs" (p. 15). In meeting these standards the statement of intent says that students should be exposed to patients "whose medical, physical, psychological, or social situations may make it necessary to modify the normal dental routines in order to provide dental treatment for that individual" (p 15). Notwithstanding the unfortunate implication of that last statement that the treatment for such patients may in some way be considered "abnormal," it is clear that graduates are at least expected to effectively treat such vulnerable patients.

In fact, dental schools always and inevitably instill certain attitudes about justice. It is simply impossible for a school to be ethically neutral. As with all values and attitude-based concepts, the moral tenets of the school and even more so the moral views of the faculty inevitably influence students. The basic concepts of professionalism, including justice-related principles and norms, are taught easily and naturally – sometimes explicitly, sometimes implicitly. The profession's moral values and normative beliefs are inevitably communicated to students by their faculty. It is that way now, and it has always been so. It is the nature of dental education and indeed all professional education.

Dental school takes only four years, which is about one-tenth of the total length of the professional lives of dentists. Yet the indelible stamp of the profession's culture occurs first and foremost then, not during the long years of practice. The experiences of professionals during their practice years serves to reinforce, sometimes modify, but rarely overthrow the basic ideals of professionalism that are introduced and hugely imprinted in professional school (Kultgen 1988, p. 86-90). Day after day, week after week, month after month, year after year, students spend almost all of their time in the company of dentists, hygienists and dental assistants. The educational program is offered by faculty, department chairs, and deans, most of whom are trained as dentists. There is no other period in their lives, neither preceding dental school nor afterwards, that the indoctrination is so effective. If we grant that dental schools inevitably partake in the ethical and political formation of their graduates, they may as well do so in a conscious, explicit, and programmatic manner.

Problems in Achieving Effectiveness

Dental school mission statements vary widely in length and in content. For example, some but not all, contain statements that list both technical excellence and high standards of professional ethics as essential to the educational experience (e.g., University of North Carolina). Some mission statements are silent on issues of social justice (e.g., University of Louisville), while others (e.g., Baylor College of Dentistry) emphasize student participation in community-based training programs and the importance of college-based outreach activities. Still others (e.g., University of Illinois) have goals for oral care that is patient-centered and "comprehensive and compassionate for a culturally diverse population." In general, when dental schools choose to write mission statements that deal with social justice, they tend to focus on how the institution approaches these problems through its outreach or educational programs. Little is written on what dental schools want their graduates to become. It is one thing for an institution to proclaim, for example, that it will strive: *To address community and regional healthcare needs through outreach initiatives, educational programs, and consultative and referral services.* It is quite something else to replace the opening words of this statement ("*To address…*") with "*To graduate practitioners who will address….*" The execution of such practitioner-oriented outcomes with respect to social justice is much more difficult to manage effectively.

There is general acknowledgment that dental graduates must gain understanding of the various oral health disparities and their causes; they must be able to correctly diagnose the conditions of these underserved patients and the factors contributing to their conditions; and they must be able to design and implement a treatment plan that is tailored to the needs of these patients, and that is effective and satisfactory yet affordable. The 2001-2007 *Pipeline, Profession and Practice: Community Dental Education* program (supported financially by the Robert Wood Johnson Foundation, the WK Kellogg Foundation and the California Endowment), is intended to reduce health disparities by impacting dental student education. This program, which amounts to the single largest privately funded dental education project ever in the US, involves 15 dental schools. The funding enables an increase in the number of underrepresented minority and low-income students, a didactic program for all students, and sixty days of treatment by students of underserved patients in community clinics (for a more detailed description, see Bailit et al. 2005).

The results of the Pipeline program are not yet known. According to a preliminary assessment by Anderson and colleagues (2005), under-represented minority students report a greater need for instruction in cultural competency and the social and behavioral determinants of health than white students, and the same students are also more likely to report an improvement in their ability to care for diverse groups as a result of the extramural experiences. This is remarkable because one can reasonably assume that these minority students are culturally *more* competent than whites and thus have *less* to gain from the extramural experiences. The findings seem to imply that white students *overestimate* their cultural competency, which in turn may reflect a lack of motivation on the part of these students to invest in oral health care for underserved populations.

On a more positive note, Anderson's study also shows that most senior students appreciate the extramural experiences. The question arises, however, whether these students upon graduation will continue treating underserved patients. These educational experiences may increase students' clinical competencies to treat underserved patients but that, in and of itself, does not necessarily ingrain in students a permanent motivation to treat such patients. Dental students already treat many underserved patients during their years in dental schools, yet upon graduation, relatively few of these students – now dentists – continue to treat poor patients (e.g., those on Medicaid), special needs children, or other such vulnerable patients.

Knowing what to do and how to do it does not yet warrant that it actually will be done and done rightly. If clinicians are to manage oral health disparities, we submit that dental schools cannot limit themselves to clinical competencies, or more specifically the "technical" aspects thereof (from the Greek "techne" meaning craft, proficiency or practice). In addition to these important *technical competencies*, dental students must also acquire *moral competencies*.

In its *Standards for Predoctoral Dental Education* the ADA's Commission on Dental Accreditation (1998) includes the following three competencies under the header "Ethics and Professionalism":

1. Graduates must be competent in applying ethical, legal and regulatory concepts to the provision and/or support of oral health care services (standard 2-20).
2. Graduates must be competent in the application of the principles of ethical reasoning and professional responsibility as they pertain to patient care and practice management (standard 2-21).
3. Graduates must recognize the role of lifelong learning and self-assessment in maintaining competency (standard 2-22).

Despite the ethical context of these definitions, their wording has primarily a technical flavor. Thus, before students graduate, they must know *how* to do certain things. After graduation, however, dentists must choose *whether* to do those things. Society hopes and expects that they will. That is why it trustingly authorizes professional discretion and autonomy for dentists. Whether or not dentists fulfill that trust depends not only on their scientific knowledge and technical competencies, but on their attitudes. Thus, moral competencies, unlike other competencies, deal not with skills but with habitual, attitude-based decisions about their application. Clinicians must be able to discern the needs and concerns of diverse categories of underserved patients; appreciate the predicament of these patients; and see themselves as caring, thoughtful practitioners who want to participate in the resolution of these problems. It is our belief that dental schools, by fostering a culture of justice, can play an important role in the formulation of this self-image.

The Impact of Dental Education on the Development of Moral Competencies

Dental schools are not the only institutions that warrant the public's trust in the competence of dentists. Licensing boards and professional associations play an important role as well. But dental schools certainly have the greatest impact on the competency development of dentists. Indeed, all dental schools are acutely aware of the leadership role they play in securing future generations of qualified dentists as well as moving the science of dentistry forward into the future.

It is one thing for dental schools to acknowledge and accept this educational responsibility. It is quite another to act on it. Wotman and colleagues remind us that in most schools, the curriculum is driven by the need to render matriculating students technically competent to independently practice dentistry by the time they graduate, a mere four years later (Wotman et al. 2003, p. 407).

In our chapter included in the first part of this book, we have argued that moral competencies are indeed competencies. They are complex attitudinal abilities. Most assuredly, when students arrive at the dental school, they bring twenty or more years of raising and education. They bring mature moral sensitivities and values. But that does not mean they have already mastered the moral competencies that are specific to the professional practice of dentistry. DePaolo reminds us that even the most mature students will undergo a process of professionalization while in dental school that will change them. Hence, "dental education should provide an environment that positively reinforces societal values and professional norms" (DePaolo 1994, p. 37). Referencing a 1993 report of the Wingspread group on higher education entitled *An American Imperative: Higher expectations for higher education,* DePaolo warns that "there is anecdotal evidence suggesting there is too little attention on too few campuses to the responsibility to transmit the compelling core values any society needs to sustain itself" (DePaolo 1994, 36).

For example, the years in dental school for most dentists constitute the last period of their lives in which they are forced daily to cope with unyielding otherness: colleagues who were chosen for them; administrators, faculty, and staff members who wield extensive power; patients who are assigned; treatments that are mandated. And there is the experience of becoming another person, a dentist. For no amount of information gathered prior to enrollment in dental school can truly prepare the student for the revolutionary years ahead. Hence, dental school is a crucial time to cultivate the moral competence of tolerance (see our earlier chapter on this and various other moral competencies).

Given that dental schools are the bulwarks of scientific advancement and the prime agents in moving the profession forward to ever higher levels of technical competence, they also carry much responsibility to make sure that graduates are morally competent to manage those advances well. There is a delicate balance to be struck between demanding excellence from students and overtaxing them with an expectation of perfection. Dental school faculty must develop and model temperance.

Likewise, dental school faculty have an extended opportunity to assist students in developing the moral competency of integrity. By role modeling integrity and by sharing their practical wisdom with students, faculty members can foster the moral growth of students. By the same token, however, four years of dental school also allows for bad habits to become ingrained. If students are exposed to conflicts over an extended period of time, such as the conflict between performing certain numbers of procedures on patients to meet educational requirements versus providing only those treatments that best serve the patients' own needs (VanDam & Welie 2001), bad faith and self-deception may set in.

Unfortunately, there is more evidence that the years in dental school may also render dental students, or at least some of them, less instead of more morally competent. Wotman and colleagues worry that some dental students are extremely skeptical and unconvinced about the role of the profession in social responsibility (Wotman et al. 2003, p.411). And the 2005 study by Sherman and Cramer in which dental students were shown to progressively become more cynical and less caring during their years in dental school, does not bode well either.

Citing once again the 1993 report of the Wingspread group on higher education, DePaolo therefore challenges each dental school to ask itself "what it proposes to do to assure that next year's entering students will graduate as individuals of character, more sensitive to the needs of the community, more competent in their ability to contribute to society, and more civil in their habits of thought, speech and action" (as cited by DePaolo 1994, p. 36). Referencing yet another report on higher education, written by Bragg and published by the American Association for the Study of Higher Education in 1986, DePaolo lists six strategies: "1) selecting students; 2) isolating students from outside influences; 3) consistency of institutional or program goals; 4) explicitness of values and role models; 5) providing opportunities for practicing responses; and 6) providing both positive and negative sanctions as feedback to students" (DePaolo 1994, 37; reference to: Bragg 1986). This list makes clear that the school must "go beyond development of formal courses – as important as they may be – to establish an environment, a community, that can serve as a paradigm for social responsibility" (Mandel

1997, p 134). Wotman and colleagues even more boldly assert that "placing greater emphasis on professional responsibility to the community requires a reexamination of the educational philosophy of the dental school" (2003, p. 407).

Factors beyond the Scope of This Chapter

The charge to the schools of dentistry is clear. It is a most laudable task. It is also a very difficult one. Ludmerer has already pointed out that medical education is limited in its ability to produce doctors who are caring, socially responsible, and capable of behaving as patient advocates (1999, xxi). In the remainder of this chapter, we will discuss several possible strategies. However, there are certain factors known to impact the moral competency development of dental students that we will not address here.

First and foremost is the issue of the rising cost of dental education. More than a decade ago, DePaolo already pointed to the paradoxical development that dental educators are devoting increasing resources to reach the lower socioeconomic sector of society, yet at the same time the increasing cost of dental education is rendering such an education inaccessible for that very segment of society (1994, p. 36). To make matters worse, the increase in student indebtedness may well steer ever more dental graduates away from that lower socioeconomic sector, catering instead to the wealthier patient populations. Indeed, there now is ample evidence that younger dentists are less willing to treat Medicaid patients than are older dentists, a trend that is most likely driven at least in part by graduates' indebtedness.

Second, in this chapter we do not address the issue of attracting a more ethnically and racially diverse student population. To be sure, this is a very important issue. Minority graduates are more likely to care for minority patients (Brown et al. 2000; Solomon et al. 2001). Attracting more minority students thus will help reduce at least one disparity, that is, the disparities among minority patient populations. However, we are not certain that this strategy will bring about the kind of systemic change we are seeking. There is the paradoxical risk that this strategy – increasing oral health care services for minority populations by training more minority dentists – actually reinforces the systemic problem underlying the staggering oral health disparities. For instead of changing the system by encouraging and training all dentists to take on their fair share of such care, we leave the task of caring for minority patients to minority dentists.

Finally, we emphasize that the call for an increased social awareness and connectedness does not mean that dental schools should become social services agencies. Dental schools must remain true to their core mission of being academic institutions. The ADEA has already pointed out that "the role of academic dental institutions as a safety net should not diminish their academic purpose. Academic dental institutions have the unique role in society of educating oral health professionals, generating new knowledge, conducting and promoting basic and applied research, and providing patient care to advance education, research, and service to their communities. If forced to choose between their academic mission and their role as a safety net for the underserved, academic dental institutions must put more effort into their academic mission than in improving access. As a safety net for the underserved, academic dental institutions can be supported and even replaced by nonacademic providers and institutions. What others cannot replace is the defining academic purpose that dental schools and advanced dental education programs play in our society" (Haden et al. 2003, p. 9).

Another way of making the same point is to say that when a dental school engages in social justice, it must do so precisely as a dental school. The backbone of any academic institution, dental schools included, is its faculty. Whereas students come and go, the faculty stays. It is the faculty that develops the educational offerings, and it is the faculty that undertakes research. Although good teachers always learn from their students, the students are first and foremost the recipients of the intellectual production by the faculty. And most importantly, the faculty are the mentors and the role models for the students. Unless the former underwrite and abide by a particular practice standard or professional norm, the latter will not adopt it. The ethics instructor may lecture about the importance of informed consent to the students, but if the clinical faculty do not reinforce this lesson by incorporating it into the practice of dentistry, by showing students how to obtain a genuine informed consent, and insist that they take this ethical norm seriously, students will not come to accept the importance of informed consent and will not develop a habit obtaining it from each and every patient. Conversely, it only takes a few instances of clinical faculty members' making light of informed consent or simply failing to make that extra effort to set students on a paternalistic course.

The same is true for the issue of social justice. If the core faculty of the dental school do not endorse such ideals and do not themselves seek to become and remain connected and engaged in the profession, the community and society at large, service-learning, community outreach and other such educational programs aimed at students will have a modest impact at best or none at worst. Even the 60 days of community-based educational programs that were required for schools to receive a Pipeline grant from the Robert Wood Johnson Foundation – a significant number of hours in an already over-packed dental curriculum – still amounts to a fraction of the typical four year dental curriculum. Thus any moral lessons learned during such outreach programs are easily outdone during the remaining time spent in the dental school itself if its faculty members do not wholeheartedly endorse the same values and reinforce those lessons in their lectures and clinical instructions.

The Scope of Planning for Moral Competencies

The plan presented below focuses on the need for "connectedness" in the professional lives of dentists. Ultimately, we wish to encourage each dental school to define the kind of professional person each of its graduates should be, and we provide some practical suggestions for achieving that ideal. We need to emphasize, however, that moral competencies, much like technical competencies, are not hammered in stone. As the science of dentistry changes, so do the technical competencies that dentists are required to master. As the values change that shape the profession and society at large, so must the moral competencies. In our earlier chapter in this book, we have described how in the course of history, many partially overlapping, partially diverging classifications of virtues have been proposed. The differences generally were not the result of fundamental theoretical disagreements but rather of the specific historical and socio-cultural contexts. In the same vein, we recommend that each dental school ask itself the fundamental question: What kind of dentists do we want our graduates to be? The answer to this question will differ for different schools, reflecting, amongst others, national differences, regional oral health needs, the religious affiliation of the university, the history of the school, and the specific academic strengths of its faculty.

The list of competencies presented in our earlier chapter can and must likewise be adjusted. Hopefully it will jump-start discussions, and the same is true for the various strategies we discuss here.

Because issues of justice always generate diverse and significant political and moral controversy, the project is one that must be undertaken with careful and realistic planning. An essential component must be a collaborative discovery process shared by a diverse group of people including not only faculty, but also students, established members of the profession, and the community at large. This broad base of involvement is important because of the social contract that exists between the public and the profession and the key role played by the dental schools in executing that contract. Breadth is essential in that what is sought involves systemic, cultural changes that will result in different perspectives on how dental professionals think about their broad relationships with each other and with other segments of society. Hence, the process is far broader than the development of an elective course, a new outreach program, or even a new curriculum.

An example of such a systemic reorientation from the world of health care is Bon Secours Health System, Inc. (BSHSI) of Marriotsville, Maryland. The BSHSI's newly developed Ethics Quality Plan (2005) is "intended to take BSHSI to a higher level of ethical awareness, expertise and behavior." Among its goals are insuring (i) that "excellence in ethics" is a BSHSI hallmark, both in the clinical and the organization arena; (ii) that the institution "is capable of meeting the challenges of [the] future; and (iii) that both "leadership and co-workers develop a suitable understanding of ethical issues and consistent habits of acting ethically." What distinguishes this Plan from many other such declarations on institutional ethics is BSHSI's readiness to implement it into practice. BSHSI actually uses its Ethics Quality Plan as a guideline for the *everyday* function of its health care system. Its mission and values statements are posted in various places around all of the BSHSI institutions. The values are discussed with each new employee and reviewed annually in department meetings either by the chair or by a member of the hospital administration. During merger talks with other institutions, the value statements are a constant frame of reference and their acceptance by the merger-partner are a necessary component of the agreement. Generally speaking, the values are utilized throughout the various decision-making processes of the institution, including the making of budgets (Personal communication, James DeBoy, Vice President, Mission, BSHSI. June 6, 2005).

Leadership and Key Players

The most important leadership must come from the office of the dental school dean. Without the sustained support and active involvement of the dean and the other top administrators, such a systemic undertaking will fail. The same can be said for the involvement of department chairs or section heads. This does not mean that success is possible based simply on an executive decision followed by a memorandum to all subordinates. In professional education, everyone has a role to play in creating a successful outcome.

The transmission of values in dental schools and in all professional schools occurs when knowledge and skills are administered day-by-day, subtly presented in the context of values and beliefs, in endless contact with one member of the profession after another. Thus, while leadership cannot come from the grassroots, the day-to-day execution of any new concepts must do so. For this reason, crucially important contributions must come from the cadre of both full time and part-time faculty. Steps must be taken to encourage their investment in this process and to increase their own "connectedness" with the school and its core beliefs.

Support of a different kind is required from the various components of the profession. Professionally based support should be enlisted from such sources as the dental association, the state board of dental examiners, and the American College of Dentists, as well as from individual interested practitioners. Without their positive involvement, there is a risk of mistrust and misunderstanding that could severely undercut the process.

Planning for Endorsement, Support, or Commitment?

In planning this project, the school's leadership must keep in mind that the project's outcomes depend in large part on how everyone involved feels about what is being attempted. Even if the outcomes are positive, such feelings will range from endorsement to support to commitment. All three are better than apathy and rejection, but there are big differences among them. The amount of work required to secure endorsement, for example, is very much different from that required for active support.

Endorsement represents the lowest positive level of affirmative response. It implies that a person or an organization approves of something. Approval is not necessarily accompanied by action. But the words are there, and the approval now is publicly known. Sometimes this is the only level of buy-in that can be achieved, particularly at the outset. And sometimes, this is the only level that is actually needed to successfully progress. However, it is important not to plan (and settle) for endorsement when what is really needed is support or commitment.

Next up the line is *support*. A supporter not only proclaims approval, he or she actively promotes it or at least helps the cause in some way. In most projects requiring action, the bulk of the work is done by supporters. Hence it is important early on in the planning stage to identify those who are needed to support the project and then plan carefully to provide them with adequate information to convince them that the project deserves their support. Supporters are much harder to secure, but without them the project is bound to fail, particularly a project with the systemic scope and impact proposed here.

Finally there are the *committed* few who provide a project with its core of sustenance and viability. The committed are those who pledge to devote themselves to a specific person or cause. A project such as the one under discussion does not require many such committed persons, but a few at different points along the way are surely essential. It is the leader's job to find such people and help them develop to their maximum effectiveness.

General Organizational Considerations

The organizational structure required for this project is that which is effective for any such effort: a steering committee, a standing committee, various subcommittees. As suggested previously, the committees need breadth. Members should be selected from the administration, department or section leaders, full time and part time dental faculty, dental hygiene faculty, dental students, dental assistants, and other staff, as well as representatives of the broader university community. Externally, representation from dental associations, the licensing board, and the state department of dental health is needed along with selected practitioners, patient advocates, and community representatives.

Prior to the accumulation of any required information, the project's leadership needs to create opportunities for its discussion in general forums. The goal of these discussions is to educate faculty (and others) to the mission of the school and to convince them that the project is worthy of their endorsement, their active support, perhaps even their commitment. Similar opportunities can be offered to external participants in the project.

Throughout the project, from its earliest planning stages to its implementation, it is crucially important that a unified message of institutional commitment is conveyed to all members of the school's community, but particularly those who have frequent contacts with students. The messages from the dental faculty who work with students on a day-to-day basis in the lecture halls, the laboratories, and the clinics are especially important. They are the daily role models, and collectively their enculturating effect during the four years of formal education is enormous. However subtle their messages might be, it is this group that needs to be most aware of the importance of their position as role models. As stated previously, inevitably their values will be collectively transmitted to their students, whether explicitly or implicitly stated. Furthermore, given the current critical shortage of full-time faculty, the understanding by part-timers of their vital function as role models cannot be understated.

The Process of Establishing the Moral Competencies

Possibly the most important component in this process is the collection of data that will enable the establishment of the various moral competencies that will define any given school and its graduates. The data collection phase can begin once the organizational framework is established and the process of acquiring internal and external support is well established. Indeed, the remainder of the project depends upon the nature and quality of the collected information.

To acquire the data, questions should be asked of dentists about the things that are important to them in their lives as professionals. Collectively, the questions would help the institution define its vision of how dentists should function as professionals in their interaction with their profession, their community, and society in general.

The data are best collected through tape-recorded small group discussions, perhaps patterned after a focus group format. Individual institutions may or may not need professional assistance in the leading of focus group discussions. Those who comprise the discussion groups should include the same array of people previously mentioned – from deans to janitors, from community dentists to state board members, and from patient advocates to town council members. In the discussions, it is important to create a climate in which people can present their views, even unpopular ones, without the risk of disapproval. The goal is to determine what the respondents believe about how dentists should interact with their patients, and particularly with the community, their profession, and society at large.

Below are examples of questions that might be used, though each institution must devise its own set of questions. In all instances, besides any general responses, examples should be requested, along with the reasons for their beliefs. When members of the group disagree, discussion leaders should determine what constitutes the point of departure. Discussion leaders should also attempt to summarize the conversation on each question. When disagreements occur, an informal vote may be taken, not to settle the moral disagreement but rather to assess the degree of division.

We organize our questions by the three levels of connectedness we outlined in our earlier chapter included in part 1 of this book: connectedness to the profession of which all dentists have chosen to be part, to the community in which they will be practicing, and to the society at large with which the profession has an implicit contract.

Regarding their chosen profession

• Should local, state, and national dental societies be involved in oral health issues of social justice? How about general health issues? Should they be concerned and involved in general community issues?

• If dental societies should be involved in such activities, in what way should the membership participate? Financial support? Direct care through their offices? Involvement in community clinics?

• With respect to colleagues who are incompetent, how should colleagues interact with them upon learning of a problem? Is it the same with impaired colleagues? Under what circumstances, if any, should dentists act as whistleblowers against incompetent, dishonest, or impaired colleagues?

• What is the role, if any, of professional peer review committees in fostering fiduciary and effective and relationships between the profession of dentistry and the community? Should dentists be willing to engage in and submit to constructive multi-disciplinary peer review activities among and with their colleagues?

• What is the role, if any, of state boards in the kinds of issues listed above?

Regarding the community in which they are be practicing

• Should dentists be involved in community activities? Why or why not? If so, to what extent? What kinds of activities?

• More specifically, what is the extent of a dentist's duty to help reduce the problem of access, to care for groups of citizens who experience oral health disparities? Is it equal or more extensive than that of the average citizen? Is this duty impacted by the degree of dental student debt at graduation?

• How should the duty to help reduce oral health disparities be manifested?

• Are dentists obligated to participate in issues of general community health and if so how?

• Are dentists obligated to participate in community activities that are not health-related? If so, are some kinds of activities more important than others? And what kinds of competencies would be expected of dentists in this regard?

Regarding society at large with which the profession has an implicit contract

• Should dentists feel obligations to involve themselves with societal concerns of a general health nature? If so, is there any reason to consider acting primarily with oral health initiatives, rather than those of general health, or of non-health origins?

• Should dentists feel obligation to be engaged in public causes, such as gender or racial discrimination, environmental issues, or global projects in developing countries?

• If dentists were to be involved in politics, given their membership in a helping profession, is their influence best placed in certain categories of activity?

In addition to the various questions about the connectedness of dentists to the profession, community, and society at large, information about role models is important because it will help determine effective approaches in the day-to-day contact between faculty and students. Dentists and dental students should be asked if they have experienced people in their lives who were role models for them and who helped them define the kind of person they would like to become. For those with positive responses, how did their role models convey the values that were important to them? By example? During conversation? Finally dental students, dentists, and faculty should be asked if is important for faculty to become involved in worthy causes?

Based on all the information that is collected, a series of guiding statements should be developed, followed by a series of concrete illustrations. The statements collectively define the kind of professional the institution wants its graduates to become. However, it is important to emphasize yet again that these statements are developed specifically for each institution in its particular historical and ethical context.

These statements can be phrased initially as the "value statements" of the profession. However, at some point these value statements have to be translated into the "moral competencies" that students must attain in order for these values to be realized. Moral competencies express most directly the concept of striving to be a better dentist.

Once selected, each competency must be defined and a descriptive interpretation must be added that has clear practical applicability. For example, a particular school may come to conclude that the moral competency of altruism is part of its identity, define it as "placing the interest of the other above your own," and next specify: "We recognize our own interests, but strive to keep them in perspective as we recognize the vulnerability of our patients. We especially recognize the interests of those who need care and with our colleagues look for appropriate ways to contribute to their well being."

It would also be prudent at this early stage of selection, definition and interpretation to pay attention to the issue of evaluation. Dental schools not only must enable students to gain certain competencies. They are also charged by the public to provide evidence that graduates have in fact gained those competencies. Technical competencies are evaluated, and it is equally important to look for appropriate ways of evaluating students' moral competencies. As pointed out earlier, however, there are crucial differences between the technical competencies and the moral competencies. Hence, the evaluative standards and methods will have to differ as well. Though not completely uncharted, the evaluation of moral competencies is certainly a new domain. Dental schools are encouraged to think of creative ways of assessing the before-and-after effect of any proposed educational programs on the attitudes, beliefs, and behaviors of faculty, staff, and students – and ultimately of the professionals they become.

Expanding the School's Culture at the Core

The next step is to put the plan into action. In some respect this involves a recapitulation of the process by which information was gathered (Harkness, James A, Retired former Director of Mission Development, Bon Secours Health System, Inc. Personal communication. June 11, 2005). Through a series of meetings involving first the upper and middle levels of administration and then all aspects of the organization, all employees and students need to be informed about the program and the institution's commitment thereto. In addition, the same attention needs to be given to any of the dental school's extramural affiliations. Three approaches are necessary to convey and express its program or moral competencies, all of which are essential for its success.

(i) *Day-to-Day Actions.* In the context of dental schools, the translation of the value statements and related moral competencies into daily custom must take place at every level and with everyone's support, including professionals, students, and staff. The kinds of activities to be undertaken will of course depend on each institution's own list of moral competencies and hence differ per institution. The subsequent list is therefore but a series of examples.

• Promote active involvement by full and part time faculty and by students in local and state dental society affairs and stimulate these organizations to taking on social causes (see also Rule & Bebeau 2005, Chpt 8).

• Encourage participation in other dental organizations with special interests, such as care for the handicapped.

• Encourage faculty to be willing to engage in and submit to constructive multidisciplinary peer review activities among and with colleagues.

• Promote the understanding among faculty about the impact they have on students, both individually and collectively. In the context of justice, the point here is that if students experience the treatment they receive as unjust, even though it is sanctioned by the school, they are unlikely to be motivated to view the world through the lens of justice to others.

• Encourage faculty to guard against conflicts between educational competency requirements and the health care needs or choices of the patient (DePaolo 1994; VanDam & Welie 2001). When such situations inevitably arise, faculty need to show by example the respect due the patient.

• Create ways for faculty to continuously remind students of the contributions that poor patients make to dental education.

• Encourage faculty to treat students in a collegial manner – explaining rather than commanding.

(ii) *Systems/Policies/Procedures which promote and specify value based activities.* Not only is the demonstration of values important on an individual level, it is necessary at the organizational level as well (BSHSI 2005). For example, budgetary and other resources should appropriately support the program. Recruitment of faculty, students, and staff ought to take into consideration evidence of support and acceptance of the values program. New employees and students ought to receive orientation to the values program, and values training should be provided to existing personnel. Examples of specific interventions include but are not limited to:

• Reduce the isolationism that characterizes many dental schools by formulating policies that foster participation in multi-disciplinary scholarship, collaborative research, co-teaching; and increased involvement in general university administration. As Cohen points out, "There is ample evidence to show that, with a few notable exceptions, dental and medical educators generally do not co-teach nor do they do research together.... Only a few members have *university* involvement in terms of teaching and research" (Cohen 2002, p. 370; italics in the original).

• Encourage research towards the reduction of oral health disparities. For as Mandel concluded, "the research enterprise has not been going far enough in the quest for social justice in research" (Mandel 1997, p. 135).

• Develop policies that will specifically attract part time faculty who share the interests of this program.

• Promote the demonstration and communication of values during regular faculty meetings.

• Foster or support issues that affect general societal welfare, including public health initiatives and other societal measures of merit, such as those involving public nutrition, environment, ecology, or racial discrimination (Rule & Bebeau 2005, p. 7-17 & 19-30).

• Foster or support issues that affect global society, such as that created in Haiti by Dr. Jeremiah Lowney (see Rule & Bebeau 2005, Chpt. 7).

• Select matriculating students who exhibit a willingness to be connected and specifically a commitment to justice in oral health care.

• Foster students' personal growth and understanding of the world in which they will be practicing through involvement with nondental community outreach groups. Examples include big brother or big sister groups or those with focus on HIV, juvenile diabetes, church outreach, or soil conservation. These outreach activities need not (all) be oral health or even health related. As Rubin notes, "by developing experiences in public health services that are unrelated to dental services, students at the University of Pittsburgh, School of Dental Medicine, through S.C.O.P.E. (Student Community Outreach Program and Education) project, gained new insights and attitudes that reflected personal growth and helped them in attaining the … school-specified competencies" (Rubin 2004, p. 461). He gives three reasons for the program's success. "First, this program for preclinical students was modeled after programs in other health care professional schools and was designed to link public health, medicine and dental care. There was a perceived need to develop multiple attributes including cultural competence. Empathy, multiculturalism, etc, and therefore a broad spectrum of community service was an important element. Second, dental school provides abundant dental-related experiences but often fails to give students a non-dental perspective on health issues. Third, working outside of dentistry provided a broad scope of patient, family, and community desires and demands" (p. 462).

• Provide service-learning opportunities. The ADEA has recommend that dental schools "encourage graduates to pursue a year of service and learning that would not only make the students more competent to provide increasingly complex care, but also serve to improve access to oral health care" (Haden et al. 2003, p. 8). Indeed, "there is evidence that (clinically based) service-learning helps develop cultural literacy, improve citizenship, enhance personal growth, and foster a concern for social problems, which leads to a sense of social responsibility and commitment to public/human service" (Rubin 2004, p. 460-461).

• Create opportunities for students to reflect on and discuss their role in dealing with health disparities and other justice related issues.

• Create repeated reminders of the importance of professional commitment during important steps in the educational process (orientation; white coat ceremony; graduation). But in so doing, have no ceremony without meaningful preparation. For example, prepare for a white coat ceremony with seminars on themes of professionalism. These could include: discussions of the meaning and significance of any oath to be taken; the taking of an oath before a judge to symbolize the profession's contract with society; reflective writings by students with commentary from exemplary dental leaders; luncheon discussions with the dean and other members of the faculty and professional community.

• Increase the effectiveness of all educational activities by understanding the process of professional identity formation (e.g., Kegan 1982; Bebeau & Lewis 2003).

(iii) **Grand Gestures.** These are special activities that show to people within and outside the institution that the values in the program are an integral component of what it stands for. Examples of Grand Gestures include:

• Develop periodic "literature and dentistry" seminars that explore themes of "connectedness" with society at large.

• Organize discussions among students that would identify important role models and the contributions they have made to their development and to the kind of person they would like to become.

• Encourage and celebrate student participation in local community causes, especially those involving the neighbors of their institution.

• Encourage and celebrate faculty leadership in worthy causes.

Concluding Remarks

This chapter has emphasized five important points. (i) The mandate for leadership in improving the problems of oral health disparities must be assumed by the profession itself. New position papers from the ADA suggests that this mandate is now being met by a commitment to this essential component of professionalism. (ii) Even though professionalization develops throughout all stages of the lives of dentists, the paradigm patterns of professionalism are presented first and most powerfully in dental school. How dentists view themselves, their profession, and their role in society is incorporated into their core attitudes and beliefs during those four years far more profoundly than at any other time. It is simply in the nature of professions that this is true. Thus, it is usually during the process of formal education that professionals develop certain moral competencies and develop a particular vision of their future working life that may or may not include a sense of obligation to care for the underserved according to their personal talents and circumstances. (iii) While dental schools are historically mandated and generally committed to this cause, there is evidence that the results of the existing educational competency listings, programs, and policies have not been effective in fostering a greater commitment to justice in oral health care among graduates. (iv) This lack of success is due, at least in part, to the overwhelming curricular emphasis on technical competencies at the detriment of moral competencies. Dental schools therefore are challenged to pay greater attention to the latter competencies. (v) But unlike technical competencies, the moral competencies of graduates cannot be increased simply by adding courses, laboratory sessions or clinical requirements to the curriculum. Rather, a systemic change is needed that impacts the very culture of the school. Given that proposals even for minor curricular adjustments tend to meet with heavy opposition, such a systemic change will not be achieved overnight. Inclusive but decisive leadership will be needed, and lots of inventiveness and patience. It is, however, a challenge that cannot be neglected much longer, for the lack of connectedness threatens the profession at many fronts, most seriously in the area of oral health disparities.

Bibliography

American Dental Association. *State and Community Models for Improving Access to Dental Care for the Underserved – A White Paper*. Chicago: American Dental Association, 2004

ADA-CODA (American Dental Association Commission on Dental Accreditation). *Accreditation Standards for Predoctoral Programs*. Chicago: American Dental Association, 1998; revised 2004. On-line at http://www.ada.org/prof/ed/accred/standards/predoc.pdf (access verified on 10/31/05)

Andersen RM, Davidson PL, Atchison KA et al. Pipeline, Profession, and Practice Program: Evaluating Change in Dental Education. *Journal of Dental Education* 2005, 69(2): 239-248

Bailit HL, Formicola AJ, Herbert KD, Stavisky JS & Zamora G. The Origins and Design of the Dental Pipeline Program. *Journal of Dental Education* 2005, 69(2): 232-238

Bebeau MJ & Lewis P. *Manual for Assessing and Promoting Identity Formation*. Minneapolis: University of Minnesota Center for the Study of Ethical Development, 2003

Brown LJ, Wagner KS & Johns B. Racial/ethnic variations of practicing dentists. *Journal of the American Dental Association* 2000, 131:1750-1754

Bragg AK. *The Socialization Process into Higher Education. AAHE-ERIC Research Report*. Washington DC: American Association for the Study of Higher Education, 1986

BSHSI – Bon Secours Health System, Inc. *Bon Secours Ethics Quality Plan*. Marriotsville AD, BSHSI, 2005. On-line at http://www.bshsi.com/strategic-direction/lead-in-catholic/ethics-purpose.htm (access verified on 10/31/2005)

Cohen MM. Major Long-Term Factors Influencing Dental Education in the Twenty-First Century. *Journal of Dental Education* 2002, 66(3): 360-373

DePaolo DP. Higher Education and Health Professions Education. Shared Responsibilities in Engaging Societal Issues in Developing the Learned Professional. *Journal of the American College of Dentists* 1994, Fall/Winter: 34-39

DePaola DP. *Beyond the University: Leadership for the Common Good*. Presentation at the 75th Anniversary Summit Conference of the American Dental Education Association "Leadership for the Future: The Dental School in the University," October 12-13, 1998. On-line at: http://www.adea.org/DEPR/Summit/depaola.pdf

Haden NK, Bailit H, Buchanan J, et al. *Improving the Oral Health Status of All Americans: Roles and Responsibilities of Academic Dental Institutions. Report of the ADEA President's Commission*. Washington DC: American Dental Education Association, 2003

Kegan R. *The Evolving Self: Problem and Process in Human Development.* Cambridge MA: Harvard University Press, 1982

Kultgen J. *Ethics and Professionalism.* Philadelphia: University of Pennsylvania Press; 1988

Ludmerer K. *Time to Heal. American Medical Education from the Turn of the Century to the Era of Managed Care.* Oxford: Oxford University Press, 1999

Mandel ID. Oral Health Research and Social Justice: The Role and Responsibility of the University and Dental School. *Journal of Public Health Dentistry* 1997, 57(3): 133-135

Rubin RW. Developing Cultural Competence and Social Responsibility in Preclinical Dental Students. *Journal of Dental Education* 2004, 68(4): 460-467

Rule JT & Bebeau MJ. *Dentists Who Care: Inspiring Stories of Professional Commitment.* Quintessence Publishing Company: Chicago, 2005

Rule JT & Veatch RM. *Ethical Questions in Dentistry* (2nd ed.). Quintessence Publishing Company: Chicago, 2004

Sherman JJ & Cramer A. Measurement of changes in empathy during dental school. *Journal of Dental Education* 2005, 69(3): 338-345

Solomon ES, Williams CR, Sinkford JC. Practice Location Characteristics of Black Dentists in Texas. *Journal of Dental Education* 2001, 65: 571-578

US Public Health Service. *Oral Health in America: A Report of the Surgeon General.* Washington DC, 2000. Available on-line at http://www.surgeongeneral.gov/library/oralhealth/ (access verified on 11/3/05)

VanDam S & Welie JVM. Requirement-driven dental education and patients' right to informed consent. *Journal of the American College of Dentists* 2001, 67(3): 40-47

Wotman S et al. Reexamining Educational Philosophy: The Issue of Professional Responsibility, "Cleveland First." *Journal of Dental Education* 2003, 67(4): 406-411

Michelle Henshaw

Service-learning, Oral Health Disparities and the Shift in Dental Education

Oral Health Disparities and the Community Responsive Dentist

Oral health disparities are prevalent in the United States and dental caries remains the most common chronic childhood disease, despite the fact that caries is entirely preventable. Contributing to the disproportionate burden of oral disease experienced by racial and ethnic minority groups is the unequal access to preventive care experienced by underserved populations. One way that the dental profession can take an active role in eliminating oral health disparities is for dentists to expand access to preventive services, on an individual and more importantly on a population level.

A necessary step toward engaging private practitioners in population-based prevention efforts and providing care to underserved populations is to have a dental workforce that views these activities as its civic and professional responsibility. Dentists must also possess the knowledge and expertise necessary to provide these services. However, dental education traditionally has not provided dental students with these skills nor had as a goal to instill this type of civic and professional responsibility in their students. Instead, the emphasis has been on the surgical treatment of disease, with a primary focus of providing for the needs of private practice patients. Unfortunately, in the United States, those with the greatest burden of disease are the same populations that have difficulty accessing private dental services.

A change in the traditional dental school curriculum is needed. In addition to training students to treat disease, dental students should be prepared to take an active role in promoting population-based disease prevention and health promotion activities. Service-learning is an educational methodology that could be incorporated into the curriculum to provide students the opportunity to develop these skills. More importantly, it can engender within students a greater sense of civic responsibility, a desire to participate in service activities and to provide care to underserved populations. This is accomplished by introducing students to the needs of a community, engaging them in addressing these needs through service and providing a connection between what they learn in the classroom and what they experienced during their service activities.

The Call to Action

Dental educators have already recognized the need to look beyond the walls of their own institutions. During the past decade, there has been an increased focus on community-based education in dental schools, mirroring a fundamental shift seen throughout other health professional schools. External forces that have spurred these initiatives include: (1) concerns about the quantity, quality, composition and distribution of the dental workforce; (2) limited learning opportunities within the walls of dental schools; (3) enhanced institutional commitment to the community; and (4) increased barriers to oral health care and oral health, disparities experienced by vulnerable populations.

This shift has been supported by many calls for change in health professional education, including the 1988 report *The Future of Public Health* by the Institute of Medicine, the 1989 report *Healthy America: Practitioners for 2005* by the PEW Health Professions Commission, *Dental Education at the Crossroads* (Field et al. 1995), and the *1995 Report to Congress* by the Council on Graduate Medical Education. The Pew report addresses the competencies for practitioners in the 21st Century, underscoring the importance of population-based care and civic responsibility. According to the Pew report, dentists shall be able, amongst others, to:

- Embrace personal ethic of social responsibility and service
- Rigorously practice preventive care
- Integrate population-based care and service into practice
- Improve access to care
- Provide culturally sensitive care
- Advocate for policy that promotes health
- Work in interdisciplinary teams

Most recently, in 2003, the American Dental Education Association's report entitled *Improving the Oral Health Status of All Americans: Roles and Responsibilities of Academic Dental Institutions* issued the following recommendations:

1. Teaching and exhibiting values that prepare the student to enter the profession as a member of a moral community of oral health professionals with a commitment to the dental profession's societal obligations

2. Developing cultural competencies in their graduates and an appreciation for public health issues

3. Serving as effective providers, role models, and innovators in the delivery of oral health care to all populations

4. Assisting in prevention, public health, and public education efforts to reduce health disparities in vulnerable populations.

In addition to the aforementioned reports, there have been several national initiatives that have assisted in the translation of these recommendations into action by promoting community-based education, including: (i) Kellogg Community Partnerships in Health Professional Education and Community-Based Public Health, (ii) the Robert Wood Johnson Foundation Pipeline, Profession and Practice: Community-based Dental Education, (iii) the CDC Bridges to Healthy Communities and (iv) the CNS/Pew Health Professions Schools in Service to the Nation.

Given the compelling internal and external forces, most dental schools have adopted some form of experiential education, most commonly in the form of community-based education. In these rotations dental students provide clinical care in community-based settings such as community or rural health centers, Veterans Administration Medical Centers, public health clinics, or other similar settings, usually under the supervision of community-based dentists (Henshaw, unpublished results). The incorporation of these activities exposes dental students to a wider variety of patients, procedures and settings that they may not experience within their own institution (Bailit 1999), and increases access to dental care for underserved populations. Dental schools have reported that upon completion of their community-based experiences students are more efficient and confident practitioners and that there is an immediate benefit of increased services delivered to underserved populations. However, few schools have assessed the impact of these programs on dental graduates' practice patterns. While it is possible that these programs have the potential to increase dental students' willingness to provide care to underserved populations and to work in public health settings, to date there is only anecdotal evidence that community-based dental education has such a positive long-term impact.

When we look to the education of other health professionals, it has been shown that an educational strategy that deliberately incorporates learning objectives as part of a non-clinical activity, so-called service-learning, is superior to community-based education when it comes to enhancing students' civic engagement. There is also a growing body of research showing that service-learning enhances students' academic performance as well as personal, social and professional development (Astin & Sax 1998; Driscoll et al. 1996; Eyler & Giles 1999). These domains are now reflected in the Accreditation Standards for Dental Education Programs from the Commission on Dental Accreditation. For example, there are competencies related to providing patient-centered care, managing diverse patient populations, successfully functioning in a multicultural work environment and serving as a leader of an oral health care team (ADA-CODA 1998). Service-learning can assist dental and dental hygiene students to gain competency in these areas. Unfortunately, to date service-learning has largely been ignored as a strategy in dental education.

A Definition of Service-learning

Service-learning is an educational methodology that has its roots in undergraduate education. It is relatively new to health professional education; although, it has been successfully incorporated into medical and nursing education (Seifer et al. 2000; Norbeck et al. 1998). There are dozens of definitions of service-learning, ranging from the very broad definition of

> any carefully monitored service experience in which a student has intentional learning goals and reflects actively on what he or she is learning throughout the experience (National Society for Experiential Education 1994),

to the much narrower definition of a method under which students learn and develop through thoughtfully organized service that:

• is conducted in and meets the needs of a community and is coordinated with an institution of higher education, and with the community;

• helps to foster civic responsibility;

• is integrated into and enhances the academic curriculum of the students enrolled;

• and includes structured time for students to reflect on the service experience (American Association for Higher Education 1993).

However, all definitions of service-learning share two common elements: (1) a structured learning activity in which community service is combined with academic objectives; and (2) the students' learning experiences are supplemented by structured reflection activities which allow the students to critically think about the service they performed and its impact on the community's needs.

Most descriptions of service-learning also stress the balance between the benefits to the community and the benefits to the students. Many feel that this is the true distinguishing feature between service-learning and community-based education. In the purest form of service-learning, the students not only provide service to the community, but the activities are structured in such a way that (a) the students gain an understanding for the context in which these activities are delivered, (b) the activities have a greater relevance to students' didactic course work, and (c) the students are provided with an opportunity to critically evaluate their social responsibility as citizens and as health professionals. When this balance is achieved, the service enhances the learning and the academic content enhances the service (Furco 1996). Moreover, the experiential aspect of service-learning allows students to apply what is presented in classroom settings. This application and critical reflection on their activities gives students the opportunity to translate information into true knowledge and skills. It also gives greater relevance and a deeper understanding of the academic concepts learned in the classroom.

An example of service-learning from nursing education can be found in North Dakota State University, where nursing students participated in the North Dakota State Diabetes Screening Program. The rate of diabetes in North Dakota is over twice that of the general United States population. As a result of this tremendous community need, this statewide screening project was developed by the Dakota Heartland Health System under the direction of a certified diabetic educator. The screening program consists of stations including admitting/history, height and weight, blood pressure, blood glucose, visual acuity, and foot examination. Nursing students staff the stations only after working with School and community-based personnel to ensure that the students have a solid academic foundation in diabetes and an orientation to the event's activities. The students have the opportunity to work at the various screening stations over multiple screening days so they can learn the different skills.

These service-learning activities include four reflection exercises designed to assist the students in making the link between the service and the academic course content. The first writing assignment is designed to prepare the students for their service and they are asked to describe the agency (mission, goals, funding, activities, etc.), the target population, their personal learning objectives and the activities they expect to be engaged in that will help them meet those objectives. The second reflection assignment is a journal which chronicles their service activities, as well as the links they have drawn between their service and academic coursework and their personal observations. The third written assignment is a paper summarizing the experience, what they learned and what they could have done to improve the experience. The final assignment is completed in small group seminars in which the students present their significant learning experiences to their classmates. Since not all students participate in the same service activities, students find this sharing a very useful exercise that allows them to benefit from all the service-learning opportunities.

According to the students' reflections the following student outcomes were observed: (1) learned to establish a rapport with clients in a short time span; (2) enhanced their abilities to admit clients, orient clients to a new setting and provide health education; (3) deepened their understanding of diabetes management and complications; (4) gained an appreciation for what it is like to live with a chronic disease and its affect on quality of life; (5) learned how individual differences in culture, values and knowledge impact the management and treatment of diabetes; and (6) increased self confidence as a health care provider (Cohen 1998).

Contrast with Traditional Community-based Education

Although both are forms of experiential education, service-learning differs from traditional community-based education in several significant ways (Furco 1996; Seifer et al. 2000):

Balance between service and learning. On one end of the spectrum, traditional community-based education often has as the primary focus the education of the dental student, with little emphasis on the needs of the community in which the education is taking place. Volunteerism is at the other end of the spectrum where the needs of the community are paramount and there is little significance placed on students' education. Service-learning creates a balance between these two priorities so that the needs of both parties are met, ensuring a mutually beneficial partnership.

Integral involvement of community partners. Rather than just serving as a site for community-based experiences, in service-learning the community partner actively engages in the planning, implementation and evaluation of the community-based experience.

Emphasis on reciprocal learning. In service-learning the distinction between teacher and student is blurred. The students bring knowledge from their academic training to the sites, often providing new insight to their community-based preceptors, while the community-based preceptors provide the students with the wealth of their vast experience in working with the community.

Emphasis on reflection. Reflection is an integral component of service-learning. Thus, the emphasis is not only on what occurs during the community-based rotation. There is also a structured reflective component that can take many forms including journal entries or discussions that help to make connections between the students' community-based experiences and their didactic and "traditional" clinical work.

Emphasis on developing citizenship skills. A concerted effort is made to assist students consider their roles as health professionals and citizens in the larger societal context.

Critical Components of Service-Learning

There have been many attempts to characterize "best practices" in service-learning. Howard's list of ten good practices provides an overview
of the fundamentals in designing a service-learning course (Table 1).

Table 1. Ten Principles of Good Practice for Service-learning

1. Academic Credit is for Learning, Not for Service
2. Do Not Compromise Academic Rigor
3. Set Goals and Learning Objectives for Students
4. Establish Criteria for the Selection of Service Placements
5. Provide Educationally Sound Learning Strategies to Harvest Community Learning
6. Prepare Students for Learning from their Community Experiences
7. Minimize the Distinction Between the Students' Community Learning and Classroom Learning
8. Rethink the Faculty Instructional Role
9. Be Prepared for Variation in, and Some Loss of Control with Student Learning Outcomes
10. Maximize the Community Responsibility Orientation of the Course

Adapted from Howard, Jeffery, ed., Michigan Journal of Community
Service-learning: Service-Learning Course Design Workbook,
University of Michigan: OCSL Press, Summer 2001, pp. 16-19.

However, there are critical components of service-learning implementation that warrant additional exploration.

Partnerships: Partnerships with community-based organizations
form the foundation for all forms of experiential education. In service-
learning, the partnerships are of critical importance because successful
learning experiences build upon the needs, resources, and abilities of the
community organization and its congruence to the academic institution's
mission, goals, resources and needs. Moreover, community partners
play critical roles in the design, administration, and evaluation of the
service-learning activities. They may sit on steering committees, design
curricula, evaluate outcomes or teach portions of the didactic courses.
Considerable effort must be expended when establishing and nurtur-
ing these partnerships, and the resultant service placements, to ensure

that the goals and expectations are clear, that roles and responsibilities are understood and that a clear and open mode of communication is established.

Preparation. No dental school would send students to community-based clinical rotations without adequate preclinical and clinical preparation because without preparation the rotation would be of no benefit to the student or the patients. The same is true for service-learning. In order for the students and community to benefit from the activities, students must have a solid foundation on which to build. The nature of the preparation will be directly related to the service activity and the course learning objectives. If service-learning or community-based education is new to your institution, then the students would also benefit from activities that would prepare them for assuming the role of learner in an experiential educational setting. This type of active learning is very different than what most students are used to and some may need guidance in the transition. The students may need to know about the community, social determinants of oral disease, oral health disparities, the community's culture, and specific knowledge related to the service provided. To expand on the previous example, if the students' service activity is to develop a presentation on the importance of oral health in diabetics for a community health center's diabetes support group, then the students must have at minimum a thorough understanding of diabetes, the culture of the target population and the relationship to diabetes, other chronic diseases and the overall health care system, the link between diabetes and oral health, as well as the evidence base for these findings.

Service. First and foremost, the service provided must be linked to the academic course work. The learning experiences that the community partner provides must challenge the students intellectually. The experience should intentionally test some of their preconceptions, biases and stereotypes that every individual brings to any situation. Although individuals often feel uncomfortable when exploring these issues, it is important for students to understand that everyone views an event from a unique perspective that has been shaped by their past experiences, culture and knowledge. Many students may not even be aware of the impact of these determinants on their interpretation and reaction to experiences. One of the true benefits of service-learning is that it guides students through the process of challenging these preconceptions and gives them the opportunity to reframe their perspective.

By design, even the most prescribed service activities will have variations in their daily implementation as a result of varying interpersonal interactions between students, staff and service recipients. Given the unique perspectives of each participating student, reports of personal student experiences of the same service situation will differ greatly with respect to their individual interpretations. Service-learning benefits from these individual differences; in fact, these differences are what make service-learning so successful. It is when students are faced with experiences that challenge their beliefs or expectations that they can engage in active cognition and true learning. This can be most readily accomplished when students are placed in situations that differ from their cultural, social or economic backgrounds. Once the students are faced with this challenge, the reflective activities are the vehicle that facilitates the personal exploration and growth.

Reflection. Reflection activities are the most important component of service-learning, in that it is the vehicle by which the actual learning occurs. Reflection activities can take many forms (Table 2) and it is the

Table 2. Types of Reflection

Academic Questions. At predefined intervals, the student writes a response to a theoretical or conceptual question. Their answer draws upon their experiences participating in service.

Descriptive Journal. Journal writing varies greatly, however, most commonly it is utilized for students to reflect on their personal responses to their experiences.

Journal Questions. Students respond to instructor generated questions, relying on their experiences when developing their responses.

Critical Incident Journal. Critical incident journal includes detailed analysis of incidents which had an effect on the students' personal or professional goals or their perceptions of their service activities.

quantity and more importantly the quality of the reflection that has been associated with deeper understanding and better application of subject matter, increased knowledge, increased complexity of problem solving and civic engagement.

Institutionalization. By definition, service-learning needs to be integrated into an academic activity, usually a course, but the more that service-learning is truly integrated into the fabric of the institution and is given equivalent levels of importance as the didactic and clinical activities, the more successful the outcomes. The institutionalization needs to be on multiple levels. Supportive administration is critical to the long term success of service-learning within an institution. However, often it is one or two motivated faculty members that introduce service-learning to an institution. If these members of the faculty are successful in linking service-learning to the school's mission and strategic goals, this is an effective way to gain the administrative support necessary to develop and sustain the service-learning curriculum. Another important component of institutionalization that is often overlooked is the development of a mechanism for faculty and staff rewards. The most common and effective reward mechanism is the incorporation of service-learning and community outreach activities into the faculty promotion and tenure criteria.

Evaluation. Evaluation of student performance in the academic course should focus on the learning that occurs and not the service that is provided. The strategies utilized in evaluating the students are dependent upon the course learning objectives and need not differ from traditional student assessment techniques. Service-learning courses often utilize essays, papers and oral presentations.

Evaluation activities should extend beyond student academic performance and should be related to the ultimate goals of service-learning. Effective program evaluation is a structured, ongoing process that provides a more thorough understanding of the program being evaluated (W. K. Kellogg Foundation Evaluation Handbook 1998). In the case of service-learning programs, it enables an understanding of the impact of the program on students, faculty, community partners, and the academic institution as well as how the program is influenced by internal and external factors. Evaluation also demonstrates what has been successful and determines areas where new directions or approaches may be beneficial, thus allowing for improvement. For example, if one of the goals of service-learning at a particular dental school is to instill a commitment to service in students, then program evaluation would include measurement of the amount of community service performed by students while in dental school, service provided after graduation, and students' and graduates' attitudes toward service.

Outcomes

Since service-learning is new to dental education, relatively little is known about the impact of service-learning on dental students. However, many studies have been done among undergraduate and other health professional students. At first glance the results are mixed. The variations in impact are probably due, at least in part, to the great variability in the rigor of the service-learning activities that are being implemented and in turn evaluated. While many academic courses say that they include service-learning activities, these activities range from true, integrated service-learning, to service activities with little connection to their didactic studies, to simply providing community-based clinical rotations. Studies evaluating true service-learning experiences show that these programs reduce students' stereotypes and biases, and improve cultural and racial understanding, sensitivity to diversity, leadership, and clarification of values (Eyler 2001). Service-learning has also been demonstrated to positively impact students' sense of social responsibility, citizenship skills and commitment to service (Astin 1998).

Clearly more research needs to be conducted on the long term impact of behavior change in dental students, and some of that research is currently underway. However, if we learn from the experience of medicine and nursing, there are many and varied opportunities to incorporate meaningful service-learning activities within the traditional dental school curriculum that will have the potential to make a tremendous impact on the dental education, the dental profession, and the community.

Status of Service-learning in Dental Education

In a 2001 Survey of United States dental schools, 90 percent of responding dental schools participated in some form of community-based clinical education activities as defined as rotations outside of the dental school where the dental students act as primary dental care providers. Nearly as many, 82 percent, reported some form of non-clinical community-based education activities. However, in contrast with the clinical community-based activities which were most often required and took place in the fourth year, the non-clinical activities were most often voluntary and were distributed equally throughout all four years.

When asked to self report on their familiarity with service-learning, 71 percent of respondents rated their familiarity as good, very good or excellent and only 29 percent reported fair or poor familiarity with service-learning. Sixty-six percent of those who had non-clinical community-based activities stated that at least some of these activities fulfilled all components of service-learning and 64 percent considered at least some of their clinical activities fulfilling all components of service-learning. When describing the methods used to evaluate the students' activities, less than half of respondents indicated the use of activities that are typically utilized for reflection such as essays, journals or oral presentations These results demonstrate that most dental educators are familiar with the concept of service-learning, but may still lack understanding of the important differences between service-learning and community-based education. However, some dental schools have successfully incorporated service-learning activities into their curriculum (Henshaw, unpublished results).

Examples of Service-learning in Dental Education

Boston University School of Dental Medicine (BUSDM). The School has central to its mission the provision of service to the community. The School recognizes its responsibility to foster in its students a sense of civic responsibility and an understanding that active citizenship is an essential component of professionalism. Although the majority of BUSDM students will enter private practice after graduation, it is one of BUSDM's goals to have their graduates actively engage in treatment and preventive service activities that improve the overall health and well being of underserved populations.

In an effort to graduate a community responsive dentist, one of BUSDM's newest service-learning activities is a 10-week community-based clinical externship rotation, integrated within the fourth and final year of study. In order for the students to gain a deeper understanding of the community they serve, BUSDM believes that the students must be completely immersed within that community. BUSDM hence requires that the students live in the community for which they provide clinical care. In addition to the clinical care provided, a distinct, but integral component of the BUSDM Externship program is the new service-learning requirement that the students complete a public health project.

The project is built around a community need that is defined by the community itself. The students then devote at least four hours per week throughout all 10 weeks of the rotation to a project that is designed to meet that community need. The purpose of the project is to enhance the students' understanding of the individual and community needs and how those needs impact health. The project gives the students the opportunity to plan, implement and evaluate population-based health promotion efforts while building capacity within the community. Prior to the rotation, the students receive didactic lectures on cultural competence, health disparities, individual and community risk factors, social determinants of disease, health care delivery systems, and population-based prevention. In addition, each student participates in a mandatory orientation designed to provide students with an overview of their sites, the population served and the public health project expectations.

The students are given the option of participating in an ongoing project sponsored by their Externship site or one of its partners, enhancing a project begun by a previous BUSDM student or developing a new project. To support the service and learning activities, the student is assigned a faculty mentor at the dental school and at his or her Externship site to guide their work on the public health project. The students participate in three written reflection exercises. In the first exercise the students must submit a brief one half page description of the project and what they hope to learn from their participation in the service activity. The second reflection activity provides an overview of the project, including the institution they are working with, the name of their project, what problem the project is designed to address, what are the factors contributing to the problem, and how this program will address those factors. They are also asked to describe one incident that happened during their first five weeks that impacted their understanding of the community or made them reexamine their beliefs, values or personal or professional goals. The final paper includes an additional critical incident reflection as well as an assessment of what they learned from the overall experience and the impact on them as citizens and professionals. Analysis of the reflection activities show that the students gained:

- Greater understanding of the community's needs and the role of a community health center
- Enhanced communication skills
- Enhanced leadership and organizational skills
- Greater sense of professionalism

- Increased motivation to learn
- Increased commitment to population-based health
- Greater awareness of oral health disparities and lack of access for disadvantaged populations
- Better preparation to treat a wider range of dental disease and patient populations.

University of Illinois at Chicago (UIC). A new Dean, Dr. Bruce Graham, arrived at the College of Dentistry (COD) in the spring of 2000. One of his earliest activities was to have the faculty develop new vision and mission statements. The Vision Statement became "By the year 2010, the University of Illinois at Chicago College of Dentistry will be recognized as a world leader." One leadership area identified stressed a broad perspective with "patient-centered, evidence-based clinical care founded on the preventive and public health sciences."

The Mission statement became "to promote optimum oral and general health to the people of the State of Illinois and worldwide through excellence in education, patient care, research, and service." Included among the goals were to "provide patient-centered care that is comprehensive and compassionate for a culturally diverse population; provide student-oriented education programs that prepare individuals for the thoughtful, ethical practice of dentistry and life-long learning; and address community and regional healthcare needs through outreach initiatives, educational programs, and consultative and referral services."

These statements provided new directions for the College, which were implemented in such ways as hiring diverse faculty and staff. A very important hire was that of a Health Educator with an educational background in Community Health, who makes sure that the school's philosophy, as specified in the mission and vision statements, transcends clinical teaching and skills.

One specific example is the *Introduction to Community-Based Education* (CBE) program, which occurs in the first semester of the first year of dental education. This course was first implemented in the Fall 2003 for the Class of 2007, the class that will be the first UIC-COD class to provide the Robert Wood Johnson Foundation Dental Pipeline initiative aim of at least 60 days of community clinical care. The goal of the course is that "Dental students will understand oral health education as an integral component within an interdisciplinary approach to patient care." The learning objectives, of this first dental school experience in working collaboratively with communities, are to:

• recognize the characteristics and demographics of a given community;

• list and discuss individual and community risk factors/social determinants of health;

• apply appropriate educational techniques and provide relevant information to audience/individuals (i.e., appropriate language and grade level of communication, choice of written, oral, or audiovisual format, use of media or other methods);

• implement proper communication skills while educating children about their levels of risk from real or potential hazards;

• interact sensitively and effectively with persons from diverse cultural, socioeconomic, educational and professional backgrounds, and with persons of all ages and lifestyle preferences; and

• collaborate effectively as a team (with peers) as well as with faculty, elementary school teachers, and children.

The CBE program is one piece of a large course known as *Comprehensive Care* and contributes 15 percent of that course grade. The CBE program is provided in five three-hour sessions. The class of about 65 students is divided into 6 groups. The first and fifth sessions include the entire class, with the middle three sessions being rotations for the 6 groups. The content of each of the five sessions is provided in Table 3.

The first session introduces the dental students to the big picture elements concerning the use of and context for service-learning. The second enables the students, with guidance of the Health Educator, to explore their own creativity in preparing a lesson plan for elementary school students coming from diverse groups of children, for example, who may be African American, Spanish-speaking, recent immigrants, or deaf. The third is the actual community school presentation, with the classroom teacher present in the room and the health educator walking among the classrooms to observe, followed by a brief time of discussion for group reflection. In the fourth session, each of the student groups work together to integrate their community experience and knowledge of disparities for presentation in the fifth session. The last session enables the students to compare and contrast their experiences, plus have additional guidance in seeing how their efforts fit into the community with comments and questions from community and

Table 3. Content of UIC "Introduction to Community-Based-Education Sessions"

Session One: Introduction
• Overview of health education as a key component of oral health care
• Oral health disparities in the nation, the state, and the local areas
• Methodology of service-learning
• Knowing your audience and presentation skills

Session Two: Community Preparation
• Overview of health education standards as they relate to oral health; health literacy and readability; lesson planning; visual aids
• Preparation of lesson plans for elementary school oral health education presentations
• Preparation of "goodie bag" for each child (containing oral care products, and bilingual English/Spanish information for caregivers)

Session Three: School Presentations
• Off-campus presentations at elementary schools
• Post-presentation group reflection

Session Four: Project Preparation
• Student-led group project preparation
• Completion of peer evaluation
• Submission of individual reflection paper

Session Five: Student Group Presentations
• Review of semester activities and concepts
• Groups present finding and experiences to one another, COD faculty members and invited community reactors
• Completion of course evaluation

faculty reactors. In addition to the group presentations and discussions, written reflections were also required. Quotes from the dental student reflections include:

• After our presentation, one of the kids mentioned that he thought dentists were cool and he wanted to be one someday. That comment made me think about how important our visit was to kids as a means of exposing them to different career opportunities;

• I think it is important to instill these values of service in dental students before we become too concerned with running our own practices;

• I believe that although they may have seen violence or heard gunshots at night while trying to fall asleep, which are things I have never experienced, there was a connection between us;

• This project does not only attempt to cover this new generation, but in fact addresses the gaps of the past and lays groundwork for the future generations as well;

• I've been thinking about writing a letter to the board of education and possibly to my congressman suggesting to expand the grammar and high school health education programs to include more dental health care; and

• I did not realize until that moment that I was no longer a kid. That these kids looked to me as a doctor and that I had a degree of responsibility about their education.

Useful, practical feedback was provided by the school teachers, in addition to their very positive views of the experience for their classrooms:

• It was educational for me as well as for my students.

• I would like to see more supplementary activities or pre-visit information or activities or worksheets or follow-up activity.

• Special needs students do better with one-on-one.

• Maybe hold onto the pencils and toothbrushes until the end. Their instinct is to drum with them. It's always hard to regroup. Maybe use a raised hand signal or use 'Stop. Look here. Listen.'

A written, structured course evaluation was provided at the end of the course. The two years of course evaluations yielded encouraging findings. The vast majority (92%) of these first year dental students reported that the course experience improved their perception of community-based education, with 82 percent rating the course as good or excellent. The only consistently mentioned negative element concerned "time." For example, in the Fall 2004 experience, administrative scheduling required that the Student Group Presentations occur during finals week. One student's reflection provides interesting insight: "This activity should have a priority in our schedules. Thus our curriculum needs to be adjusted to enable us to continue to do this."

Indiana University School of Dentistry (IUSD): Increasingly, students applying for dental school are asking what civic engagement opportunities IUSD offers. They are looking for a school where they can participate in community-based programs. This commitment was evidenced when the idea emerged to take portable dental equipment to homeless shelters that house children, and provide sealants for the kids on the four Wednesday evenings during Children's Dental Health Month.

Some IUSD faculty were skeptical about the possibility of getting 40 IUSD students, 10 students per week, to volunteer when they would receive no clinic credit for the effort. When 110 students volunteered on the first day of recruitment, it was apparent that great potential for community service existed at IUSD.

Since that time, numerous community-based programs have been developed with emphasis on providing a variety of settings and populations to be served. There is an attempt to balance local, state and international opportunities for service and learning so that students internalize the ethic of helping at home while also embracing a global perspective.

IUSD is also committed to encouraging community service because policymakers and citizens nowadays expect community responsiveness and accountability, especially from publicly funded institutions. In 2002, Indiana legislators showed their support for service-learning by passing a concurrent resolution urging private, and especially public institutions of higher education in Indiana to adopt service-learning as a central form of engagement, civic outreach and citizenship education.

One of the most popular service programs, the shelter sealant program, involves a cross-section of IUSD, including students of all programs and class levels, staff and faculty. On a monthly basis, students from all classes, staff and faculty volunteer to take portable dental equipment to Indianapolis homeless shelters and shelters for victims of domestic violence. Combining service and learning is the key to making the experience meaningful and educational for students. In the service-learning methodology, students are helped to understand the link between their educational goals and the service that they are providing. Students participate in both structured preparation exercises prior to the service and reflection activities after their experience. In the shelter sealant program, prior to the service visit, students participate in an orientation that enables them to learn more about the population they will be serving, about the portable equipment they'll be using, and about appropriate infection control protocol in public health settings. After the visit, through reflection, students gain a greater depth of understanding about the situations in which they are working. They are forced to look at issues, such as homelessness or lack of access to dental care for low-income children, and have a greater understanding of the complexities of the situations.

Another key component of service-learning is that it creates a reciprocal learning experience whereby community partners become teachers. Social workers responsible for adults who are developmentally disabled and working in Goodwill Industries' sheltered workshop became teachers for dental students who are providing dental services for their clients as part of a fourth year elective. The volunteer mentors from Goodwill Industries authoritatively teach topics that they grasp much more profoundly than IUSD faculty who do not work exclusively with this population. They effectively lead discussions about deaf culture, autism, sign language, needed resources for people with disabilities, sensitively handling seizure disorders, pertinent legislative issues, and how to communicate with people with disabilities.

Seal Indiana is IUSD's state-wide mobile dental sealant program. The program has been in operation since March 2003. With the endorsement of Indiana Dental Association's Board of Trustees, Seal Indiana has provided services for more than 6,000 children from low-income families. Fourth year dental students and second year dental hygiene students have required service-learning rotations. Dental students serve three day rotations and dental hygiene students provide one day of required service and many of them volunteer for additional days. Students prepare for this experience by completing Web-based assignments including health policy and demographic searches. Following their rotation, students go back to the Web-site to reflect in writing on their experience, and complete a post-rotation survey and evaluation.

The objective of the students' preparation is to help them have a better grasp of the processes that shape laws and budgets that have a tremendous impact on oral health and the practice of dentistry. Federal and state policy makers control funding for dental schools, oral health research, community health centers, Medicaid reimbursement, fluoridation, dental practice acts and more. In addition, the present fourth year dental student will be expected to participate in the first annual IUSD Health Policy Day that is being planned in cooperation with Indiana Dental Association representatives Ed Popcheff and Jay Dziwlik. This day will be dedicated to enhancing students' knowledge about the health policy process and give them an opportunity to meet and talk with their legislators about health issues. The Seal Indiana rotation aims to help students understand their role in being an advocate for healthful public policy.

Conclusion

Dental schools have embraced the concept of community-based clinical education and have successfully integrated these activities into their curriculum. Although community-based education and service-learning have some common elements, and increasingly in dental education the two terms are being used interchangeably, the underlying focus and the instructional design employed in these two educational methodologies are significantly different. Despite the fact that many dental educators have heard of service-learning, few schools have integrated genuine service-learning activities into the curriculum.

While at first glance it appears that making the shift from community-based education to service-learning would be simple, it is actually a complex transition requiring an investment in resources, most importantly an investment in faculty development and time. However, as more undergraduate institutions are incorporating service-learning into their curricula, more students entering the health professional schools are going to be well versed in this educational approach and may well seek out dental schools that have embraced service-learning.

With all of the external pressures on the health professions as a whole and dental education in particular, a key question remains: Should dental education actively pursue service-learning? After all, this educational strategy is so new to dental education that there is little evidence that it makes a difference in the dental graduate. Moreover, the dental school curriculum is so densely packed that dental education is more often trying to decompress the curriculum, rather than add additional courses and student responsibilities.

Although there are barriers to making curricular changes in all institutions, it is important to remember that service-learning is not intended to be a stand alone course. The more integrated service-learning activities are with students' existing course of academic study, the more relevance and importance will be given to the service activities by both the faculty and students. There is no doubt that service-learning will take more of the students' time outside of the traditional classroom setting and more faculty resources. But these resources are well-spent if indeed these service-learning activities successfully promote the skills of critical thinking, life long learning, and evidence-based practice, while simultaneously facilitating the students' mastery of the course material. Of course, the benefits of service-learning are much greater than just improving critical thinking skills and reinforcing academic concepts. The uniqueness of service-learning is that it can accomplish this while at the same time fostering a broader sense of professionalism and civic responsibility and providing students the skills to deliver population-based care. Hence, the key question to be asked perhaps is more appropriately phrased: "Can dental education afford not to invest in service-learning?" In order to answer that question, individual dental schools and dental education as a whole must ask what the next generation of dental professionals should aspire to, and whether, as a profession, we see it as our obligation to reduce oral health disparities and make available effective oral health care to all in need of such care.

Bibliography

American Association for Higher Education: Series on Service-Learning in the Disciplines. 1990. National and Community Service Act of 1990

Astin AW & Sax LJ. How Undergraduates Are Affected By Service Participation. *Journal of College Student Development* 1998, 39(3): 251-263

Bailit H. Community-based clinical education program. Major findings and recommendations. *Journal of Dental Education* 1999, 63(12): 981-989

Bringle R & Hatcher J. A Service Learning Curriculum for Faculty. *The Michigan Journal of Community Service Learning*, 1995, Fall: 112-122

ADA-CODA (American Dental Association Commission on Dental Accreditation). *Accreditation Standards for Predoctoral Programs.* Chicago: American Dental Association, 1998; revised 2004. On-line at http://www.ada.org/prof/ed/accred/standards/predoc.pdf (access verified on 10/31/05)

Council on Graduate Medical Education. *Report to Congress.* Washington DC: Government Printing Office, 1995

Driscoll A, Holland B, Gelmon S & Kerrigan, S. An Assessment Model for Service-Learning: Comprehensive Case Studies of Impact on Faculty, Students, Community, and Institutions. *Michigan Journal of Community Service Learning* 1996, 3: 66-71

Eyler JS. Reflection: Linking Service and Learning –Linking Students and Communities. *Journal of Social Issues* 2002, 58(3): 517-534

Eyler JS & Giles DE Jr. *Where's the Learning in Service-Learning?* San Francisco CA: Jossey-Bass, Inc., 1999

Eyler JS, Giles DE, Jr, Stenson C & Gray C. *At A Glance: What We Know about The Effects of Service-Learning on College Students, Faculty, Institutions and Communities, 1993-2000: Third Edition.* Campus Compact, 2001

Field MJ (Ed.). *Dental Education at the Crossroads.* Washington DC: National Academy Press, 1995

Furco A. Service learning: A balanced approach to experiential education. In Raybuck J & Taylor B (Eds.). *Expanding Boundaries: Service and Learning.* Washington DC: Corporation for National Service, 1996

Haden, N., Catalanotto F., Alexander, C. et al. *Improving the Oral Health Status of All Americans: Roles and Responsibilities of Academic Dental Institutions: The Report of the ADEA President's Commission*, 2003.

Henshaw MM, Frankl CS, Bolden AJ, Mann ML, Kranz SM, Hughes BL. Community-based Dental Education at Boston University School of Dental Medicine. *Journal of Dental Education* 1999, 63(12): 933-937

Howard J (Ed.). *Michigan Journal of Community Service Learning: Service-Learning Course Design Workbook.* University of Michigan: OCSL Press, 2001; pp. 16-19

Institute of Medicine. *Dental Education at the Crossroads: Challenges and Change.* Washington DC: National Academy Press, 1995

Mofidi M, Strauss R, Pitner L & Sandler E. Dental Students' Reflections on Their Community-Based Experiences: The Use of Critical Incidents. *Journal of Dental Education* 2003, 67(5): 515-23

National Society for Experiential Education. *Parital List of Experiential Learning Terms and Their Definitions.* Raleigh NC: National Society for Experiential Education, 1994

Norbeck JS, Connolly C & Koerner J (Eds.). *Caring and Community: Concepts and Models for Service-Learning in Nusring.* Washington DC: American Association for Higher Education, 1998

Pew Health Professions Commission. *Recreating Health Professional Practice for a New Century: the Fourth Report of the Pew Health Professions Commission.* San Francisco: Pew Health Professions Commission, December 1998

Seifer SD, Hermanns K & Lewis J (Eds.). *Concepts and Models for Service-Learning in Medical Education.* Washington DC: American Association for Higher Education, 2000

Pamela Zarkowski

Oral Health Disparities:
A Proposal for Educational Change

Introduction

Addressing oral health disparities and improving the oral health status of all citizens of the United States requires a multifaceted approach. Dental professional education, including predoctoral, graduate and allied dental education, must refocus its approach to the entire spectrum of the educational process. Prior to outlining recommendations for a change in educational approaches, it is important to briefly review the current status of oral health in the United States.

A landmark publication, *Oral Health America: A Report of the Surgeon General* (US Dept. of Health and Human Services 2000), provides a valuable summary of the current status of oral health in the United States. The report reveals that the burden of oral diseases "is disproportionate among the U.S. population. Certain ethnic and racial minorities, elderly, disabled and medically compromised have a disproportionate amount of the disease." The Report provides epidemiological and other data to support its findings (see Table 1, next page).

In addition to the Surgeon General's Report, other entities interested in assessing the current oral health status in the United States utilize the concept of "grading" the fifty States. During 2000-2003, Oral Health America evaluated the 50 states and the District of Columbia on their performance in prevention of oral health disease, access to dental care, and health status. The report states: "States with straight-A potential are struggling to advance" (Oral Health American 2003, p. 4). Oral Health America determined that the overall grade for all states was average, in the C range. The report card for the three-year period improved from a C – earned in 2000 to a C grade in both 2002 and 2003.

There certainly had been concerns about the oral health status of the citizens of the United States prior to 2000 and the publication of the Surgeon General's Report. Attempts were made to address oral health

Table 1: Major findings of "Oral Health America: A Report of the Surgeon General"

- Oral diseases and disorders in and of themselves affect health and well being throughout life.
- Safe and effective measures exist to prevent the most common dental diseases-dental caries and periodontal diseases
- Lifestyle behaviors that affect general health such as tobacco use, excessive alcohol use and poor dietary choices affect oral and craniofacial health as well.
- There are profound and consequential oral health disparities within the US population
- More information is needed to improve America's oral health and eliminate health disparities.
- The mouth reflects the general health and well-being.
- Oral diseases and conditions are associated with other health problems.
- Scientific research is the key to further reduction in the burden of diseases and disorders that affect the face, mouth and teeth.

Source: U.S. Dept. of Health and Human Services. Oral Health in America: A Report of the Surgeon General. Rockville, MD: USDHHS, NIDCR, NIH, 2000.

disparities on local, regional, and national levels through legislation, education, and the efforts of community focused advocacy groups and health professions associations. However, the impact on oral health status was limited. Following the publication of the Surgeon General's Report, a number of new initiatives to address oral health disparities have occurred. Examples include national legislation such as The Healthcare Safety Net amendments as well as individual state initiatives and legislative efforts. Collaborative partnerships with educational institutions, industry and community-based groups are also evident. There has been financial support through the efforts of philanthropic groups such as Robert Wood Johnson Foundation and dental association sponsored programs. Conferences and professional meetings have chosen oral health as a primary theme as demonstrated by the 2000 conference titled *Face of the Child.*

Various reports and publications continue to outline goals on improving oral health status. *Healthy People 2010* provides a list of objectives related to oral health with specific outcomes stated. Another outgrowth of the Surgeon General's Report is the 2002 publication National Call to Action (US Department of Health and Human Services 2003). National Call emphasizes six action elements to address the oral health disparities problem. The National Call lists the elements and strategies to meet the "action" recommendations. The five action elements (Table 2) are proposed to stimulate a response from individuals and groups best positioned to act.

Table 2. A National Call to Action To Promote Oral Health

Action 1: Change Perceptions of Oral Health
Action 2: Overcome Barriers by Replicating Effective Programs and Proven Effects
Action 3: Build the Science Base and Accelerate Science Transfer
Action 4: Increase Oral Health Workforce Diversity, Capacity and Flexibility
Action 5: Increase Collaborations

Source: US Department of Health and Human Services. A National Call to Action To Promote Oral Health. Rockville, MD: US Department of Health and Human Services, Public Health Service, Centers for Disease Control and Prevention and The National Institutes of Health, National Institute of Dental and Craniofacial Research. NIH Publication No. 03-5303, May 2003

Those targeted to respond include community leaders, volunteers, health care professionals, research investigators, policy makers and public and private agencies.

A publication by the American Dental Education Association (ADEA) in March 2003 also addresses the issue of oral health disparities from an educational perspective. The publication, *ADEA Commission on Improving Oral Health Status of All Americans: Roles and Responsibilities of Academic Institutions*, reviews an educational institution's obligations from an ethical and moral viewpoint. The report emphasizes two guiding principles for academic institutions. The first is the obligation to contribute to the common good and the second is the dental profession's obligation as a moral community. Common good, as it relates to access to care, requires replacing the ethic of individual rights with an ethic of the common good (Callahan 2003). As professionals we must challenge ourselves, as members of the same community, to further those goals we share in common. The interest in achieving those goals recognizes and respects the freedom of individuals to pursue their own goals. The common good requires having the social systems, institutions, and environments that work in a manner that benefits all people. The ADEA report cited DePaola's recommendation to educational institutions to contribute to the common good (1998). DePaola's emphasized expanding the community capacity for enhancing wellness; expanding community-based education and clinical care, which is, taking dental education into the community. He also challenged dental institutions to engage in health care reform debate to accomplish change. An additional recommendation was partnering with community leaders, the private sector, and state and city government to attack socioeconomic, psychological environmental determinants of health and assist in empowering the community to self-actualization. Recognizing the importance of research in the mission of all institutions, he highlighted the need to conduct research programs that model social responsibility.

Referencing medical ethicist Edmund Pellegrino, the report also described the dental profession's membership as part of a moral community. The members of a moral community are bound to each other by a set of commonly held ethical commitments whose purpose is to something other than mere self-interest (Bulger & McGovern 2001). Pellegrino's recommendations to medical care providers ring true to dental providers as well. He suggests that as members of a moral community, health care providers must recognize the vulnerability of the patient and the inequality in the relationship. Based on these two factors, the provider has a professional responsibility to protect the patient. The relationship is also influenced by the interaction between the provider and patient and the nature and complexity of medical decisions. The interface between the professional's technical skills and recognition of the patient's moral beliefs and requests is a key element in the health care decisions that are made. Pellegrino suggests that because of the specialized knowledge and training characteristic to medicine, specific obligations must be fulfilled. The obligation to care for the ill flows from the fact that society traditionally funds the educational experience. Thus, the learner is obligated to provide care to benefit society, guided by accreditation and other standards to safeguard the public. Moral complicity is the final safeguard of patient's well-being.

How does the discussion of common good and membership in a moral community, focused on improving the well-being of patients, apply to dental and allied dental education? The student must be prepared to enter the oral health care profession as a member of the moral community. The principles guiding the education of a dentist or allied dental professional are based on the concept that access to basic oral health care is a human right and the oral health care delivery system must serve the common good. In addition, the oral health care needs of vulnerable populations have a unique priority. In addition to possessing the appropriate knowledge and skill set, there is an obligation to have a diverse and competent workforce. Thus, the role of dental education is to implement changes in educational approaches, and change the next generation of practitioners. This can be accomplished by refocusing education to serve the interests of the public in education, research, and service mission of institutions. For example, if we assume that dental and dental hygiene professionals must strive to contribute to the common good, the skill set of dental providers must be expanded to better contribute as a member of an interdisciplinary provider team. Oral and general health delivery models cannot be isolated educationally or in practice. Stronger linkages among primary care dentistry, medicine, and public health are necessary to allow both interdisciplinary and cross-disciplinary training. Scholarly journals and other sources of lifelong learning opportunities must also provide a source of evidence that is "cross trained." Most importantly, dental professionals must recognize their obligation to lead in changing educational models, professional perspectives and political environments.

Addressing oral health disparities issues, while satisfying the need to contribute to the common good, requires educational institutions to embrace mission synthesis as a guiding framework for outcomes planning. Mission synthesis involves intellectual growth accompanied by the acquisition of social and emotional life skills. The emphasis on these skills provides the basis for meaningful and constructive consequences in the lives of students and the communities of which they are members. The demands of good citizenship, aimed at the common good, and the demands of a professional career are similar. They both require social and emotional maturity, capacity to communicate well and an ability to work with others toward a common purpose.

Educational institutions traditionally highlight three aspects in their mission: research, teaching, and service. In order to accomplish mission synthesis, three different concepts are proposed: *discovery, learning, and engagement.* Discovery encompasses community-based scholarship and the development of new knowledge. Learning links educational goals with professional life skills. The emphasis is on service-learning and problem based learning using community-based models and issues. Engagement refers to community-institutional alliances and partnerships to meet educational and service goals and objectives.

To accomplish the task of redirecting the educational experience of dental and allied dental students, one must consider the entire spectrum of the professional students' experience and practice, that is, consider selecting students with an interest in community-based care and seek to engage practitioners, throughout their professional careers, in contributing to the common good. A moniker capturing this suggestion would be "from prerequisite to obit," that is, from the recruitment and acceptance to dental school, to the endpoint of one's professional career.

As mentioned, redirecting professional education and its outcomes requires first of all rethinking the applicant assessment process. The criteria for the appropriate selection of incoming students in professional schools must be evaluated and potentially expanded. Candidates could be assessed using different assessment tools. For example, a candidate could be asked to respond to an essay topic emphasizing outreach or community-based activities. Interview questions could include seeking information about skill and interest in contributing to the common good. Recruitment literature could highlight the institution's commitment to recruit and retain professional students interested in utilizing their talents and expertise to better serve the community. Campus visits may include a visit to outreach clinics or shadowing of students currently providing care in community-based clinics or sites. Orientation activities would begin the student's introduction to the theme of contributing to the well-being of a community through various activities including cultural competence and sensitivity training. A White Coat ceremony, in addition to emphasizing a welcome to the profession, could review the professional obligation to be part of a moral community of health care providers. Potential and incoming students must observe the institution's commitment to diversity. In addition to a diverse faculty that can serve as mentors and role models, community-based practitioners can also be linked to the institution to assist the students in their academic program and community focused education.

The environment of the educational institution provides an additional avenue for supporting the institution's commitment to a mission synthesis that includes discovery, learning, and engagement. Educational institutions must model interdisciplinary interactions. Faculty recruitment and retention, for both full – and part-time faculty, should attempt to identify and hire individuals with goals similar to the institutions as it relates to community and the common good. Faculty assessment and recognition should be rethought to include rewards for discovery and community engagement. Community advisors, including non-dental personnel, can be included as members of appropriate committees or task forces, to assist the institution to better educate and thus serve the community. Simply stated, there is a need to show institutional commitment to the common good as a consistent thread in recruitment of students, curriculum planning and implementation, committee and faculty appointments, school sponsored programs, research if applicable, and annual reports and alumni events.

Curriculum change is needed as well. Traditionally, dental and allied education includes biomedical, clinical, and behavioral sciences. The 2001-2002 American Dental Association (ADA) dental curriculum clock hour report highlights that the largest percentage of clock hours focused on operative dentistry at 612.6 whereas community dentistry/public health had an average of 157.1 clock hours. Suggestions for curriculum reform should consider community-based sciences in addition to the three traditional areas of biomedical, dental, and behavioral sciences. The community-based sciences, with the integration of a socio-behavioral and cultural curriculum, would satisfy the need to keep a community focus care threaded throughout the educational experience. The focus on recognition that oral health can be achieved with patient engagement and interventions, rather then solely relying on surgical and pharmacological approaches would reinforce the diverse approaches to patient assessment and care that are important to professional student development. The idea of refocusing the emphasis of education on community-based themes is apparent in health professions literature and should be considered by dental and allied dental educational institutions.

As educational institutions consider curriculum reform, a review of the Competencies for the 21st Century, as suggested by the Pew Health Professions Commission (O'Neil 1998), provides an important source of recommendations highlighted in Table 3. The Pew Health Professions

Commission suggestions were published almost a decade ago and remain important in today's health care environment (Table 3). The competencies

Table 3. Competencies for the 21st Century

• Embrace a personal ethic of social responsibility and service
• Exhibit ethical behavior in all professional activities
• Provide evidence based, clinically competent care
• Incorporate the multiple determinants of health in clinical care
• Apply knowledge of the new sciences
• Demonstrate critical thinking, reflection and problem solving skills
• Understand the role of primary care
• Rigorously practice preventive health care
• Integration population based care and service into practice
• Improve access to health care for those with unmet needs
• Practice relationship centered care with individuals and families
• Provide culturally sensitive care to a diverse society
• Partner with communities in health care decisions
• Use communication and IT effectively and appropriately
• Work in interdisciplinary teams
• Ensure care that balances individual professional, system and societal needs
• Practice leadership
• Take responsibility for quality of care and health outcomes on all levels
• Contribute to the continuous improvement of the health care system
• Advocate for public policy that promotes and protects the health of the public
• Continue to learn and to health others to learn

Source: O'Neil, EH and The Pew Health Professions Commission Recreating Health Professional Practice for a New Century, Fourth Report of the Pew Health Professions Commission, Executive Summary, San Francisco, CA Dec. 1998

highlight personal qualities including an ethical commitment to social service. The Pew Health Professions Commission suggests educational strategies important to the development of culturally competent skilled practitioners, capable of collaboration in order to provide needed oral health services. There is also an expectation that the health professional is competent in assessing and contributing to improving the quality of health care and the health care delivery system.

Redirecting the dental curriculum will require decompression to allow the introduction of new skill and knowledge sets. To accomplish the education of a 21st century dental provider, the focus must be on both patient and family centered care with an emphasis on health promotion in oral and general health. This is supported by an increased understanding of oral-systemic health linkages and behavioral and social determinants of health outcomes. As part of the strategies to provide interdisciplinary care, cross-training is necessary (e.g., pediatric dentistry training for non-pediatric professionals). Non-traditional providers must be considered as a source of assessment and care, especially rethinking the roles of allied personnel and their role in oral and general health delivery. Educational strategies should include service-learning, education about injury prevention, cultural competence, social sensitivity and ethics. Educational modules addressing health beliefs and practices, as well as an introduction to basic skills of languages other than English must be found in all curricula. These new developments in dental education must also be paralleled in medical education. Medical education must expand the oral health knowledge and skills of all primary care practitioners as well as provide opportunities for dental students and dental hygiene students to participate in clerkships in areas of medicine related to oral health or oral health delivery. Most assuredly, each of these suggestions requires a shift in the current educational paradigm and, in some instances, radical change. However, change is necessary to meet the unmet needs.

Of course, the outlined changes in competency listings must also be implemented, which is potentially even more difficult than listing them. Implementation strategies must be supported on multiple levels including altering accreditation standards, educational and assessment mechanisms, outcome priorities, continuing education requirements, and professional codes of ethics. The theme of addressing oral health disparities and access to care issues must be a common thread in multiple aspects of professional education and lifelong learning. Examples of promising successful strategies are:

• Develop and support of new models of oral health care delivery which may include expanding the knowledge and skill base of allied dental professionals and non-dental personnel

• Educate dental and allied dental professionals to assume new roles in prevention, detection, and early recognition of broad range of complex diseases
• Make service-learning integral to all educational programs
• Change accreditation standards to reflect a new emphasis with an updated set of standards
• Change professional codes to better reflect a commitment to addressing access issues as an ethical obligation
• Publish and disseminate facts with specific suggestions about the role of practitioners in addressing unmet needs
• Change state continuing education requirements and licensure renewal obligations to include service and education to underserved

So far, our focus has been on dental education. However, it is also important to consider the potential role of allied dental professionals and rethink how they might contribute to the access issue in collaboration with their dental colleagues. Allied dental education is characterized by a curriculum that prepares graduates in the traditional skills and knowledge necessary to practice dental hygiene. If we are committed to rethinking the model of oral health care delivery, allied dental professionals are a source of "personpower" not to be ignored. Dental hygienists could be trained to become mid-level practitioners (as already implemented in countries other than the United States) with the appropriate skill set to provide needed oral health services, including basic restorative care not requiring doctoral level training. Educating such a mid-level allied dental professional will require innovative curricular changes, possibly including the kinds of externships that are part of the medical curriculum.

The changes in the education of the allied dental professional may include the incorporation of a series of educational tracks, developed within the dental hygiene program, requiring the student to have educational experiences in collaboration with public health and community-based entities, medicine, government, and industry. Career pathway choices for the allied dental professional might include that of:

• *Provider*: preventive and simple restorative skills
• *Community focused*: knowledge of community-based approaches to assessment, planning, and provision of care as well as the economic, political, legislative implications

• *Interdisciplinary health team member*: education and experiences as part of the "wellness" team

• *Educators/mentors*: both in the classroom/clinic/outreach setting and in "practice"

• *Researcher*: contributing to the community-based research knowledge base

• *Change agent/advocate*: politically aware and astute to contribute to legislative and policy changes necessary to address oral health disparities and future issues

Depending on the track taken, a more appropriate professional title for such an allied practitioner may be Oral Health Specialist (OHS).

A change as dramatic as the development of a mid-level practitioner, or oral health specialist, requires purposeful curriculum assessment, change, and implementation. In addition to modifications in how and what allied health professionals are taught, such a change in the skill and knowledge set of what was perceived, as a "traditional dental hygienist" will also demand a redefinition of the dental team members' roles and responsibilities. Finally, changes will be necessary in accreditation requirements and licensure requirements. But if oral health disparities are to be addressed, the potential role of a "different" type of allied dental professional cannot be ignored.

As proposed earlier, to address the demands of oral health care delivery, the commitment must be from prerequisite to "obit." Thus, alumni and professional organizations are a critical resource to educate and motivate licensed oral health care providers to join in the task. A commitment to serving the underserved must be evident post graduation and consistently throughout the professional's career and even into retirement. The potential for both practicing and retired oral health care providers to contribute is immense. However, it is important that all dental graduates, and particularly those not yet exposed to such a revised curriculum, participate in lifelong learning opportunities to enhance and update their competencies. This should include continuing education courses that highlight changing patterns of disease, cultural competence, health belief models and other topics that sensitize the practitioner to the broad and diverse patient population requiring care. Continuing education requirements could also be expanded to include credit for volunteer service to underserved populations. Various "levels" of community service with appropriate recognitions for attainment of each level could be developed. Either a professional association or alumni association could institute these levels. Alternatively, codes of ethics, whether nationally or by state, could require an ethical requirement to provide "pro bono" service to patients (similar to existing requirements in legal codes of ethics). This change would codify the requirement to provide care to those who otherwise could or would not seek it from traditional private practice settings.

Finally, educational change must be complimented by efforts for public action that results in policy change. Dental health care professionals, in their educational experiences and as licensed professionals, must be aware of the impact of government activism that is necessary to achieve equity in care (Edelstein 2002). Political activism can address issues of workforce, licensing, insurance coverage, oral and general health service integration and reimbursement, disease surveillance, research funding and ultimately, professional education. Public action strategies and the roles and responsibilities of the oral health professional to actively advocate for change can be included in educational programs, alumni and continuing education programs and through the efforts of professional organizations. Strategies to encourage successful policy change and political activism could include a wide range of activities, including redirecting funding support for oral health services and research, building an effective health care delivery infrastructure, and focusing on public health initiatives to combat oral health diseases. Using previously successful models to bring the public and political attention to the impact of oral health diseases, prevention and health promotion, like those used to drive immunization programs, are also a consideration.

Conclusion

A number of concepts and recommendations were made in this presentation. The basis for the proposals is the obligation of the dental profession to contribute to the common good as part of a moral community. Educators, clinicians, advocates, and others have given thoughtful consideration to directions that the health professions can and should take to address oral health disparities. Dental and allied dental education, as well as accreditation groups, licensing and regulation bodies and professional associations must consider their potential to make changes and act on that potential in a decisive and deliberate manner. It has been suggested "There is a special place in hell reserved for the morally indifferent and the safety neutral." There is a need to take the "next steps" and as dental professionals, lead to action, to truly make addressing oral health care needs a life long commitment, from prerequisite to obit, for all members of the dental team.

Bibliography

Bulger RJ & McGovern, JP (Eds.). *Physician Philosopher, the Philosophical Foundation of Medicine – Essays by Dr. Edmund Pellegrino.* Charlottesville VA: Carden Jennings, 2001

Callahan, D. Individual Good and Common Good: A Communitarian Approach to Bioethics. *Perspectives in Biology and Medecine* 2003, 46(4) 496-507, p. 297

DePaola D. Beyond the University: Leadership for the Common Good. In Haden NK & Tedesco LT. (Eds.). *Leadership for the Future: The Dental School in the University.* Washington DC: American Association of Dental Schools [now the American Dental Education Association], 94-102, 1999

Edelstein BL. External forces impacting on US health care: implication for future dental practice. *Journal of the American College of Dentists* 2002, 69(3): 39-43

Haden NK, Bailit H, Buchanan J et al. *Improving the Oral Health Status of All Americans: Roles and Responsibilities of Academic Dental Institutions. Report of the ADEA President's Commission.* Washington DC: American Dental Education Association, 2003

Oral Health America. *Keep America Smiling: The Oral Health America National Grading Project 2003.* Chicago: Oral Health America, 2003. Available on-line at: http://www.oralhealthamerica.org/pdf/2003ReportCard.pdf (access verified on 10/31/05)

O'Neil EH & The Pew Health Professions Commission Recreating Health Professional Practice for a New Century. *Fourth Report of the Pew Health Professions Commission, Executive Summary.* San Francisco, 1998

U.S. Dept. of Health and Human Services. *A National Call to Action to Promote Oral Health.* Rockville, MD: US Department of Health and Human Services, Public Health Service, Centers for Disease Control and Prevention and The National Institutes of Health, National Institute of Dental and Craniofacial Research. NIH Publication No. 03-5303, May 2003

U.S. Dept. of Health and Human Services. *Oral Health in America: A Report of the Surgeon General.* Rockville, MD: USDHHS, NIDCR, NIH, 2000. Available on-line at: http://www.surgeongeneral.gov/library/oralhealth/ (access verified on 11/3/05)

Part IV

Appendices

Appendix 1

American Dental Education Association

Improving the Oral Health Status
of All Americans:
Roles and Responsibilities
of Academic Dental Institutions

This report was first published in the *Journal of Dental Education*, 2003, 67(5): 563-583. It is also available on-line at: http://www.jdentaled. org/cgi/reprint/67/5/563.pdf. The Report has been republished here integrally with the kind permission of the American Dental Education Association. Because of repagination of the Report in this book, we urge those wishing to cite the Report to reference either of the two aforementioned original versions instead.

Association Report

Improving the Oral Health Status of All Americans: Roles and Responsibilities of Academic Dental Institutions

The Report of the ADEA President's Commission*

N. KARL HADEN, PH.D. ~ FRANK A. CATALANOTTO, D.M.D.

CHARLES J. ALEXANDER, PH.D. ~ HOWARD BAILIT, D.M.D., PH.D.

ANN BATTRELL, R.D.H., B.S. ~ JACK BROUSSARD, JR., D.D.S.

JUDITH BUCHANAN, PH.D., D.M.D. ~ CHESTER W. DOUGLASS, D.M.D., PH.D.

CLAUDE EARL FOX III, M.D., M.P.H. ~ PAUL GLASSMAN, D.D.S., M.A., M.B.A.

R. IVAN LUGO, D.M.D., M.B.A. ~ MARY GEORGE, R.D.H., M.ED.

CYRIL MEYEROWITZ, D.D.S., M.S. ~ EDWARD R. SCOTT II, D.M.D.

NEWELL YAPLE, D.D.S. ~ JACK BRESCH, M.A.L.S.

ZLATA GUTMAN-BETTS, M.A. ~ GINA G. LUKE, B.S.

MYLA MOSS, M.A., M.S.W. ~ JEANNE C. SINKFORD, D.D.S., PH.D.

RICHARD G. WEAVER, D.D.S. ~ RICHARD W. VALACHOVIC, D.M.D., M.P.H.

Abstract: Academic dental institutions are the fundamental underpinning of the nation's oral health. Education, research, and patient care are the cornerstones of academic dentistry that form the foundation upon which the dental profession rises to provide care to the public. The oral health status of Americans has improved dramatically over the past twenty-five to thirty years. In his 2000 report on oral health, the Surgeon General acknowledges the success of the dental profession in improving the oral health status of Americans over the past twenty-five years, but he also juxtaposes this success to profound and consequential disparities in the oral health of Americans. In 2002, the American Dental Education Association brought together an ADEA President's Commission of national experts to explore the roles and responsibilities of academic dental institutions in improving the oral health status of all Americans. They have issued this report and made a variety of policy recommendations, including a Statement of Position, to the 2003 ADEA House of Delegates. The commission's work will help guide ADEA in such areas as: identifying barriers to oral health care, providing guiding principles for academic dental institutions, anticipating workforce needs, and improving access through a diverse workforce and the types of oral health providers, including full utilization of allied dental professionals and collaborations with colleagues from medicine.

*The commission was appointed in 2001 by ADEA President Pamela Zarkowski and continued its work through 2002 with Dr. David Johnsen as ADEA President. The commission was chaired by Dr. Frank A. Catalanotto.

Dr. Haden is Associate Executive Director and Director, ADEA Center for Educational Policy and Research; Dr. Catalanotto is Professor, Department of Pediatric Dentistry, University of Florida College of Dentistry; Dr. Alexander is Associate Dean for Student Affairs, University of California, San Francisco School of Dentistry; Dr. Bailit is Professor Emeritus and Director, University of Connecticut Health Policy Center; Ms. Battrell is Director, Dental Hygiene Education, American Dental Hygienists Association; Dr. Broussard is a general dentist in South Pasadena, CA; Dr. Buchanan is Associate Dean for Academic Affairs, University of Pennsylvania School of Dental Medicine; Dr. Douglass is Chair, Oral Health Policy and Epidemiology, Harvard School of Dental Medicine; Dr. Fox is Director, Johns Hopkins Urban Health Institute; Dr. Glassman is Associate Dean for Information and Education Technology and Director, Advanced General Dentistry Residency, University of the Pacific School of Dentistry; Dr. Lugo is Associate Dean for Institutional Relations and Community Affairs and Acting Chair, Department of Dental Informatics, Temple University School of Dentistry; Prof. George is Director, Allied Dental Educational Programs, University of North Carolina-Chapel Hill School of Dentistry; Dr. Meyerowitz is Chair and Director, University of Rochester School of Medicine and Dentistry; Dr. Scott is Immediate Past President, National Dental Associaton and a general and cosmetic dentist in Tallahassee, FL; Dr. Yaple is an oral and maxillofacial surgeon and Past President, AADE; Mr. Bresch is Associate Executive Director and Director, ADEA Center for Public Policy and Advocacy; Ms. Gutman-Betts is Program Manager, ADEA Center for Educational Research; Ms. Luke is Director, State Government Relations and Advocacy Outreach, ADEA Center for Public Policy and Advocacy; Ms. Moss is Director, Congressional Relations, ADEA Center for Public Policy and Advocacy; Dr. Sinkford is Associate Executive Director and Director, ADEA Center for Equity and Diversity; Dr. Weaver is Associate Director, ADEA Center for Educational Research; and Dr. Valachovic is ADEA Executive Director. Direct correspondence to Dr. N. Karl Haden, ADEA, 1625 Massachusetts Ave, N.W., Washington, DC 20036; 202-667-9433 phone; 202-667-0642 fax; hadenk@adea.org.

Academic dental institutions are the fundamental underpinning of the nation's oral health. As educational institutions, dental schools, allied dental education, and advanced dental education programs are the source of a qualified workforce, influencing both the number and type of oral health providers. As centers of discovery, academic dental institutions ensure that oral health practice evolves through research and the transfer of the latest science. As providers of care, academic dental institutions are a safety net for the underserved, centers of pioneering tertiary care, and contributors to the well-being of their communities through accessible oral health care services. The interlocking missions of education, research, and patient care are the cornerstones of academic dentistry that form the foundation upon which the dental profession rises to provide care to the public.

The oral health status of Americans has improved dramatically over the past twenty-five to thirty years. Successive cohorts of the population by age are experiencing less dental disease. The mean number of decayed, missing, or filled surfaces of teeth of U.S. children ages five to seventeen has declined from 7.1 to 2.5. Approximately 55 percent of children five to seventeen have had no tooth decay in their permanent teeth,[1] and the number of school-aged children receiving dental sealants has increased in recent years.[2] The mean number of teeth present in adults ages eighteen to seventy-four has trended upwards in all age groups. The percent of all adults who are edentulous has fallen from 14.7 to 7.7 percent.[1] Over the past twenty years, deaths resulting from oral and pharyngeal cancers have declined by nearly 25 percent, and new cases have declined by 10 percent.[1] Community water fluoridation is hailed as one of the great public health achievements of the twentieth century.

Oral Health in America: A Report of the Surgeon General, published in the year 2000, is a landmark in the history of oral health. For the first time, the Surgeon General of the United States identified oral health as integral to general health, saying: "Oral health is a critical component of health and must be included in the provision of health care and the design of community programs."[1] Table 1 provides a summary of the report's major findings. The Surgeon General acknowledges the success of the dental profession, but juxtaposes this success with profound and consequential disparities in the oral health of Americans.

As indicated in the Surgeon General's report, the burden of oral diseases and conditions is disproportionate among the United States population

(Appendix 1). Other recent reports corroborate these findings.[2,4-6] Underserved individuals and families living below the poverty level experience more dental decay and are more likely to have untreated teeth than those who are economically better off. Black/African Americans and Hispanic/Latinos have higher proportions of untreated teeth than their white counterparts. A higher proportion of lower income individuals, at all ages, have evidence of gingivitis and periodontal disease than do middle or higher income individuals. A higher percentage of individuals below the poverty level are edentulous than those above. Elderly, disabled, and medically compromised populations have a disproportionate amount of oral disease, from dental caries to periodontal disease and oral cancer. Oral cancer is the sixth most common cancer in U.S. males and ranks as the fourth most common cancer among African American men.[7] While water fluoridation is a proven means to reduce dental caries, many areas of the country remain unflouridated, resulting in poorer oral health in those communities. Moreover, dental caries are far from eradicated even in fluoridated communities.

While the adequacy of the aggregate number of dentists to meet the nation's oral health needs is unclear, disparities are prominently reflected in the geographical distribution of dentists. The number of Dental Health Professions Shortage Areas designated by the U.S. Health Resources and Services Administration (HRSA) Bureau of Health Professions has grown from 792 in 1993 to 1,895 in 2002. In 1993, HRSA estimated that 1,400 dentists were needed in these areas; by 2002, the number of dentists needed had grown to more than 8,000. More than 40,122,000 people live in Dental Health Professions Shortage Areas.[8]

State legislatures are increasingly turning to alternatives to the current delivery system to address access issues for underserved populations. For example, the California legislature has mandated that the State Board of Dental Examiners certify foreign dental schools so their graduates can take the state licensing examination.[9] More recent legislation in California mandates that the state board bring Mexican dentists into California to work in underserved settings.[10] Over the past decade, many states have addressed access by increasing the use of dental hygienists, permitting hygienists to provide care in specific settings under unsupervised practice or less restrictive supervision.[11]

In 2002, the American Dental Education Association (ADEA) brought together a commission of national experts to explore the roles and responsibilities of academic dental institutions in improving the oral health status of all Americans. This report is based upon their deliberations. While not intended to provide an exhaustive analysis of the plethora of issues and studies related to the growing access to oral health care problem, this report provides the background for the Statement of Position and other policy recommendations proposed by the commission to ADEA.

The report is organized around the following major themes:

1. Need and Demand: Identifying Barriers to Oral Health Care
2. Access to Oral Health Care: Guiding Principles for Academic Dental Institutions
3. Anticipating Workforce Needs
4. The Patient Care Mission of Academic Dental Institutions
5. Improving Access Through a Diverse Workforce
6. Removing Barriers to a More Diverse Workforce
7. Types of Oral Health Providers

In its conclusion, the report contains a series of recommendations in five different areas with the purpose of focusing academic dentistry on a common set of strategies to improve the oral health of all Americans, especially the underserved.

Table 1. Major findings of the surgeon general's report

• Oral diseases and disorders in and of themselves affect health and well-being throughout life.

• Safe and effective measures exist to prevent the most common dental diseases—-dental caries and periodontal diseases.

• Lifestyle behaviors that affect general health such as tobacco use, excessive alcohol use, and poor dietary choices affect oral and craniofacial health as well.

• There are profound and consequential oral health disparities within the U.S. population.

• More information is needed to improve America's oral health and eliminate health disparities.

• The mouth reflects general health and well-being.

• Oral diseases and conditions are associated with other health problems.

• Scientific research is key to further reduction in the burden of diseases and disorders that affect the face, mouth, and teeth.

Need and Demand:
Identifying Barriers to Oral Health Care

The Surgeon General's Report demonstrates the need for oral health care and the impact of poor oral health on individuals, communities, and society at large (Appendix 1). As the term is used in this report, *need* for oral care is based on whether an individual requires clinical care or attention to maintain full functionality of the oral and craniofacial complex. The disproportionate burden of oral diseases and disorders indicates that specific population groups are in greater need of oral health care. *Demand* is generally understood as the amount of a product or service that users can and would buy at varying prices. The extent of oral health care disparities clearly indicates that many of those in *need* of oral health care do not *demand* oral health care. While universal access to oral health care is frequently identified as an admirable goal, practical considerations often lead to the conclusion that it is, in fact, unattainable given present resources. Currently in the United States, the provision of health care services, including oral health care services, is treated like a manufactured commodity, with access, price, and quality subject to the incentives that dictate a competitive marketplace. In such a marketplace economy, the variety of factors influencing demand gives way to one major factor: the ability to pay for services rendered.

Health care, and by implication, oral health care, should be treated differently than marketplace commodities. First, oral health is a part of general health. Health is a human good experienced by all humans, vital to human flourishing and basic to the pursuit of life, liberty, and happiness. Secondly, the science and knowledge about oral health is not the property of any individual or organization; rather, society grants individuals the opportunity to learn at academic dental institutions with an assumed contract that this knowledge will benefit the society that granted the opportunity to obtain it. Thirdly, the practice of all health care is based on the commitment to the good of the patient. To ensure that those in need receive care, attention must focus on the variety of barriers that limit access to oral health care and thereby negatively affect demand, barriers such as:

Knowledge and Values

- Those in need of oral health care lack knowledge about the prevention of oral health diseases and awareness of their clinical need.[1,4]
- The general public often does not appreciate the importance of oral health and perceives it as independent from and secondary to general health.[1,4]
- Many public policymakers do not understand or value oral health as a part of general health and healthcare, thereby marginalizing oral health to a policy issue of lower priority.[1,4,13]

Availability of Care

- Many in need do not have access to a provider within their community due to the maldistribution of dentists, the consequent geographic disparity of oral health providers, and other factors as noted below.[1,5,8,14]
- Many underserved population groups cannot secure an appointment with an oral health provider because some oral health providers are unwilling to care for the underserved due to low reimbursement rates, lack of insurance, insufficient practice capacity to accept additional patients, and other factors.[15-17]
- Much of the oral health workforce is unprepared to render culturally competent care to racially and ethnically diverse populations, to people with complex medical and psychosocial conditions or developmental and other disabilities, to the very young, and to the aged.[17-19]

Ability to Pay and Lack of Insurance

- Because of their economic status, some under-served are unable to pay for oral health care services.[20-23]
- Most underserved groups lack dental insurance.[1,4,21,22]
- Low reimbursement rates for public programs such as Medicaid and the State Children's Health Insurance Program (SCHIP) dissuade providers from rendering care to the poor and to children.[20-25]
- Nearly 75 percent of dentists do not treat Medicaid-insured patients.[26]
- Because dental care is not covered by Medicare, many of the elderly are deterred from seeking oral health care.[19,24,25]

Regulatory Considerations

+ Most state laws and regulations restrict access to care by limiting the type of practice settings and imposing restrictive supervision requirements on allied dental personnel, limits and requirements that are incommensurate with the education and experience of many allied dental professionals.[6,27,28]

Systemic Barriers within Health Care Delivery

+ The underlying barrier to good oral health for the underserved is an oral health care system that has changed little over the past century. The traditional model of oral and dental care, namely that of the solo practice dentist assisted by allied dental personnel providing care under the dentist's supervision, is no longer adequate to address the nation's oral health needs.[1,23]

As academic dental institutions, the dental profession, policymakers, and other stakeholders reconsider the delivery system, the traditional model of oral and dental care will continue to serve an important role in meeting the nation's oral health needs; but a number of other models must be supported, developed, and employed to ensure oral health care for all Americans. The separation of oral health from systemic health in the U.S. health care system has resulted in a disciplinary chasm between oral health providers and the rest of medical care to the detriment of the patient, especially the underserved. This system must be challenged and changed. Academic dental institutions provide not only an alternative model through their clinics, but they also play a basic role in developing new models and recruiting future providers to work within these practice settings.

Access to Oral Health Care:
Guiding Principles for Academic Dental Institutions

The goal of ensuring access to oral health care for all Americans follows from the concept of the American society as a good society, from the role of academic dental institutions in meeting the common good, and from the moral responsibilities of the professional community of oral health providers. The good society can be understood as one that relies on a moral infrastructure—families, schools, faith communities, and other institutions—and informal social controls to promote substantive values.[29,30] Members of the good society are expected to contribute to causes that improve all of society rather than merely acting out of self-interest. Social institutions such as family and schools help to form the backbone of the good society. While the United States does not always meet these expectations, arguably it was the intention of the Founders and remains a national purpose that both our leaders and other members of society fulfill social responsibilities for the good of the whole.

As noted, schools play a fundamental role in the good society. In reflecting on the history of higher education in the United States, Rudolph observes that "The American college was conceived as a social investment. . . . Social purpose might also be defined as national purpose. A commitment to the republic became a guiding obligation of the American college."[31] As professional schools, including academic dental institutions, became a part of universities, they too accepted the responsibility to serve the common good.[32] In recent years, this social purpose has come under scrutiny from the public who often perceive the university's self-interest as outweighing the concern for the public good.[33-35] DePaola attributes the lack of an identifiable, public good agenda as one reason for the public's loss of confidence in higher education. He observes that both the university and the dental school, and by implication, other academic dental institutions, must establish goals for the common good, which include improving access to oral health care.[36]

At the 1998 American Association of Dental Schools Leadership Summit Conference, Hershey used the metaphor of the dental school as the "front porch" to the university, a component of the university that has extensive contact with the public and substantial potential for public service.[37] As the front porch of their parent institutions, academic dental institutions improve the oral health of all Americans by providing patient care, teaching prevention in community settings, conducting and translating research to the benefit of their communities and the nation, partnering with community leaders, including those in organized dentistry, to promote and provide care, and advocating for oral health at the local, state, and national levels. The most obvious role of academic dental institutions in meeting community, state, and national oral health needs is educating future oral health professionals. However, a major aspect of the educational process is sometimes overlooked or at least underemphasized, namely, teaching the values that prepare the student to enter a morally responsible profession.

Pellegrino refers to the medical profession as a "moral community." By implication, the dental profession, including allied dental groups, also constitutes a moral community, "one whose members are bound to each other by a set of commonly held ethical commitments and whose purpose is something other than mere self-interest." Pellegrino maintains that moral purpose arises from the nature of the activity in which the members of the community engage. He delineates four aspects of medicine, *which apply equally to dentistry*, as a special kind of human activity that gives moral status to individual members and collectively to the profession:[38]

1. **Vulnerability and inequality.** The vulnerability of the sick person and the consequent inequality that it produces into the provider-patient relationship is a fundamental result of illness. Without access to special knowledge and skill, the person in need loses freedom to pursue life's goals, to make his or her own decisions, and to help oneself. The provider has a professional and moral obligation to protect the patient in this vulnerable condition and to act in the best interest of the patient.

2. **The nature of medical decisions.** Medical decisions, including those made by dental professionals, are both technical and moral. In seeking the patient's good, the provider must respect the patient's moral beliefs and requests. At times, the provider is confronted with a conflict between the patient's physical well-being and the patient's values. Providing culturally competent care is an example of the unique interaction between technical skill and personal values that belong to the healing professions.

3. **The nature of medical knowledge.** The nature of medical knowledge creates an obligation in those who acquire and possess it. First, it is practical knowledge for the express purpose of caring for the sick. Secondly, through health professions education, especially that in the context of clinical care and its accompanying risks and opportunities, society grants the health professional the privilege to obtain special knowledge. Society also funds health professions education in unique ways, substantially different from its funding of other areas of higher education and professional education. There is an assumed contract between the learner and society that this knowledge will benefit the society that granted the opportunity to obtain it. Lastly, as with the medical professions, the dental professions manage knowledge and its application through accreditation and by establishing standards and institutions that safeguard the public.

4. **Moral complicity.** Pellegrino observes, "No order can be carried out, no policy observed, and no regulation imposed without the physician's assent. . . . He is inescapably the final safeguard of the patient's well being. The

physician is therefore de facto a moral accomplice in whatever is done that adversely affects his patient."[38] In the realm of oral health care, such moral complicity also characterizes the place of the dentist.

What do these four aspects mean for academic dentistry? Academic dental institutions are a part of this moral community. In the teacher-student relationship, academic dental institutions play a fundamental role in inculcating values that frame the dental profession's societal obligations. Academic dental institutions must prepare students to enter the oral health care profession as a member of a moral community. Being a part of this community not only means placing the interest of the patient above economic self-interest, but also participating in the organized profession.

While each dentist and each allied dental professional has a role to play in improving access, the organized dental and allied dental profession, including dental academia, must assume the leadership role in addressing access to oral health care for all Americans. Acting as a moral community, the organized professions of oral health providers have tremendous influence on state and federal policymakers, community leaders, industry, and other stakeholders to help the profession fulfill its moral duties. As part of fulfilling this public trust, the American Dental Association (ADA) in its Code of Ethics and Professional Conduct expresses the concept that "the dental profession should actively seek allies throughout society on specific activities that will help improve access to care for all."[39] The Pew Health Professions Commission in its list of competencies for the twenty-first century emphasizes a personal ethic of social responsibility and service as part of the larger issues of professional responsibility and social justice essential to improving the health of all groups of society.[40]

Recent activities by the ADA such as Give Kids a Smile National Children's Dental Access Day[41] and advocacy for dental access legislation are examples of how organized dentistry can improve care for the underserved.[42-43] New Mexico enacted legislation to improve access through "collaborative practice," allowing dental hygienists to treat patients in a variety of settings according to a protocol with a consulting dentist.[44] Another example, the Robert Wood Johnson Foundation (RWJF) $19 million Pipeline, Profession, and Practice: Community-Based Dental Education project is a partnership between a private foundation and dental schools to expand existing initiatives and to develop new ones for long-term impact on access to oral health care.[45] Academic dental institutions have a responsibility to develop the next generation of leaders for organized dentistry and the organized allied dental professions so that such efforts continue and grow in frequency and impact.

Guiding principles as a philosophy of oral health care have an enduring quality that transcends immediate problems and issues to shape the beliefs and values of the academic dental community and the professionals it educates. The following general principles are proposed to guide academic dental institutions in pursuit of their missions of education, research, and outreach to improve the oral health status of all Americans:

+ **Access to basic oral health care is a human right.** A human right is a claim that persons have on society by virtue of their being human. In the good society, individuals have a moral claim to oral health because oral health is a necessary condition for the attainment of general health, well-being, and the pursuit of other basic human rights acknowledged by the society as its aims and to which, therefore, the society is already committed. The corollary of a right is a duty. The duty to ensure basic oral health for all Americans is a shared duty that includes federal, state, community, public, and private responsibilities. The dental profession, including academic dental institutions, as the moral community entrusted by society with knowledge and skill about oral health, has the duty to lead the effort to ensure access for all Americans.

+ **The oral health care delivery system must serve the common good.** Society grants the health professions a large degree of self-regulation and governance. In return, there is an implicit contract and obligation to serve the public good. Professionalism demands placing the interest of patients above those of the profession. Economic market forces, societal pressures, and professional self-interest must not compromise the contract of the oral health provider with society. The objective of the oral health care system should be a uniform basic standard of care accessible to all.

+ **The oral health needs of vulnerable populations have a unique priority.** Every person has intrinsic human dignity. Oral health professionals must individually and collectively work to improve access to care by reducing barriers. The equitable provision of oral health care services demands a commitment to the promotion of public health, prevention, public advocacy, and the exploration and implementation of new models that involve each oral health professional in the provision of care.

✦ **A diverse and culturally competent workforce is necessary to meet the oral health needs of the nation.** The workforce of the future must be prepared to meet the needs of a diverse population. Academic dental institutions, as the source of oral health professionals, have a distinct responsibility to educate dental and allied dental professionals who are competent to care for the changing needs of our society. This responsibility includes preparing providers to care for an aging population, a racially and ethnically diverse population, and individuals with special needs. In so doing, academic dental institutions can anticipate and address unmet oral health needs in underserved populations.

These guiding principles are reflected in the major considerations that follow for improving the oral health status of all Americans.

Anticipating Workforce Needs

The ADA, in its 2001 report on the *Future of Dentistry*,[46] projected that the ratio of professionally active dentists to population would continue to decline from its peak of 60.2 per 100,000 in 1994 to 54.2 per 100,000 in 2020. However, the ADA report stated that due to expected annual increases in the productivity of the dental workforce, "The national supply of dental services is likely to increase . . . that a major increase in the aggregate number of dentists is probably not necessary at this time."[46] Added to this projection is an expectation that, with changing disease patterns and continuing improvements in the oral health of the population, fewer dentists will be required to manage the oral health care needs of even an expanding population.

Responding to a 1994 ADA-projected decline in the dentist to population ratio, the Institute of Medicine (IOM), Committee on the Future of Dental Education, in its 1995 report *Dental Education at the Crossroads*, stated that it found no compelling evidence that would allow it to recommend with confidence that dental school enrollments be increased.[47] The committee concluded that workforce planning would have to proceed with caution: that while the ratio of dentists to population was declining, there was an unestimated inherent productive capacity within the dental sector to meet increases in demand. It was also acknowledged that the history of stimulating the supply of health care providers showed little effect on reducing shortage areas or improving access to care by special or underserved populations.

The conclusions reached in the ADA and IOM reports reflect aggregate workforce numbers and capabilities. Missing from these aggregate efforts and conclusions is the evident issue that a sizable portion of the population has difficulty availing itself of needed or wanted oral health care, regardless of the current or projected number of dentists or of current or projected levels of their productivity. Missing from the various workforce scenarios is an ostensible concern in fulfilling a public trust: the professional obligation and responsibility to provide competent care for a diverse population and to improve the oral health of all groups of society.

Over the past forty years, dental schools have responded to federal construction and capitation grants, perceived shortages and surpluses of dentists, and increases and decreases in dental school applicants. The number of graduates rose almost 81 percent from 3,181 in 1965 to a peak of 5,756 in 1984. But by 1993, the number of graduates had fallen by over 34 percent to stand at 3,778 graduates, a decline that can be attributed in large part to the closure of six private dental schools between 1984 and 1994. In 2001, Northwestern University graduated its last class and closed its dental school. Two new dental schools have opened since 1997, bringing the total to fifty-five accredited dental schools, with another dental school planned to open in 2003. Through the two new dental schools and increases in dental school enrollments, the number of graduates has grown almost 16 percent from a low of 3,778 in 1993 to 4,367 in 2001.

Dental schools are located in thirty-four states, plus the District of Columbia and Puerto Rico. While sixteen states are without a dental school, many schools have agreements to accept students from those states. The source of qualified oral health workforce extends beyond dental schools. Academic dental institutions are located in every state. For example, at present there are 731 residency training programs, 348 at dental schools and 383 at nondental school sites such as hospitals. These programs include 417 dental specialty programs, 230 General Practice Residency programs, and eighty-four Advanced Education in General Dentistry residency training programs in the United States. There are over 260 dental assisting and over 260 dental hygiene programs across the nation. As of 1999/2000, there were thirty-three dental laboratory technology programs accredited by the ADA Commission on Dental Accreditation in twenty-three states.[48]

What are the responsibilities of academic dental institutions, in particular, dental schools, in ensuring a workforce of quality, size, composition, and distribution such that it has the capability of meeting the oral health requirements of all groups of society? While dental schools are a national resource, individually, the schools have a tendency to supply specific states with their dental workforce. Thus dental schools manage the supply of dentists and influence the availability of care and access to care primarily in the areas they supply with dentists. Anticipating and meeting workforce requirements and addressing disparities in access to care can best be approached by schools if they understand the workforce requirements of the areas they primarily supply, anticipate the resources necessary to fulfill expectations, and give leadership to the initiatives essential to achieving workforce goals over which they have a sense of responsibility and control. Allied dental education programs are likewise positioned to monitor workforce requirements in the areas they serve. Dental specialty programs and advanced programs must give careful attention to national trends, working closely with their parent institutions, the practicing community, accrediting bodies, and other stakeholders to meet the need for providers.

Traditionally, the primary focus of dental education has been to prepare students to enter a private practice dental office. As academic dental institutions consider future workforce requirements, the curriculum should be examined in the light of different points of entry into dental practice. Such a process should include education about the needs of special groups such as the very young, the aged, and the mentally and physically disabled, the medically compromised, and the underserved. Increased attention must be given to rendering culturally competent care. The process should involve strong guidance in the professional socialization of future practitioners and should encourage students to practice in underserved areas and to participate in outreach programs and community service.[49] Learning about public health issues and the development of public health competencies are important components of the educational experience.[17] Practical steps include exposing students to the delivery of care in a community-based setting as early as possible in the educational process. Ideally, these community-based programs are a part of an integrated health system involving dental teams and non-traditional providers such as primary care physicians and nurses.

The Patient Care Mission of Academic Dental Institutions

Patient care is a distinct mission of academic dental institutions. Academic dental institutions—dental schools, hospital-based and other advanced dental education programs not based in dental schools, and allied dental education programs—have played and will continue to play a vital role in reaching the underserved. A 1998 survey by the ADA confirmed dental schools as leaders in providing care to underserved populations. The mission of nearly 97 percent of the schools who responded to the survey included service to the community. Approximately 41 percent of patients seen in dental school clinics, including school-based and community-based clinics, were under the age of fourteen. Fifty percent of dental school clinic patients were covered by a public assistance program such as Medicare or Medicaid, and another 32 percent did not have private insurance. The majority of patients came from families whose annual income was estimated at $15,000 or below. The most frequently reported special population group receiving care at dental school clinics was low-income individuals, followed by individuals with mental, medical, or physical disabilities.[50]

Residency training clinics are a major source of dental services for underserved populations. The regulations that govern Graduate Medical Education (GME) funding for the training and education of dental residents in outpatient clinics also allow funding for stipends, benefits, and teaching costs for residents that work in community clinics. Currently, there are electronic distance education curricula under development that would allow community clinics to offer accredited programs without the need to develop a complementary didactic program, creating additional residency positions. Dental schools should encourage graduates to pursue a year of service and learning that would not only make the students more competent to provide increasingly complex care, but also serve to improve access to oral health care. ADEA should work with other organizations to advocate for a requirement that all dental graduates participate in a year of service and learning in an accredited PGY-1 program.

If regulatory bodies move further toward legislation that supports a year of postdoctoral education, as has recently happened in the state of New York, most of the new residency positions are likely to be created in community health centers, including rural health clinics, county health departments, and similar public health programs. These entities are a major source of oral health care for underserved populations. Dental education leaders must frequently inform and remind state legislatures of the importance of residency training in clinics where traditionally underserved populations seek care. ADEA, other organized dental associations, and academic dental institutions must continue to advocate for funding to increase dental residency positions and for loan forgiveness to ease the financial burden for dental graduates participating in these programs.

Oral health care at academic dental institutions has grown from care incidental to students gaining clinical competence in a variety of entry-level procedures to the institutions serving as providers of comprehensive dental care. As with medical schools and other parts of the academic health center, efficiently delivered patient-centered care is necessary for academic dental institutions to compete for and retain a patient pool for students and residents and to improve clinic and institutional productivity and revenues. At many academic dental institutions, patient care is a mandated responsibility of the parent institution as they are expected to contribute more directly to the benefit of the community as a whole, in part as exchange for the amounts of public dollars received from state and federal sources and in part of fulfilling the public trust society has granted the health professions. Academic dental institutions have moved to more efficient patient management systems, to greater use of off-site clinic facilities and community-based programs of care, and an increased responsiveness to societal priorities.

As academic dental institutions consider their patient care mission, there is one important caveat that they, the dental profession, policymakers, and other stakeholders must carefully consider: academic dental institutions alone cannot solve the access to care problems. Partners in addressing access must necessarily include the private practice community, community health centers, and state and federal policymakers. The role of academic dental institutions as a safety net should not diminish their academic purpose. Academic dental institutions have the unique role in society of educating oral health professionals, generating new knowledge, conducting and promoting basic and applied research, and providing patient care to advance education, research, and service to their communities. If forced to choose between their academic mission and their role as a safety net for the underserved, academic dental institutions must put more effort into their academic mission than in improving access. As a safety net for the underserved, academic dental institutions can be supported and even replaced by nonacademic providers and institutions. What others cannot replace is the defining academic purpose that dental schools and advanced dental education programs play in our society.

Improving Access Through a Diverse Workforce

The race and ethnic composition of the U.S. population is projected to change significantly over the next fifty years. By the middle of this century, the Black/African American population will increase from 12.1 to 13.6 percent, and the Native Americans will increase from 0.7 to 0.9 percent. Asian/Pacific Islanders will increase from 3.5 to 8.2 percent. The most significant increase will be in the Hispanic/Latino population, from 10.8 to almost 25 percent of the U.S. population. The White/Caucasian population will decline from about 73 to 53 percent.[51] Currently, about 14 percent of professionally active dentists are non-white: almost 7 percent are Asian/Pacific Islander; 3.4 percent are Black/African American; 3.3 percent are Hispanic/Latino; and 0.1 percent are Native American. About 30 percent of dentists under the age of forty are non-white. However, less than one-half of these minority dentists under forty years of age are Black/African American, Hispanic/Latino, or Native American.[52]

With these projected demographic changes, our society will need to take measures to ensure that the health care workforce is prepared to care for a more diverse population. That we are currently ill prepared to take care of the needs of an increasingly diverse society is reflected in a recent study by the Institute of Medicine (IOM). The IOM study found that racial and ethnic minorities generally receive lower quality health care than whites do, even when they have comparative insurance, income, age, and severity of conditions.[53] These findings go beyond conclusions about the impact of lower socioeconomic status on the health care of minorities found in the Surgeon General's report on oral health and Healthy People 2010 to signify a much larger problem.[1,2] Possible reasons for these disparities include an inequitable health care system, cultural differences resulting in different rates of utilization, and lack of cultural competence among providers to care for a diverse patient pool.

Physician studies have shown that minority physicians can improve access to medical care and are more likely than white physicians to practice in communities where physician shortages exist and to treat minority and poorer patients.[54] Data from the ADA corroborate that minority dentists are more likely to care for minority patients (Table 2). Presumably, minority patients are more comfortable seeing providers of the same ethnic and racial group. Perhaps this level of comfort is found in the ability of minority providers to give more culturally sensitive care. Assuming that increasing the number of minority health care providers will increase the use of health care services by minority groups,[54-57] actions must be taken to secure the oral health of the nation in the decades to come through a diverse workforce.

While the percentage of minority dental students has significantly increased since 1980, from about 13 to 34 percent, this increase is primarily due to the growth in the number of Asian/Pacific Islander students. The number of Asian/Pacific Islander students grew from 5 percent of first-year enrollees in 1980 to nearly 24 percent of the 1999 first-year enrollees. The number of underrepresented minorities, defined as racial and ethnic populations that are underrepresented relative to the number of individuals who are members of the population involved,[58] has grown less than three percentage points during the same time period. Year 2000 saw slight increases in the underrepresented minority student enrollment for both Black/African American (4.79 percent from 4.68 percent in 1999) and Hispanic (5.33 percent from 5.28 percent in 1999) students.[59] The only group that approached parity with its representation in the U.S. population is Native Americans. In 2000 this group was 0.65 percent of dental enrollment and 0.7 percent of the U.S. population.

Converting the percentage of minority composition of first-year enrollment to the actual number of minority first-time enrollees presents an alarming trend in minority student representation. During the decade of the 1990s, there was a 15 percent decline in the number of underrepresented minority first-year students. In particular, the number of Black/African American students fell 19 percent, from 215 to 174. The number of Hispanic/Latino students fell 16 percent, from 245 to 205. This trend, juxtaposed with the projected racial and ethnic demographics of the United States in fifty years, indicates urgent measures are needed to build a diverse oral health workforce.

Table 2. Dentists and patients by race/ethnicity				
Patients:	White	Hispanic	Black	Asian
Dentists:				
White	76.6%	8.5%	10.5%	3.2%
Hispanic	43.6%	45.4%	9.8%	3.0%
Black	27.0%	7.9%	61.8%	2.3%

Source: ADA, 1996 Dentist Profile Survey

Removing Barriers to a More Diverse Workforce

Current ADEA policy strongly endorses the continuous use of re-cruitment, admission, and retention practices that achieve excellence through diversity in American dental education.[60] However, in spite of concerted efforts to recruit underrepresented minorities to careers in dentistry, there has been little increase in the size of the underrepresented minority dental applicant pool over the last ten years. The challenge is made difficult because of a lower proportion of underrepresented minorities in post-secondary institutions, which in turn is caused by lower high school completion rates, attendance at primary and secondary schools with poor academic standards, lack of preparation in science and math, too few mentors, and the lack of access to other educational and career opportunities.

There are a myriad of other factors that create barriers for under-represented minorities to enter dentistry. For example, the number of Black/African American and Hispanic/Latino oral health profes-sionals, including dentists and allied dental personnel, is so small as to provide little exposure to the dental profession and even less chance for mentorship at an early age. Because many Black/African American, Hispanic/Latino, and Native American families are unfamiliar with the dental profession, the image of dentistry as a career fails to attract young people from these ethnic and racial groups. Competition is keen among all the professions for academically qualified underrepresented minori-ties, resulting in aggressive recruitment for the best students. The small number of minority faculty combined with little-to-no Black/African American, Hispanic/Latino, and Native American representation in many dental education schools and programs dissuades some potential students. The cost of dental education is also a barrier for many. In 2001, the average indebtedness of dental graduates, $113,000,[61] exceeded that of medical graduates, approximately $104,900.[62] Admissions requirements sometimes create unnecessary barriers because they have traditionally been based upon restrictive policies rather than policies that are predictive of the diversity of practitioners needed to meet the needs of a diverse population. Future admissions practices should be consistent with sustaining a commitment to a diverse student body, diversity in the health professions, and thereby to ensuring access to oral health care for all Americans.[59]

ADEA is currently pursuing a variety of strategies to increase the recruitment and retention of underrepresented minority students and faculty. The 2002 $1 million grant from the W.K. Kellogg Foundation to administer the W.K. Kellogg/ADEA Access to Dental Careers (ADC) Program is an exemplary partnership to increase underrepresented minority representation in dental schools. The ADC program will provide institutional grants to RWJF Pipeline, Profession, and Practice Program: Community-Based Dental Education grantees and will supplement the underrepresented minority recruitment and retention component of the RWJF program.[45,63] Hopefully, other foundations will consider funding similar initiatives. ADEA, the ADA, the National Dental Association, the Hispanic Dental Association, and the Society of American Indian Dentists must work collaboratively to secure more funding from federal sources as well. For example, federal funding for Title VII programs including the Faculty Loan Repayment Program and the Minority Faculty Fellowship Program should be increased. Partnerships with business and industry to develop scholarships, loan forgiveness, and recognition awards provide additional opportunities.

Among the strategies that require more attention are the early identification and development of students who are likely to pursue careers in the health professions. Major efforts are needed to strengthen the academic pipeline. National organizations must explore the development of a database of students who are successful achievers in math and science. Model programs such as the National Science Foundation program that focuses on strengthening math and science skills of middle and high school students should be duplicated. The Bureau of Health Professions' Health Careers Opportunity Program (HCOP), Centers of Excellence (COE), and the Kids into Health Careers Program provide excellent opportunities to inform minority and economically disadvantaged students and parents about careers in the health professions. Ultimately, these programs should improve overall access to health for underrepresented minorities and other disadvantaged populations by increasing the minority applicant pool for health professions education. Academic dental institutions can promote dentistry through outreach and involvement of children and youth in their communities through early contact programs.

Each academic dental institution can help identify and share strategies in mentoring, recruitment, minority faculty development, admissions process review, and cultivating a better image of oral health professions among minority youth. Academic dental institutions and national dental associations in cooperation with partnering organizations, including other health professions organizations at the national, state and local levels, private foundations, special interest and advocacy groups such as the National Congress of Black Churches, the Congressional Hispanic Caucus, the Congressional Black Caucus, the National Association for the Advancement of Colored People, public education, and the federal and state governments must continue to promote the value of diversity as related to quality of care, to inform minority groups about the opportunities and rewards of a career in oral health care, and to encourage minority youth to prepare for and apply to dental school and other academic dental programs. Finally, as academic dental institutions, the practicing community, other stakeholders in the delivery of health care, and their national organizations interact with policymakers at both the state and federal level, there continues to be a need to reframe the argument for affirmative action based on serving the common good.

Types of Oral Health Providers

According to the Bureau of Labor Statistics, dental assistants held about 229,000 jobs in 1998.[64] The U.S. Department of Health and Human Services estimates that there are nearly 141,000 licensed dental hygienists in the United States.[65] The National Association of Dental Laboratories' "mid-range estimate" is 48,000 for the number of dental laboratory technicians.[66] The Center for Health Workforce studies projects nearly a 30 percent growth rate in health care occupations between 2000 and 2010. However, the growth rate for dentists during this time is projected at only 5.7 percent; in contrast, dental hygienist jobs are predicted to grow by 37 percent.[67] As policymakers consider future dental workforce needs in the light of growing access to oral health problems, they will invariably look to the declining dentist to population ratio and new roles for both traditional and nontraditional providers of oral health care.

The current oral health workforce has reserve productive capacity through the utilization of allied dental professionals. As the ratio of dentists to population declines and as the demand for or need of dental services increases, in the national aggregate or through programs to underserved population groups or areas, there will be a need to draw upon this reserve capacity and even expand productive capacity through a more extended use of allied dental professionals. Tapping into this reserve capacity must not only include a more intensive utilization of allied dental personnel, but the examination of new roles and responsibilities, in a less restrictive delivery system, that would further augment the output of the dental team and extend the availability of oral health care. As has been well documented, extended utilization of allied health personnel is one way to increase the efficiency of health care delivery and the availability of care.[26,68-73]

Regulatory Considerations for
Improving Access to Oral Health Care

Forty-nine states allow dental hygienists to provide services under general supervision in some settings. General supervision requires that a dentist authorize a dental hygienist to perform procedures, but his or her presence is not mandatory in the treatment facility during the delivery of care. With the variation in individual state practice acts, the definition of general supervision varies widely, as do the services that dental hygienists are allowed to perform. In some states, dental hygienists can practice only under direct supervision, that is, a dentist must be present in the facility while the dental hygienist provides care. In fourteen states, dental hygienists may provide care in certain settings under various forms of unsupervised practice and less restrictive supervision.[11]

In California, dental hygiene practice is expanded through special license designations of a Registered Dental Hygienist in Alternative Practice (RDHAP). Unsupervised practice means that dental hygienists can assess patient needs and treat the patient without the authorization or presence of a dentist.[27] RDHAPs are indicative of a new type of oral health care provider. Special requirements for RDHAPs include a bachelors degree or equivalent, three years clinical practice, and completion of a 150 clock hour special course and exam. Other states with less restrictive supervision are instructive of ways in which allied dental professionals, especially dental hygienists, can provide oral health care in underserved settings (Table 3).

One of the major challenges to full utilization of allied dental professionals is state laws and regulations that limit practice settings and impose restrictive supervision requirements. The level of supervision should reflect the education, experience, and competence of the allied dental professional. At present, many state practice acts do not reflect what allied dental professionals have been educated to do competently. While academic dental institutions cannot themselves effect a change in the laws and regulations, they are often positioned to influence the elimination of regulatory language that unnecessarily restricts the services provided by allied dental professionals. More specifically, the leadership of academic dental institutions is positioned to inform legislative leaders and state board members about ways that dental assistants, dental hygienists, and dental laboratory technicians can contribute to alleviating the access to oral health care problems in their communities and states.

To ensure the competence of allied dental professionals, the academic dental education community must continue to support accredited programs, nationally recognized certification for dental assistants and dental laboratory technicians, and licensure for dental hygienists.

As pressure mounts on policymakers to improve access to oral health care, it is likely that state practice acts will become less restrictive, especially for dental hygienists who have graduated from accredited programs and are licensed. Academic dental institutions, including those community and technical colleges, should monitor how these developments are evolving in the states they serve. Educational programs should anticipate these changes so that allied dental graduates will be prepared to provide expanded care in unconventional settings.

Table 3. Examples of states with less restrictive supervision for dental hygienists

California. RDHAPs may work as an employee of another RDHAP who is an independent contractor or sole proprietor of an alternative dental hygiene practice. An RDHAP may practice in residences of the homebound, schools, residential facilities, and other institutions, as well as in dental health professional shortage areas. New legislation (California SB1589) would authorize RDHAPs to be an employee of a primary care clinic or specialty clinic, a clinic owned or operated by a public hospital or health system, and a clinic owned and operated by a hospital that maintains the primary contract with a county government.

Colorado. Dental hygienists may engage in unsupervised practice in all settings for all licensed dental hygienists for prophylaxis and several other services, including: removal of deposits, accretions, stains, curettage, application of fluorides and other recognized preventive agents, oral inspection and charting, and topical anesthetic.

Connecticut. Dental hygienists with two years experience may practice without supervision in institutions, public health facilities, group homes, and schools. Services include: complete prophylaxis, removal of deposits, accretions and stains, root planing, providing sealants, and assessment and treatment planning.

New Mexico. Collaborative practice is permitted based on a written agreement between the dental hygienist and one or more consulting dentists. Dental hygienists may treat patients according to an agreed-upon protocol of care with the collaborating dentist. The protocol is equivalent to standing orders that permit the dental hygienist to provide such services as preliminary assessment, x-rays, prophylaxis, and fluoride treatment. Case-by-case approval is given for procedures such as sealants and root planing.

Oregon. Dental hygienists may initiate service for patients in limited access settings such as extended care facilities, correctional facilities, facilities for the disabled or mentally ill, schools and preschools, and job training centers. The dental hygienist with a limited access permit can perform all dental hygiene services, with the exception of several services that must be authorized by a dentist.

Washington. Unsupervised practice by dental hygienists is permitted in hospitals, nursing homes, home health agencies, group homes for the elderly, handicapped, or youth, state institutions under department of health and human services, jails, and public health facilities, provided that the hygienist refers to a dentist for dental treatment and planning.

Source: American Dental Hygienists' Association, Division of Governmental Affairs, July 2002

For example, dental hygienists should be prepared to assume new roles as oral health educators, providing educational services, oral health training programs, and oral health screenings without supervision. Dental hygienists have new roles to play in the treatment of periodontal disease. Dental assistants should carry out extended functions that can further increase the productivity of the dental team and facilitate access to oral health care. Dental laboratory technicians must be prepared for emerging roles in the light of scientific advances in biomimetics and bioengineering. The evolving roles of allied dental professionals underscore the need for quality education through accreditation and the recognition of professional competence through certification and licensure.

The significance of the federally funded "Training and Expanded Auxiliary Management" (T.E.A.M.)[74] in the 1970s has largely been lost. However, even as many state practice acts change to allow less restrictive supervision, dental professionals will be most effective as they contribute to an integrated oral health team. The attitudes and behaviors of superior team performance are learned best in the context of the provision of care with other health care professionals. Interdisciplinary courses and activities, especially with dental students and even with nontraditional providers such as physicians and other primary care providers, and greater involvement in community health care delivery systems are critical steps to prepare the future allied dental workforce. Students should experience integrated care in an efficient delivery system.

Nontraditional Providers of Oral Health Care

In commenting on the need for dental education's leadership for the common good, DePaola observes, "Oral health professionals often fail to achieve improvements in the oral health of the community because they are not provided or lack the skills necessary to share their knowledge and expertise with those beyond the dental office, the dental school, or the university."[36] Reduced access to oral health care is one of the prices of professional isolation that has too often characterized dentistry. Isolation gives the impression to other health professionals, policymakers, and the public that oral health is not as important as general health. Integration into the health care system is a fundamental step toward improving access to oral health care. Dental services must be accessible, affordable, and valued by the underserved. Primary care practice is the front line for underserved populations and *potentially* serves to provide dental screening, prevention, education—and referrals to dentists and allied oral health professionals. A recent report by the HRSA Advisory Committee on Training in Primary Care Medicine and Dentistry observes that two-thirds of all Americans interact with a primary care provider every year.[75] Family physicians, pediatricians, other primary care physicians, nurse practitioners, and physician assistants should be enlisted to monitor the oral health of their patients. However, at present the medical community is neither sufficiently conversant with oral health nor adequately integrated with their dental colleagues to effect significant change on the status of oral health.

Of the fifty-five accredited U.S. dental schools, forty-four are part of academic health centers. Residency training programs, specialty programs, General Practice Residency and Advanced Education in General Dentistry programs, and allied programs are well ensconced in a variety of settings that provide opportunities for interaction with other health professions. Academic dental institutions are thus well positioned to educate other health professionals about oral health. One way to foster this integration is to provide students with clinical experiences in public dental clinics that are integrated into larger medical clinics. Dental schools could initiate interaction among dental and medical students and other primary care practitioners not merely in the basic sciences, but also in clinical practice. Not only must primary care medical practitioners learn to be a part of the oral health team; dentists must become more involved in assessing the overall health of their patients through screening, diagnosis, and referral. Meeting the access to oral health care challenge will require collaboration across the health professions.

Summary of Roles and Responsibilities

Where dental education and dental practice are today was influenced and much determined by decisions made fifteen years ago. Where dental education and dental practice will be and wish to be fifteen years from now is influenced and much determined by decisions made today. With the length of time required for developing new models of oral health care delivery, program planning, development, implementation, and training, effecting change can easily take ten years. The uncertainties of workforce requirements remain, along with the issues of workforce composition and distribution that affect the availability of and access to oral health care, which contribute to disparities of oral health status. Decisions must be made now to guide the development of dental education policy, position, and action regarding the number, diversity, and type of oral health care providers and roles and responsibilities of academic dental institutions in patient care and improving access to oral health care.

With the communities of dental education, regulation, dental practice, and other health professions working together, in conjunction with public and private policymakers and partners, the oral health care needs of the underserved will be met, thereby ensuring access to quality oral health care for all Americans. In summary, academic dental institutions can work to this end most effectively by discharging these roles and responsibilities:

- Preparing competent graduates with skills and knowledge to meet the needs of all Americans within an integrated health care system;
- Teaching and exhibiting values that prepare the student to enter the profession as a member of a moral community of oral health professionals with a commitment to the dental profession's societal obligations;
- Guiding the number, type, and education of dental workforce personnel to ensure equitable availability of and access to oral health care;
- Contributing to ensure a workforce that more closely reflects the racial and ethnic diversity of the American public;
- Developing cultural competencies in their graduates and an appreciation for public health issues;
- Serving as effective providers, role models, and innovators in the delivery of oral health care to all populations; and
- Assisting in prevention, public health, and public education efforts to reduce health disparities in vulnerable populations.

Recommendations for Improving the Oral Health Status of All Americans: Roles and Responsibilities of Academic Dental Institutions

1. To monitor future oral health care workforce needs:

1.1 As a part of each academic dental institution's strategic plan, include an assessment of the dental workforce status and requirements of the areas primarily served by the institution. Conduct of the assessment should include representation from state and local dental and allied dental societies, appropriate federal, state, and local health departments, educators from pre- and postdoctoral and allied academic dental institutions, and other strategic partners. The assessment and resulting plan should consider: the age, gender, retirement, and replacement characteristics of the current workforce; population demographics and trends; underserved populations and communities; and understaffed facilities that serve such populations and communities.

1.2 Collaborate with state and local dental and allied dental societies to advocate jointly for federal and state funds and programs that will assist academic dental institutions in meeting projected workforce number and composition requirements, along with incentives and programs designed to achieve a more equitable distribution of and access to oral health care.

1.3 Engage in health services research through the Agency for Health Research and Quality to gather information on utilization, cost, cost-effectiveness, outcomes of treatment, measurement of disease, and health outcomes. Develop measures for oral health status, including measures specific to gender, ethnic and racial groups, the elderly, children, and medically compromised patients.

2. To improve the effectiveness of the oral health care delivery system:

2.1 Develop and support new models of oral health care that will provide care within an integrated health care system. New models should involve other health professionals, including family physicians, pediatricians, geriatricians, and other primary care providers as team members. These models should also expose students to different points of entry into dental practice such as public health, hospitals, community health, academics, and other opportunities.

2.2 Educate dental and allied dental students to assume new roles in the prevention, detection, early recognition, and management of a broad range of complex oral and general diseases and conditions in collaboration with their colleagues from other health professions.

2.3 Advocate for stronger linkages among primary care dentistry, primary care medicine, and public health through interdisciplinary faculty training. Faculty development funding should be made available through dental programs under Title VII, Section 747.

2.4 Convene through ADEA a task force of health professions leaders from medicine, dentistry, the allied dental professions, public health, nursing, and related areas to develop a process for integrating didactic and clinical oral health curricula into medical and other health professions education.

2.5 Promote the adoption of the *Healthy People 2010* Oral Health Objectives in the communities of which the academic dental institution is a part. Involve community health centers, communities of faith, public school health personnel, nursing home health personnel, and local health care professionals in the pursuit of these objectives.

2.6 Encourage minority students and faculty to pursue advanced education and research training opportunities and research supplements for minority investigators through the National Institute for Dental and Craniofacial Research and other federal, state, and private programs.

2.7 Work closely with the ADA, the American Dental Hygienists' Association, the Hispanic Dental Association, the National Dental Association, and the Society of American Indian Dentists to advocate for increased funding for Medicaid and State Children's Health Insurance Programs.

2.8 Advocate for increases in federal Medicaid payments to compensate for state cutbacks, improve care, and lessen the access problems of the uninsured.

2.9 Enhance interdisciplinary education opportunities by integrating medical and dental education through problem-based learning, team building, and grand rounds involving cross disciplinary students and a variety of primary care providers.

2.10 Work closely with the ADA and other organizations to advocate for increased funding and loan forgiveness for General Practice Residency and Advanced Education in General Dentistry programs and dental specialty programs, particularly pediatric dentistry and dental public health programs, so that the number of positions and funding are sufficient for a requirement that all dental graduates participate in a year of service and learning in an accredited PGY-1 program.

2.11 Maintain and seek increased federal funding for dental Graduate Medical Education (GME), and develop relationships with hospitals to increase dental residency training positions reimbursed through the GME program.

2.12 Encourage all dental graduates to pursue postdoctoral dental education in a general dentistry or advanced dental education program and continue to monitor the feasibility of requiring a year of advanced education for all dental graduates. Work with other organizations to advocate for a requirement that all dental graduates participate in a year of service and learning in an accredited PGY-1 program.

3. To prepare students to provide oral health services to diverse populations:

3.1 Facilitate interaction between students and faculty and community leaders from different ethnic and racial backgrounds in forums to discuss the importance of oral health care and the perceptions of the respective communities.

3.2 Incorporate cultural competency concepts in all aspects of the clinical instruction curriculum.

3.3 Provide in the curriculum and in other forums opportunities to teach students about their professional obligation to serve the public good and encourage students to explore how they and the profession can ensure oral health care for all Americans.

3.4 Provide rotations in off-site clinics to deliver oral health care to underserved populations as a means to develop culturally competent oral health providers.

3.5 Encourage the ADA Commission on Dental Accreditation to add an accreditation standard addressing cultural competency and to include cultural competency in its curriculum survey so that data on outcomes can be collected.

3.6 Advocate for adequate curriculum time devoted to theoretical and practical considerations in providing care to patients with complex needs and circumstances, including those with developmental and other disabilities, the very young and the aged, and individuals with complex psychological and social situations. Include didactic and clinical educational experiences.

3.7 Foster collaboration between pre- and postgraduate educational institutions to develop a continuum of educational experiences in the care of patients with complex needs.

3.8 Work with the ADA Commission on Dental Accreditation to adopt or strengthen accreditation standards at all levels of dental education related to competency in treatment of people with special needs. Include a requirement that graduates of dental education programs be able to manage or treat, consistent with their educational level, a variety of patients with complex medical and psychosocial conditions, including those with developmental and other disabilities, the very young, the aged, and individuals with complex psychological and social conditions.

4. To increase the diversity of the oral health workforce:

4.1 Expose minorities to careers in oral health at an early age. Develop dental school programs and allied dental education programs that promote dentistry through outreach and involvement of children, youth, and undergraduate students in the community through pre-admission programs and other early contact programs. The HRSA *Kids Into Health Careers* program, Centers of Excellence, and Health Careers Opportunities programs should be supported, particularly for implementation at the local level.

4.2 Through ADEA, identify and publish best practices in the recruitment and retention of underrepresented minority students and faculty.

4.3 Explore best practices in distance learning and develop programs that will provide much of the student's education in the community in which he or she lives. Successful models currently exist in dental hygiene education that should be studied for application to other dental education programs in community and technical colleges and in dental schools.

4.4 Review and amend admissions criteria in the context of the common good and the importance of educating a diverse workforce to meet the oral health needs of an increasingly diverse society.

4.5 Expand funding for scholarships and loans for underrepresented minorities from federal, state, and private sources.

4.6 Through ADEA, work closely with the ADA, the American Dental Hygienists' Association, the Hispanic Dental Association, the National Dental Association, and the Society of American Indian Dentists to develop mentoring programs to formalize interactions between minority dentists and youth. Include outcome measures.

5. To improve the effectiveness of allied dental professionals in reaching the underserved:

5.1 Develop the knowledge and skills necessary to serve a diverse population, provide experiences of oral health care delivery in community-based and nontraditional settings, and encourage externships in underserved areas.

5.2 Advocate for statutory and regulatory reform to ensure that state practice acts do not unnecessarily restrict the care that allied dental professionals who have graduated from accredited programs and, in the case of dental hygienists, hold the appropriate license, to provide care to the public.

5.3 Continue to support accredited allied dental programs as the educational standard for entry into the profession.

5.4 In each state, monitor and anticipate changes in supervision requirements for allied dental professionals and modify the curriculum and extramural experiences of students so as to prepare them to provide more extended services in a variety of practice settings.

5.5 Engage students in the local community to provide oral health promotion and disease prevention education to children and parents in underserved groups. Settings should include schools, nursing homes, community activity centers.

Acknowledgment

ADEA thanks the William J. Gies Foundation for the Advancement of Dentistry for its generous support of the ADEA Commission on Improving the Oral Health Status of All Americans. The views expressed in this report are those of the ADEA Commission on Improving the Oral Health Status of All Americans and are not intended to represent the position of the William J. Gies Foundation.

REFERENCES

1. Oral health in America: a report of the surgeon general. Rockville, MD: National Institutes of Health, National Institute of Dental and Craniofacial Research, U.S. Department of Health and Human Services, 2000.

2. National Center for Health Statistics. Healthy people 2000 review, 1998-99. Hyattsville, MD: Public Health Service, 1998.

3. Greenlee RT, et al. Cancer statistics, 2000. Cancer J for Clinicians 2000;50;7-33.

4. Oral health: factors contributing to low use of dental services by low-income populations. GAO/HEHS-00-149. Washington, DC: U.S. General Accounting Office/Health, Education, and Human Services Division, September 2000.

5. Warren RC. Oral health for all: policy for available, accessible, and acceptable care. Washington, DC: Center for Policy Alternatives, September 1999.

6. State efforts to improve children's oral health. Issue Brief. Washington, DC: National Governors' Association Center for Best Practices, Health Policy Studies Division, November 20, 2002.

7. Kosary CL, et al., eds. SEER cancer statistics review, 1973-92 tables and graphs. NIH Pub. no. 96-2789. Bethesda, MD: National Cancer Institute, December 1995:17, 34, 542, 355, 361.

8. Division of Shortage Designation Bureau of Primary Health Care, HRSA. At: http://bphc.hrsa.gov/databases/newhpsa/newhpsa.cfm. Accessed: November 26, 2002.

9. California, 1997-98, AB 1116.

10.California, 2001-2002, AB 1045.

11.States permitting unsupervised practice/less restrictive supervision. Chicago: Division of Government Affairs, American Dental Hygienists' Association, January 2003.

12. The types of access barriers have remained relatively unchanged over the past two decades. See, for example: Barriers to attaining an effective

dental health system, proceedings of the region IX dental conference. San Francisco: U.S. Department of Health, Education and Welfare, Regional Office, 1979.

13. For example, even though the HRSA Advisory Committee on Training in Primary Care Medicine and Dentistry recommended that FY 2002 funding for the Primary Care Medicine and Dentistry health professions programs (Title VII) be increased to $15 million, dental programs received only $6 million, or 6.4 percent of total funding for these programs. President Bush's budget proposal for FY 2003 calls for the General Dentistry/Pediatric Dentistry residency training programs to be totally unfunded.

14. American Dental Association. 1998 Survey of practitioners. Chicago: American Dental Association, 1999.

15. Linn E. Professional activities of black dentists. J Am Dent Assoc 1972; 82:118.

16. Montoya R, Hayes-Bautista D, Gonzales L, Smeloff E. Minority dental school graduates: do they serve minority communities? Am J Public Health 1978;68:10.

17. National Academy of Sciences, Institute of Medicine. Unequal treatment: confronting racial and ethnic disparities in health care. Washington, DC: National Academy Press, 2002.

18. Buckley L. Why health professions need to understand the disadvantaged. In: Dummett C, ed. Community dentistry. Springfield, IL: Charles Thomas, 1974.

19. Pyle MA. Changing perceptions of oral health and its importance to general health: provider perceptions, public perceptions, policymaker perceptions. Spec Care Dentist 2002;22(1):8-15.

20. The Newshour with Jim Lehrer/Kaiser Family Foundation. National survey on the uninsured. As cited in: Uninsured in America: a chart book. 2nd ed. Menlo Park, CA: Kaiser Family Foundation, March 2000.

21. American College of Physicians-American Society of Internal Medicine (ACP-ASIM). No health insurance? It's enough to make you sick: scientific research linking the lack of health coverage to poor health, November 30, 1999. At: www.acponline.org/uninsured/index.html/html. Accessed: December 12, 2002.

22. Ayanian J, et al. Unmet health needs of uninsured adults in the United States. JAMA 2000;284:2061.

23. Amara R, et al. Health and health care 2010. Institute for the Future. San Francisco: Jossey-Bass Publishers, 2000:127.

24. Berk M, Schur C, Cantor J. Ability to obtain health care: recent estimates from the Robert Wood Johnson Foundation National Access to Care Survey. Health Aff 1995;14(3):139-46.

25. Mueller CD, Schur CL, Paramore LC. Access to dental care in the United States. J Am Dent Assoc 1998;129:429-37.
26. American Dental Association Survey Center. 2000 survey of current issues in dentistry: dentists' participation in Medicaid. Chicago: American Dental Association, 2000.
27. Bureau of Primary Health Care. Dental care access. Washington, DC: HRSA, Office of State and National Partnerships, 2001. At: http://bphc. hrsa.gov:80/OSNP/DentalCare.htm. Last revised August 6, 2002. Accessed: February 20, 2003.
28. Access to care, 2001. American Dental Hygienists' Association Position Paper. At: www.adha.org/profissues/access_to_care.htm. Accessed: November 27, 2002.
29. Etzioni A. Law in civil society, good society, and the prescriptive state. Chicago Kent Law Rev 2000;75:355-77.
30. Etzioni A. The good society. J Political Philosophy 1999;7:88-103.
31. Rudolph A. The American college and university: a history. Athens: University of Georgia Press, 1990.
32. Valachovic RW, Machen B, Haden NK. The value of the dental school to the university. In: Haden NK, Tedesco LT, eds. Leadership for the future: the dental school in the university. Washington, DC: American Association of Dental Schools [now American Dental Education Association], 1999:6-13.
33. Bok D. Reclaiming the public trust. Change, July/August 1992:13-9.
34. Alfred RL, Weissman J. Higher education and the public trust: improving stature in colleges and universities. ASHE-Eric Higher Education Research Report, No. 6, 1987.
35. Delattre EJ, Bennet WJ. Education and the public trust: the imperative for common purposes. Washington, DC: Ethics and Public Policy Center, January 1988.
36. DePaola D. Beyond the university: leadership for the common good. In: Haden NK, Tedesco LT, eds. Leadership for the future: the dental school in the university. Washington, DC: American Association of Dental Schools [now American Dental Education Association], 1999:94-102.
37. Panel discussion, 1998 AADS Leadership Summit Conference. In: Haden NK, Tedesco LT, eds. Leadership for the future: the dental school in the university. Washington, DC: American Association of Dental Schools [now American Dental Education Association], 1999:124-31.
38. Bulger RJ, McGovern JP, eds. Physician philosopher: the philosophical foundation of medicine—essays by Dr. Edmund Pellegrino. Charlottesville, VA: Carden Jennings, 2001.
39. American Dental Association. Code of ethics. At: www.ada.org/prof/ prac/law/code/interpretation.html. Accessed: November 26, 2002.

40. O'Neil EH and the Pew Health Professions Commission. Recreating health professional practice for a new century: the fourth report of the Pew Health Professions Commission. San Francisco: Pew Health Professions Commission, December 1998.

41. American Dental Association. At: www.ada.org/prof/accessinfo.html. Accessed: November 26, 2002.

42. Palmer C. Health safety net law helps expand dental access. ADA News November 4, 2002.

43. Palmer C. Congress joins ADA, historic dental access legislation nears approval. ADA News October 21, 2002.

44. Sec 61-5A-4D, rule 16.5.17. New Mexico, 1999.

45. Columbia University. At: http://dentalpipeline.columbia.edu/prog_info_pressrelease.html. Accessed: November 26, 2002.

46. American Dental Association. Future of dentistry. Chicago: American Dental Association, Health Policy Resources Center, 2001.

47. Institute of Medicine. Dental education at the crossroads: challenges and change. Field MJ, ed. Washington, DC: National Academy Press, 1995.

48. American Dental Association Survey Center. 1999/2000 survey of allied dental education. Chicago: American Dental Association, 2001.

49. "Dental education institutions and programs should: ... Provide students with formal instruction in ethics and professional behavior, and make the students aware of acceptable professional conduct in instructional and practice settings. Institutions and programs should ensure that student clinical experiences foster ethical patient care. . . . Offer programs that encourage students to serve in areas of oral health care need. . . . Encourage students to participate in outreach programs, and, upon graduation, to participate in community service." ADEA policy statements, revised and approved by the 2001 House of Delegates. J Dent Educ 2002;66:840.

50. American Dental Association Survey Center. 1998 survey of dental school satellite clinics and the 1998 dental society survey of dental school satellite clinics. Chicago: American Dental Association, 1999.

51. Bureau of the Census. Statistical abstract of the United States. Washington, DC: U.S. Department of Commerce, Economics and Statistics Administration, 1998.

52. American Dental Association Commission on the Young Professional. A portrait of minority and women dentists. Washington, DC: Decision Demographics, 1992.

53. Smedley BD, Stith AY, Nelson AR, eds. Unequal treatment: confronting racial and ethnic disparities in health care. Washington, DC: Institute of Medicine, National Academy Press, 2002.

54. Association of American Medical Colleges. Amicus brief, Grutter v. Bollinger, February 18, 2003.

http://www.aamc.org/affirmativeaction. February 28, 2003.

55. Canto JD, Miles EL, Baker LC, Barker DC. Physician service to the underserved: implications for affirmative action in medical education. Inquiry 1996;33:167-80.

56. Komaromy M, et al. The role of black and Hispanic physicians in providing health care for underserved populations. N Engl J Med 1996;334(16):1305-10.

57. Solomon ES, Williams CR, Sinkford JC. Practice location characteristics of black dentists in Texas. J Dent Educ 2001;65:571-8.

58. U.S. Health Resources and Services Administration, Federal Register, December 4, 1985.

59. Sinkford JC, Harrison S, Valachovic RW. Underrepresented minority enrollment in U.S. dental schools—the challenge. J Dent Educ 2001;65:564-70.

60. "The American Dental Education Association strongly endorses the continuous use of recruitment, admission, and retention practices that achieve excellence through diversity in American dental education. Dental education institutions should identify, recruit, and retain underrepresented minority students; identify, recruit, and retain women and underrepresented minorities to faculty positions; and promote women and underrepresented minorities to senior and administrative positions. Dental education institutions should accept students from diverse backgrounds, who, on the basis of past and predicted performance, appear qualified to become competent dental professionals." ADEA policy statements, revised and approved by the 2001 House of Delegates. J Dent Educ 2002;66:839.

61. Weaver RG, Haden NK, Valachovic RW. Annual ADEA survey of dental school seniors: 2002 graduating class. J Dent Educ 2002;66:1388-1404.

62. Medical school debt fact card. Washington, DC: Association of American Medical Colleges, October 2002.

63. American Dental Education Association, Center for Equity and Diversity. At: www.adea.org. Accessed: November 26, 2002.

64. U.S. Department of Labor, Bureau of Labor Statistics. Occupational outlook handbook. Chicago: Bureau of Labor Statistics, 2000.

65. State health workforce profiles. Washington, DC: U.S. Department of Health and Human Services, Health Resources and Services Administration, Bureau of Health Professions National Center for Health Workforce Information and Analysis, December 2000.

66. Essential facts: a dentist's guide to dental technology certification. Tallahassee, FL: National Association of Dental Laboratories, 2000.

67. Center for Health Workforce Studies. Healthcare employment projections: an analysis of Bureau of Labor Statistics occupational projections,

2000-2010. Rensselaer: University at Albany, State University of New York, School of Public Health, January 2002.

68. Chapko MK, Milgrom P, Bergner M, Conrad D, Skalabrin N. Delegation of expanded functions to dental assistants and hygienists. J Dent Hyg 1993;67:249-56.

69. Cooper MD. A survey of expanded duties usage in Indiana: a pilot study. J Public Health Dent 1984;44:22-7.

70. Sisty NL, Henderson WG, Paule CL, Martin JF. Evaluation of student performance in the four-year study of expanded functions for dental hygienists at the University of Iowa. Am J Public Health 1978;68(7):664-8.

71. Access to dental care for low-income children in Illinois—report summary. Chicago: Illinois Center for Health Workforce Studies, December 2000.

72. Distribution of the dental workforce in Washington state: patterns and consequences—project summary. Seattle: WWAMI Center for Health Workforce Studies, November 2000.

73. Benn DK. Applying evidence-based dentistry to caries management in dental practice: a computerized approach. J Am Dent Assoc 2002;133:1543-50.

74. Health Professions Educational Assistance Act of 1976 (PL-94-484), Title VII.

75. Bureau of Health Professions, U.S. Health Resources and Services Administration, Advisory Committee on Training in Primary Care Medicine and Dentistry. At: http://bhpr.hrsa.gov/medicine-dentistry/actpcmd1.htm. Accessed: November 27, 2002.

Appendix 1. *From the 2000 Surgeon General's Report on Oral Health: The Burden of Oral Diseases and Disorders*

Oral diseases are progressive and cumulative and become more complex over time. They can affect our ability to eat, the foods we choose, how we look, and the way we communicate. These diseases can affect economic productivity and compromise our ability to work at home, at school, or on the job. Health disparities exist across population groups at all ages. Over one third of the U.S. population (100 million people) has no access to community water fluoridation. Over 108 million children and adults lack dental insurance, which is over 2.5 times the number who lack medical insurance. The following are highlights of oral health data for children, adults, and the elderly. (Refer to the full report for details of these data and their sources.)

Children

+ Cleft lip/palate, one of the most common birth defects, is estimated to affect 1 out of 600 live births for Whites and 1 out of 1,850 live births for African Americans.

+ Other birth defects such as hereditary ectodermal dysplasias, where all or most teeth are missing or misshapen, cause lifetime problems that can be devastating to children and adults.

+ Dental caries (tooth decay) is the single most common chronic childhood disease—5 times more common than asthma and 7 times more common than hay fever.

+ Over 50 percent of 5- to 9-year-old children have at least one cavity or filling, and that proportion increases to 78 percent among 17-year-olds. Nevertheless, these figures represent improvements in the oral health of children compared to a generation ago.

+ There are striking disparities in dental disease by income. Poor children suffer twice as much dental caries as their more affluent peers, and their disease is more likely to be untreated. These poor-nonpoor differences continue into adolescence. One out of four children in America is born into poverty, and children living below the poverty line (annual income of $17,000 for a family of four) have more severe and untreated decay.

+ Unintentional injuries, many of which include head, mouth, and neck injuries, are common in children.

+ Intentional injuries commonly affect the craniofacial tissues.

+ Tobacco-related oral lesions are prevalent in adolescents who currently use smokeless (spit) tobacco.

+ Professional care is necessary for maintaining oral health, yet 25 percent of poor children have not seen a dentist before entering kindergarten.

+ Medical insurance is a strong predictor of access to dental care. Uninsured children are 2.5 times less likely than insured children to receive dental care. Children from families without dental insurance are 3 times more likely to have dental needs than children with either public or private insurance. For each child without medical insurance, there are at least 2.6 children without dental insurance.

+ Medicaid has not been able to fill the gap in providing dental care to poor children. Fewer than one in five Medicaid-covered children received a single dental visit in a recent year-long study period. Although new programs such as the State Children's Health Insurance Program (SCHIP) may increase the number of insured children, many will still be left without effective dental coverage.

+ The social impact of oral diseases in children is substantial. More than 51 million school hours are lost each year to dental-related illness. Poor children suffer nearly 12 times more restricted-activity days than children from higher-income families. Pain and suffering due to untreated diseases can lead to problems in eating, speaking, and attending to learning.

Adults

+ Most adults show signs of periodontal or gingival diseases. Severe periodontal disease (measured as 6 millimeters of periodontal attachment loss) affects about 14 percent of adults aged 45-54.
+ Clinical symptoms of viral infections, such as herpes labialis (cold sores), and oral ulcers (canker sores) are common in adulthood, affecting about 19 percent of adults 25 to 44 year of age.
+ Chronic disabling diseases such as temporomandibular disorder, Sjögren's syndrome, diabetes, and osteoporosis affect millions of Americans and compromise oral health and functioning.
+ Pain is a common symptom of craniofacial disorders and is accompanied by interference with vital functions such as eating, swallowing, and speech. Twenty-two percent of adults reported some form of oral-facial pain in the past 6 months. Pain is a major component of trigeminal neuralgia, facial shingles (post-herpetic neuralgia), temporomandibular disorder, fibromyalgia, and Bells' palsy.
+ Population growth as well as diagnostics that are enabling earlier detection of cancer means that more patients than ever before are undergoing cancer treatments. More than 400,000 of these patients will develop oral complications annually.
+ Immuno-compromised patients, such as those with HIV infections and those undergoing organ transplantation, are at higher risk for oral problems such as candidiasis.
+ Employed adults lose more than 164 million hours of work each year due to dental disease or dental visits.
+ For every adult 19 years or older without medical insurance, there are three without dental insurance.
+ A little less than two thirds of adults report having visited a dentist in the past 12 months. Those with incomes at or above the poverty level are twice as likely to report a dental visit in the past 12 months as those who are below the poverty level.

Older Adults

+ Twenty-three percent of 65- to 74-year-olds have periodontal disease (measured as 6 millimeters of periodontal attachment loss). Also, at all ages men are more likely than women to have more severe disease, and at all ages people at the lowest socioeconomic levels have more severe periodontal disease.

- About 30 percent of adults 65 years and older are edentulous, compared to 46 percent 20 years ago. These figures are higher for those living in poverty.
- Oral and pharyngeal cancers are diagnosed in 30,000 Americans annually; 8,000 die from these diseases each year. These cancers are primarily diagnosed in the elderly. Prognosis is poor. The 5-year survival rate for white patients is 56 percent; for blacks, it is only 34 percent.
- Most older Americans take both prescription and over-the-counter drugs. In all probability, at least one of the medications will have an oral side effect—usually dry mouth. The inhibition of salivary flow increases the risk for oral disease because saliva contains antimicrobial components as well as minerals that can help rebuild tooth enamel after attack by acid-producing, decay-causing bacteria. Individuals in long-term care facilities are prescribed an average of eight drugs.
- At any given time, 5 percent of Americans aged 65 and older (currently some 1.65 million people) are living in a long-term care facility where dental care is problematic.
- Many elderly individuals lose their dental insurance when they retire. The situation may be worse for older women, who generally have lower incomes and may never have had dental insurance. Medicaid funds dental care for the low-income and disabled elderly in some states, but reimbursements are low. Medicare is not designed to reimburse for routine dental care.

Source: U.S. Department of Health and Human Services. Oral health in America: a report of the Surgeon General. Rockville, MD: HHS, National Institutes of Health. National Institute of Dental and Craniofacial Research, 2000.

Appendix 2

FDI-WORLD DENTAL ASSOCIATION PRINCIPLES OF ETHICS

These International Principles of Ethics for the Dental Profession should be considered as guidelines for every dentist. These guidelines cannot cover all local, national, traditions, legislation or circumstances.

The professional dentist

2. will practice according to the art and science of dentistry and to the principles of humanity

3. will safeguard the oral health of patients irrespective of their individual status

The primary duty of the dentist is to safeguard the oral health of patients. However, the dentist has the right to decline to treat a patient, except for the provision of emergency care, for humanitarian reasons, or where the laws of the country dictate otherwise.

The professional dentist

– should support oral health promotion The dentist should participate in oral health education and should support and promote accepted measures to improve the oral health of the public.

FDI-WORLD DENTAL ASSOCIATION POLICY STATEMENT ON GLOBAL GOALS FOR ORAL HEALTH (JOINT FDI-WHO-IADR STATEMENT)

Goals: – To promote oral health and to minimise the impact of diseases of oral and craniofacial origin on general health and psychosocial development, giving emphasis to promoting oral health in populations with the greatest burden of such conditions and diseases;

Objectives : – To develop accessible cost-effective oral health systems for the prevention and control of oral and craniofacial diseases using the common risk factor approach; – To promote social responsibility and ethical practices of care givers. – To reduce disparities in oral health between different socio-economic groups within countries and inequalities in oral health across countries.

FDI-WORLD DENTAL ASSOCIATION POLICY STATEMENT
ON IMPROVING ACCESS TO ORAL HEALTH CARE

The FDI, as the authoritative, professional worldwide organisation for dentistry, supports the principle that all communities and people should have access to the best possible oral health care to achieve optimum oral health.

The dental profession recognises that the key to the achievement of this objective is improving access to oral health care, in particular to deprived, underprivileged communities and people. The factors that influence access include financial and social infrastructure, caries prevalence, changing disease pattern, birth rate and ageing populations. Barriers to improving oral health care may arise from the individual himself, the dental profession, society in general and the government. Lack of perceived need, inadequate resources, uneven distribution of manpower, low priorities and lack of political will are barriers of unconcern.

FDI-WORLD DENTAL ASSOCIATION POLICY STATEMENT
ON ORAL AND DENTAL CARE OF PEOPLE WITH DISABILITIES

1. The FDI Mission Statement supports the principle that all people should have access to the best possible care to achieve optimal oral health.

2. The FDI International Principles of Ethics for the Dental Profession states that the professional dentist will safeguard the oral health of patients irrespective of their individual status.

3. The FDI supports the United Nations declaration that disabled people should have access to medical treatment without discrimination.

4. Oral and dental care for people with disabilities should be offered to the same standard as for non-disabled people, mindful of the

consequences of oral disease and/or its treatment for people with disabilities.

AMERICAN COLLEGE OF DENTISTS –
ETHICS HANDBOOK FOR DENTISTS

Access to dental care.

The dentist must be aware of and comply with the laws and regulations that govern discrimination and access issues. Dentistry should be available, within reason, to all seeking treatment. ... A dentist should normally be available to address potentially health-threatening dental conditions and to ease pain and suffering. A dentist must not unlawfully restrict access to professional services. Barriers that restrict access of physically impaired individuals should be eliminated to the extent that this can be reasonably accomplished.

Obligation to treat patients

The dentist is not obligated to accept or treat everyone. However, the dentist must avoid actions that could be interpreted as discriminatory; the dentist must be aware of laws and regulations that govern discrimination. A patient in pain or at health risk from an acute dental condition should be examined, then treated, and appropriately referred.

AMERICAN DENTAL ASSOCIATION – CODE OF ETHICS

SECTION 3–Principle: Beneficence ("do good")
The dentist has a duty to promote the patient's welfare.

This principle expresses the concept that professionals have a duty to act for the benefit of others. Under this principle, the dentist's primary obligation is service to the patient and the public-at-large.

3.A. Community Service. Since dentists have an obligation to use their skills, knowledge and experience for the improvement of the dental health of the public and are encouraged to be leaders in their community, dentists in such service shall conduct themselves in such a manner as to maintain or elevate the esteem of the profession.

3.C. Research And Development. Dentists have the obligation of making the results and benefits of their investigative efforts available to all when they are useful in safeguarding or promoting the health of the public.

3.D. Patents And Copyrights. Patents and copyrights may be secured by dentists provided that such patents and copyrights shall not be used to restrict research or practice.

SECTION 4–Principle: Justice ("fairness")
The dentist has a duty to treat people fairly.

This principle expresses the concept that professionals have a duty to be fair in their dealings with patients, colleagues and society. Under this principle, the dentist's primary obligations include dealing with people justly and delivering dental care without prejudice. In its broadest sense, this principle expresses the concept that the dental profession should actively seek allies throughout society on specific activities that will help improve access to care for all.

4.A. Patient Selection. While dentists, in serving the public, may exercise reasonable discretion in selecting patients for their practices, dentists shall not refuse to accept patients into their practice or deny dental service to patients because of the patient's race, creed, color, sex or national origin.

4.A.1. Patients with Bloodborne Pathogens. A dentist has the general obligation to provide care to those in need. A decision not to provide treatment to an individual because the individual is infected with Human Immunodeficiency Virus, Hepatitis B Virus, Hepatitis C Virus or another bloodborne pathogen, based solely on that fact, is unethical.

4.B. Emergency Service. Dentists shall be obliged to make reasonable arrangements for the emergency care of their patients of record. Dentists shall be obliged when consulted in an emergency by patients not of record to make reasonable arrangements for emergency care. If treatment is provided, the dentist, upon completion of treatment, is obliged to return the patient to his or her regular dentist unless the patient expressly reveals a different preference.

AMERICAN DENTAL HYGIENISTS' ASSOCIATION –
CODE OF ETHICS FOR DENTAL HYGIENISTS

4. Basic Beliefs. We recognize the importance of the following beliefs that guide our practice and provide context for our ethics:

– The services we provide contribute to the health and well being of society.

– All people should have access to healthcare, including oral healthcare.

5. Fundamental Principles. These fundamental principles, universal concepts, and general laws of conduct provide the foundation for our ethics.

– Complementarity. The principle of complementarity assumes the existence of an obligation to justice and basic human rights. It requires us to act toward others in the same way they would act toward us if roles were reversed. In all relationships, it means considering the values and perspective of others before making decisions or taking actions affecting them.

– Community. This principle expresses our concern for the bond between individuals, the community, and society in general. It leads us to preserve natural resources and inspires us to show concern for the global environment.

6. Core Values. We acknowledge these values as general guides for our choices and actions

– Beneficence. We have a primary role in promoting the well being of individuals and the public by engaging in health promotion/disease prevention activities.

– Justice and Fairness. We value justice and support the fair and equitable distribution of healthcare resources. We believe all people should have access to high-quality, affordable oral healthcare.

7. Standards of Professional Responsibility. We are obligated to practice our profession in a manner that supports our purpose, beliefs, and values in accordance with the fundamental principles that support our ethics. We acknowledge the following responsibilities:

– Serve all clients without discrimination and avoid action toward any individual or group that may be interpreted as discriminatory.

AUSTRALIAN DENTAL ASSOCIATION –
PRINCIPLES OF PROFESSIONAL DENTAL PRACTICE

2.1 The primary responsibility of dentists is the health, welfare and safety of their patients.

3.3 Dentists should make the results of personal research freely available and should be prepared to share any scientific, clinical or technical knowledge.

AUSTRALIAN DENTAL ASSOCIATION –
POLICY STATEMENT ON THE DELIVERY OF ORAL HEALTH CARE
SPECIAL GROUPS: INDIGENOUS AUSTRALIANS

4.1 Access to affordable, culturally and emotionally appropriate and acceptable dental care is difficult for most indigenous Australians. In conjunction with research programs to guide planning and development, it is recognised that all members of the primary care workforce, and teachers, need better training and knowledge of primary oral health care.

4.2 The following workforce initiatives are supported by the Australian Dental Association Inc. [ADA]:

– identification of indigenous Australians as suitable members of the dental workforce and granting of special places for them in the vocational and higher education sectors;

– undergraduate, postgraduate and continuing education programmes to raise awareness of oral health issues in the indigenous community; and

– encouragement of the dental workforce to work within indigenous communities.

CANADIAN DENTAL ASSOCIATION – CODE OF ETHICS

Article 4: Emergencies. A dental emergency exists if professional judgement determines that a person needs immediate attention to relieve pain, or to control infection or bleeding. Dentists have an obligation to consult and to provide treatment in a dental emergency, or if they are unavailable, to make alternative arrangements.

Article 5: Provision of Duties. A dentist shall remember the duty of service to the patient and therefore is responsible to provide for care to all members of society. A dentist shall not exclude, as patients, members of society on the basis of discrimination which may be contrary to applicable human rights legislation. Other than in an emergency situation, a dentist has the right to refuse to accept an individual as a patient on the basis of personal conflict or time constraint.

Article 6: Community Activities. Dentists by virtue of their education and role in society, are encouraged to support and participate in community affairs, particularly when these activities promote the health and well-being of the public.

Article 5: Patients and Copyright. Dentists have the obligation of making the results of their investigative efforts available to all when they are useful in safeguarding or promoting the health and well-being of the public. Patents and copyrights may be secured by a dentist provided that they and the remuneration derived from them are not used to restrict research, practice, or the benefits of the patented or copyrighted material.

CHRISTIAN MEDICAL AND DENTAL SOCIETY
THE CHRISTIAN DENTIST'S OATH

With God's help, I will love those who come to me for healing and comfort. I will honor and care for each patient as a person made in the image of God, putting aside selfish interests.

With God's guidance, I will endeavor to be a good steward of my skills and of society's resources. I will convey God's love in my relationships with family, friends, and community. I will aspire to reflect God's mercy in caring for the lonely, the poor, the suffering, and the dying.

INDIAN DENTAL ASSOCIATION — CODE OF ETHICS

Section 5 : If a dentist is consulted in an emergency by the patient of another practitioner who is temporarily absent from his office, or by a patient who is away from home, the duty of the dentist so consulted is to relieve the patient of any immediate disability by temporary service only, and then refer the patient back to the regular dentist.

PHILIPPINE DENTAL ASSOCIATION – CODE OF ETHICS

Section 1. Primary Duty. – The dentist's primary duty of serving the public is accomplished by giving his professional service to the best of his capabilities and to conduct himself in such a manners as to hold his profession in high esteem.

Section 2. Emergency Service. – A dentist, when consulted in an emergency by the patient of another, shall attend ONLY to the conditions leading to the emergency. Upon completion of the treatment, he shall return the patient to his dentist of record and inform him of the conditions found and treated.

Section 7. Discoveries of Works.– In the interest of public health, the dentist must make available his discoveries, inventions or works which are useful in safeguarding or promoting health, subject to patent or copyright laws.

Section 8. Dental Health Care Program. – The dentist shall participate in programs designed for dental health education and care. He shall participate in volunteer programs for the delivery of dental health service in underserved and unserved areas.

Section 9. Leadership. – In all efforts to improved the dental health of the public, the dentist shall make available to the community his skill, knowledge, and experience, particularly in his field of specialty.

SWEDISH DENTAL ASSOCIATION – CODE OF ETHICS

A dentist: 1. shall be guided in his or her professional work by humanitarian principles and honesty. The primary consideration must always be the patient's health and well-being.

Contributors

David W. Chambers, EdM, MBA, PhD
Associate Dean for Academic Affairs & Scholarship
University of the Pacific
Arthur A. Dugoni School of Dentistry
San Francisco, California, USA

Shafik Dharamsi, MSc, PhD
Assistant Professor
Global Oral Health & Community Dentistry
Department of Oral Health Sciences
The University of British Columbia
Vancouver, Canada

Raul I. Garcia, DMD, MMedSc
Northeast Center for Research to Evaluate & Eliminate Dental Disparities
Department of Health Policy & Health Services Research
Boston University School of Dental Medicine
Boston, Massachusetts, USA

Sefik Görkey, DDS, PhD
Professor & Chair
Medical History & Ethics Department
Marmara University
Faculty of Medicine
Istanbul, Turkey

Michelle Henshaw, DDS
Associate Professor & Director of Community Health Programs
Center for Research to Evaluate & Eliminate Dental Disparities
& Department of Health Policy & Health Services Research
Boston University School of Dental Medicine
Boston, Massachusetts, USA

Sinikka Salo, DDS, PhD
Business Development Director
R&D Unit, Sendai-Finland Wellbeing Center
3-24-1, Mizunomori, Aoba-ku,
Sendai, 981-0962, Japan

Pöyry Matti, DDS, PhD,
Executive Director
Finnish Dental Association
Helsinki, Finland

Kimberly McFarland, DDS
Dental Director, State of Nebraska
Adjunct professor, Creighton University Medical Center School of Dentistry
    & Adjunct professor, University of Nebraska Medical Center, College of
    Dentistry
Lincoln, Nebraska, USA

Mary McNally, MSc, DDS, MA
Assistant Professor
Faculty of Dentistry, Dalhousie University
University Avenue
Halifax, Nova Scotia Canada

Linda C. Niessen, DMD, MPH, MPP
Vice President, Clinical Education
DENTSPLY International &
Clinical Professor, Department of Restorative Sciences
Baylor College of Dentistry
Texas A&M Health Science Center
Dallas, Texas, USA

Gunilla Nordenram, DDS, PhD
Associate Professor
Institute of Odontology
Karolinska Institutet
Huddinge, Sweden

James T. Rule, DDS
Professor Emeritus
Baltimore College of Dental Surgery
University of Maryland
Baltimore, Maryland, USA

Jos V.M. Welie, MMedS, JD, PhD
Professor of Medical & Dental Ethics
Center for Health Policy and Ethics
Creighton University Medical Center
Omaha, Nebraska, USA

Gerald R. Winslow, PhD
Professor of Ethics
Loma Linda University
Loma Linda, California, USA

Pamela Zarkowski, MPH, JD
Professor & Executive Associate Dean
University of Detroit Mercy
School of Dentistry
Detroit, Michigan, USA

Author Index

Subject Index